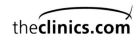

CLINICS IN
CHEST MEDICINE

Pleural Disease
GUEST EDITOR
Steven A. Sahn, MD

June 2006 • Volume 27 • Number 2

SAUNDERS

An Imprint of Elsevier, Inc.
PHILADELPHIA   LONDON   TORONTO   MONTREAL   SYDNEY   TOKYO

W.B. SAUNDERS COMPANY
A Division of Elsevier Inc.

Elsevier Inc. • 1600 John F. Kennedy Boulevard • Suite 1800 • Philadelphia, Pennsylvania 19103-2899

http://www.chestmed.theclinics.com

CLINICS IN CHEST MEDICINE	**Volume 27, Number 2**
June 2006	**ISSN 0272-5231**
Editor: Sarah E. Barth	**ISBN 1-4160-3590-7**

The Clinics in Chest Medicine (ISSN 0272-5231) is published quarterly by W.B. Saunders, 360 Park Avenue South, New York, NY 10010-1710. Months of publication are March, June, September, and December. Business and Editorial Offices: 1600 John F. Kennedy Boulevard, Suite 1800, Philadelphia, PA 19103-2899. Accounting and Circulation Offices: 6277 Sea Harbor Drive, Orlando, FL 32887-4800. Periodicals postage paid at New York, NY and additional mailing offices. Subscription prices are $195.00 per year (US individuals), $300.00 per year (US institutions), $95.00 per year (US students), $215.00 per year (Canadian individuals), $360.00 per year (Canadian institutions), $125.00 per year (Canadian students), $250.00 per year (international individuals), $360.00 per year (international institutions), and $125.00 per year (international students). International air speed delivery is included in all *Clinics* subscription prices. All prices are subject to change without notice. **POSTMASTER:** Send address changes to *The Clinics in Chest Medicine*, Elsevier Periodicals Customer Service, 6277 Sea Harbor Drive, Orlando, FL 32887-4800. Customer Service: 1-800-654-2452 (US). From outside of the US, call 1-407-345-4000.

Clinics in Chest Medicine is covered in *Index Medicus, Current Contents/Clinical Medicine, EMBASE/Excerpta Medica, Science Citation Index,* and *ISI/BIOMED.*

Printed in the United States of America.

GUEST EDITOR

STEVEN A. SAHN, MD, Professor (Medicine); and Director, Division of Pulmonary, Critical Care, Allergy, Sleep Medicine, Medical University of South Carolina, Charleston, South Carolina

CONTRIBUTORS

KHALID F. ALMOOSA, MD, Assistant Professor of Medicine, Department of Internal Medicine, Division of Pulmonary, Critical Care, and Sleep Medicine, University of Cincinnati College of Medicine, Cincinnati, Ohio

VEENA B. ANTONY, MD, Professor of Medicine, Division of Pulmonary and Critical Care Medicine, University of Florida, Gainesville, Florida

MICHAEL H. BAUMANN, MD, Professor (Medicine); and Medical Director, Respiratory Care, Division of Pulmonary, Critical Care, and Sleep Medicine, University of Mississippi Medical Center, Jackson, Mississippi

GREGORY BOHACH, PhD, Professor of Microbiology, Molecular Biology & Biochemistry; and Chairman, Microbiology, University of Idaho, Moscow, Idaho

STEPHEN J. CHAPMAN, BM, BCh, MA, MRCP, Specialist Registrar and Wellcome Research Fellow, Oxford Centre for Respiratory Medicine, Headington, Oxford, United Kingdom

ROBERT J.O. DAVIES, DM, FRCP, Reader and Consultant in Respiratory Medicine, Oxford Centre for Respiratory Medicine, Headington, Oxford, United Kingdom

PETER DOELKEN, MD, Assistant Professor (Medicine), Division of Pulmonary, Critical Care, Allergy, and Sleep Medicine, Medical University of South Carolina, Charleston, South Carolina

JOHN C. ENGLISH, MD, Department of Pathology and Laboratory Medicine, Vancouver General Hospital, Vancouver, British Columbia, Canada

JEROME ETIENNE, MD, PhD, Professor of Medicine & Microbiology, Co-Director, Centre Nationales de Reference Staphylococcques, INSERM E0230, Faculte de Medecine Laennec, Lyon, France

FERGUS V. GLEESON, FRCP, FRCR, Consultant Radiologist, Department of Radiology, Churchill Hospital, Headington, Oxford, United Kingdom

JOHN E. HEFFNER, MD, Professor of Medicine and Executive Medical Director, Center of Clinical Effectiveness and Patient Safety, Medical University of South Carolina, Charleston, South Carolina

JAY HEIDECKER, MD, Fellow, Division of Pulmonary, Critical Care, Allergy, and Sleep Medicine, Medical University of South Carolina, Charleston, South Carolina

JOHN T. HUGGINS, MD, Assistant Professor (Medicine), Division of Pulmonary, Critical Care, Allergy, and Sleep Medicine, Medical University of South Carolina, Charleston, South Carolina

MICHAEL A. JANTZ, MD, FCCP, Assistant Professor of Medicine, Division of Pulmonary and Critical Care Medicine, University of Florida, Gainesville, Florida

Y.C. GARY LEE, MBChB, PHD, FCCP, FRACP, Wellcome Advanced Fellow, Centre for Respiratory Research, University College London, London; and Honorary Consultant Chest Physician and Senior Lecturer, Oxford Centre for Respiratory Medicine, Churchill Hospital, Oxford, United Kingdom

KEVIN O. LESLIE, MD, Department of Laboratory Medicine and Pathology, Mayo Clinic Scottsdale, Scottsdale, Arizona

RICHARD W. LIGHT, MD, Professor (Medicine), Vanderbilt University, Nashville, Tennessee

GERARD LINA, MD, PhD, Associate Professor of Medicine & Microbiology, Senior Researcher, Centre Nationales de Reference Staphylococcques, INSERM E0230, Faculte de Medecine Laennec, Lyon, France

PAUL H. MAYO, MD, Associate Professor of Clinical Medicine, Albert Einstein College of Medicine, Bronx, New York

FRANCIS X. McCORMACK, MD, Professor of Medicine and Director, Department of Internal Medicine, Division of Pulmonary, Critical Care, and Sleep Medicine, University of Cincinnati College of Medicine, Cincinnati, Ohio

NAGMI R. QURESHI, MRCP, FRCR, Fellow in Thoracic Radiology, Department of Radiology, Churchill Hospital, Headington, Oxford, United Kingdom

NAJIB M. RAHMAN, BM, BCh, MA, MRCP, Specialist Registrar and Pleural Research Fellow, Oxford Centre for Respiratory Medicine, Headington, Oxford, United Kingdom

STEVEN A. SAHN, MD, Professor (Medicine); and Director, Division of Pulmonary, Critical Care, Allergy, Sleep Medicine, Medical University of South Carolina, Charleston, South Carolina

DAVID S. TERMAN, MD, former Professor of Medicine, Microbiology & Immunology; and Director, Cancer Biology Program, Baylor College of Medicine, Houston, Texas; CEO-Chairman, Jenomic, Inc., Carmel, California

FRANCOIS VANDENESCH, MD, PhD, Professor of Medicine & Microbiology, Co-Director, Centre Nationales de Reference Staphylococcques, INSERM E0230, Faculte de Medecine Laennec, Lyon, France

SOPHIE D. WEST, MBChB, MRCP, Specialist Registrar, Oxford Centre for Respiratory Medicine, Churchill Hospital, Oxford, United Kingdom

CONTENTS

The pleura and lung are intimately associated and share many pathologic conditions. Nevertheless, they represent two separate organs of different embryonic derivation and with different yet often symbiotic functions. In this article, the authors explore the pathologic manifestations of the many conditions that primarily or secondarily affect the pleura.

Pleural fibrosis can result from a variety of inflammatory processes. The response of the pleural mesothelial cell to injury and the ability to maintain its integrity are crucial in determining whether normal healing or pleural fibrosis occurs. The pleural mesothelial cell, various cytokines, and disordered fibrin turnover are involved in the pathogenesis of pleural fibrosis. The roles of these mediators in producing pleural fibrosis are examined. This article reviews the most common clinical conditions associated with the development of pleural fibrosis. Fibrothorax and trapped lung are two unique and uncommon consequences of pleural fibrosis. The management of pleural fibrosis, including fibrothorax and trapped lung, is discussed.

Imaging plays an important role in the diagnosis and subsequent management of patients with pleural disease. The presence of a pleural abnormality is usually suggested following a routine chest x-ray, with a number of imaging modalities available for further characterization. This article describes the radiographic and cross-sectional appearances of pleural diseases, which are commonly encountered in everyday practice. The conditions covered include benign and malignant pleural thickening, pleural effusions, empyema and pneumothoraces. The relative merits of CT, MRI and PET in the assessment of these conditions and the role of image-guided intervention are discussed.

Pleural Ultrasonography

Paul H. Mayo and Peter Doelken

Ultrasonography has achieved acceptance as a routine clinical tool for clinicians managing pleural disease. This article provides an overview of the field of pleural ultrasonography with an emphasis on clinical applicability and procedure guidance.

Pleural Manometry

John T. Huggins and Peter Doelken

The goals of therapeutic thoracentesis are to remove the maximum amount of pleural fluid to improve dyspnea and to facilitate the diagnostic evaluation of large pleural effusions. Pleural manometry may be useful for immediately detecting an unexpandable lung, which may coexist when any pleural fluid accumulates. Pleural manometry may improve patient safety when removing large amounts of pleural fluid. The basics of pleural space mechanics are discussed as they apply to the normal pleural space and to pleural effusion associated with expandable and unexpandable lung. This article also discusses the instrumentation required to perform bedside manometry, how manometry may decrease the risk of re-expansion pulmonary edema when large amounts of fluid are removed, and the diagnostic capabilities of manometry.

Discriminating Between Transudates and Exudates

John E. Heffner

The dichotomous classification of pleural fluid as a transudate or an exudate simplifies diagnostic efforts in determining the cause of pleural effusions. Multiple pleural fluid tests are available to discriminate between these two classes of effusions. Tests commonly used in clinical practice depend on the detection in pleural fluid of large-molecular-weight chemicals that enter the pleural space to greater degrees in conditions associated with exudative compared with transudative effusions. Considerable misclassifications can occur with all available testing strategies, so clinicians benefit from adopting a nondichotomous, bayesian approach for interpreting test results.

The Approach to the Patient with a Parapneumonic Effusion

Najib M. Rahman, Stephen J. Chapman, and Robert J.O. Davies

Parapneumonic effusion is a common clinical problem, and those that go on to develop pleural infection have high morbidity and mortality. The process of pleural infection evolution involves changes in pleural physiology that are increasingly being elucidated and understood. The microbiology of pleural infection has changed over recent years, with clear differences emerging between hospital- and community-acquired infections. Using biochemical surrogates of infection, chest drainage can be undertaken rationally for those who do not respond to antibiotics alone. Recent data suggest that fibrinolytics do not influence outcomes in pleural infection. The optimal type and timing of surgery remain controversial.

FORTHCOMING ISSUES

RECENT ISSUES

ELSEVIER
SAUNDERS

Clin Chest Med 27 (2006) xi

CLINICS
IN CHEST
MEDICINE

Dedication

This issue is dedicated to my parents, Irwin and Mildred, who continue to provide me with their wisdom and support; my wife, Claire, my soul mate, who brings me constant happiness; my children, Karen, Stacey, James, Michael, and Rachel, who continue to bring joy into my life; and my grandchildren, Turner, Sydney, Jimmy and Seve, who amaze me with their innocence, enthusiasm, insight, and unconditional love.

Steven A. Sahn, MD
Division of Pulmonary, Critical Care,
Allergy, and Sleep Medicine
Medical University of South Carolina
96 Jonathan Lucas Street
Suite 812-CSB
PO Box 250630
Charleston, SC 29425, USA
E-mail address: sahnsa@musc.edu

Clin Chest Med 27 (2006) xiii – xiv

CLINICS
IN CHEST
MEDICINE

Preface

Pleural Disease

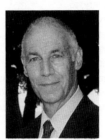

Steven A. Sahn, MD
Guest Editor

Pleural disease is truly a mirror of diseases in the thorax and systemic disease. Pleural effusions primarily form because of imbalances in hydrostatic and oncotic pressures, increased capillary permeability, and impaired lymphatic drainage. Less commonly, fluid of extravascular origin, such as cerebrospinal fluid, urine, bile, and chyle, can enter the pleural space.

In structuring this issue, I have attempted to disseminate an overview and update of the spectrum of pleural diseases. It was my hope to provide useful clinical information that can be applied directly to the pulmonologist's practice and to stimulate clinical and basic researchers to investigate unanswered questions.

The issue begins with a detailed description of the normal pleura and the pleura in disease by Drs. John English and Kevin Leslie from the Mayo Clinic, Scottsdale. A plethora of color photomicrographs augment the discussion. Drs. Michael Jantz and Veena Antony from the University of Florida in Gainesville follow with a review of the pathogenesis of pleural fibrosis. Much of this information, which is from Dr. Antony's laboratory, helps in our understanding of why pleural inflammation results in fibrosis in some individuals and normal healing without sequelae in others.

Drs. Nagmi Qureshi and Fergus Gleeson of Churchill Hospital in Oxford, England provide instructive radiographic images that help the clinician diagnos-

tically and in directing the management of patients with pleural effusions. This article is followed by a discussion of pleural ultrasound by Drs. Peter Doelken and Paul Mayo from the Medical University of South Carolina in Charleston and Mount Sinai School of Medicine in New York, respectively, which is emerging as an extremely useful diagnostic and therapeutic tool. In addition, pleural ultrasound provides an extra measure of safety in the management of these patients. The methodology and value of pleural manometry is discussed by Dr. Terrill Huggins of the Medical University of South Carolina. Dr. Huggins explains the concept of pleural elastance and the use of the pressure/volume curve of the pleural space for the diagnosis of pleural effusions and management of patients with malignant pleural effusions. The pressure/volume curve determines the likelihood of successful pleurodesis and the rationale for selecting an indwelling catheter for palliation for patients with malignant effusions.

Dr. John Heffner from the Medical University of South Carolina provides insight for the clinician who is faced with classifying patients' effusions as transudative or exudative. His Bayesian approach to this issue is clinically enlightening. Drs. Naj Rahman, Stephen Chapman, and Robert Davies from the Oxford Centre for Respiratory Medicine discuss the approach to the management of patients with parapneumonic effusions, which includes data from the

0272-5231/06/$ – see front matter © 2006 Elsevier Inc. All rights reserved.
doi:10.1016/j.ccm.2006.01.008

recently published Multicenter Intrapleural Sepsis Trial (MIST1). They appropriately stress that timing is of utmost importance in providing the most appropriate management of these patients. Dr. Jay Heidecker and I follow with a new classification of pleural effusions after coronary artery bypass graft surgery, dividing these effusions into postoperative, early, late, and persistent. These effusions encompass a spectrum of causes from atelectasis secondary to phrenic nerve injury, immunologically induced post-cardiac injury syndrome, trauma from harvesting of the internal mammary artery, and dysfunctional healing leading to lung entrapment or trapped lung. An understanding of the heterogeneous effusions that develop after coronary artery bypass graft surgery should be helpful to the pulmonologist asked to evaluate these patients.

I follow with a new classification of pleural effusions derived from extravascular origin (PEEVO). These effusions include transudates from peritoneal dialysis and urinothorax and exudates, such as chylothorax, biliothorax, and extravascular migration of a central venous catheter with infusion of total parenteral nutrition. Dr. Richard Light from Vanderbilt University in Nashville follows with his experience on the approach to the patient with an undiagnosed pleural effusion.

Dr. David Terman and I, together with collaborators from France and the United States, discuss a potentially important new treatment for malignant pleural effusions, staphylococcal enterotoxin superantigen. We report exciting preliminary studies from China demonstrating that intrapleural staphylococcal superantigen not only results in resolution of malignant pleural effusions from non-small cell lung cancer but provides a significant survival benefit compared with patients treated with talc poudrage with similar Karnofsky Performance Scale scores. Drs. Sophie West and Y.C. Gary Lee from the Oxford Centre for Respiratory Medicine and University College, respec-

tively, provide an update on the management of malignant pleural mesothelioma. Drs. Khalid Almoosa, Francis McCormack, and I discuss the impact of pleural disease in lymphangioleiomyomatosis (LAM). Much of the data presented in this article are derived not only from the previous literature but from a recent large survey of women in the LAM Foundation database. The data confirm that patients with LAM have the highest prevalence of pneumothorax of any underlying lung disease at 67% as well as an extremely high recurrence rate of approximately 70%, ipsilaterally or bilaterally. Although the prevalence of chylothorax is less common than that of pneumothorax, it provides a therapeutic challenge. We conclude with a rationale for early surgical management of pneumothorax in LAM and provide several options for controlling chylothorax. The issue concludes with a rational approach to management of spontaneous pneumothorax based on evidence and expert opinion from a consensus panel chosen by the American College of Chest Physicians and headed by Dr. Michael Baumann from the University of Mississippi.

It is my hope that this issue of *Clinics in Chest Medicine* provides the reader with a more complete understanding of the pathogenesis, diagnosis, and management of patients with pleural disease, which encompasses a significant component of the practice of pulmonary medicine.

Steven A. Sahn, MD
Division of Pulmonary, Critical Care,
Allergy, and Sleep Medicine
Medical University of South Carolina
96 Jonathan Lucas Street
Suite 812-CSB
PO Box 250630
Charleston, SC 29425, USA
E-mail address: sahnsa@musc.edu

ELSEVIER
SAUNDERS

Clin Chest Med 27 (2006) 157 – 180

CLINICS
IN CHEST
MEDICINE

Pathology of the Pleura

John C. English, MD[a],*, Kevin O. Leslie, MD[b]

[a]Department of Pathology and Laboratory Medicine, Vancouver General Hospital, Vancouver, BC, Canada
[b]Department of Laboratory Medicine and Pathology, Mayo Clinic Scottsdale, 13400 East Shea Boulevard,
Scottsdale, AZ 85259, USA

The pleura and lung are intimately associated and share many pathologic conditions. Nevertheless, they represent two separate organs of different embryonic derivation and with different yet often symbiotic functions. In this article, the authors explore the pathologic manifestations of the many conditions that primarily or secondarily affect the pleura. Given significant space constraints, an all-inclusive discussion of pleural pathologic conditions requires brevity. Further reading is suggested whenever appropriate.

Embryology and anatomy of the pleura

Three primary mesodermal body cavities form in vertebrates: the pleural cavities, the pericardial cavity, and the peritoneal cavity. These distinct spaces develop from the coelomic cavity during early embryogenesis. The lung buds grow into these cavities, becoming enveloped in a fashion analogous to pushing a fist into a balloon [1]. The portion of the coelomic cavity that directly abuts the lung bud and surrounds it is referred to later in development as the visceral pleura. Once the lung is fully developed, the space between the visceral pleura and parietal pleura (the portion of the coelomic cavity that abuts the chest wall, diaphragm, and mediastinum) becomes nothing more than two opposed pleural surfaces separated by 10 to 20 µm of glycoprotein-rich fluid. It is estimated that the normal volume of pleural fluid in the adult is proportional to body weight (0.1–0.2 mL/kg). The

normal pleural fluid has a protein concentration of approximately 1.5 g/dL [2]. The pleural fluid has a few cells under normal conditions, including rare macrophages, mesothelial cells, and lymphocytes. The entire surface area of the pleura in a male adult is approximately 2000 cm². Fig. 1 presents the pleural surfaces as viewed through the videothoracoscope.

The parietal pleura derives its blood supply from branches of the intercostal arteries [3]. The mediastinal pleura is supplied by the pericardiophrenic artery, whereas the diaphragmatic parietal pleura derives its blood supply from the superior phrenic and musculophrenic arteries. Most authorities currently believe that the visceral pleura derives most of its blood supply from the bronchial arterial system.

The lymphatic anatomy of the visceral pleura and parietal pleura is important in the homeostasis of pleural fluid volume in the normal individual. In disease, excess production or decreased absorption of lymph plays a significant role in the generation of effusions. A complete discussion of the pathologic findings and diagnosis of pleural effusions is beyond the scope of this article; suffice it to say that protein content and increased cellular components in the pleural fluid are often useful in determining disease etiology. For our purposes, one fundamental component of the lymphatic anatomy is the existence of naturally occurring pores (stomata) in the caudal portions of the peripheral parietal pleura and lower mediastinal parietal pleura [4]. These pores are capable of transferring particulate matter and cells directly into lymphatic channels for removal. Most of the fluid that accumulates abnormally in the pleural space is derived from the lung through the visceral pleura and absorbed primarily through the parietal pleura.

---

* Corresponding author.
 E-mail address: leslie.kevin@mayo.edu (K.O. Leslie).

158 ENGLISH & LESLIE

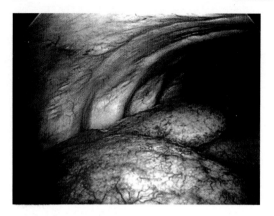

Fig. 1. Visceral and parietal pleura. The right chest cavity as seen through the videothoracoscope. The parietal pleura covers the chest wall (*upper left half*), and the visceral pleura covers the lung (*lower right half*).

The normal pleura is a thin translucent membrane and consists of five layers that may be difficult to distinguish by light microscopy (Fig. 2). These layers are (1) the mesothelium (flattened mesothelial cells joined primarily by tight junctions); (2) a thin layer of submesothelial connective tissue; (3) a superficial elastic tissue layer, (4) a second loose subpleural connective tissue layer rich in arteries, veins, nerves, and lymphatics; and, finally, (5) a deep fibroelastic layer adherent to the underlying lung parenchyma, chest wall, diaphragm, or mediastinum. Elastic tissue histochemical stains performed on tissue sections are often useful in defining these layers. A distinctive ultrastructural feature of the mesothelial cell is the presence of long slender microvilli present on the

mesothelial surface facing the pleural space. These microvilli are believed to provide increased surface area for the release of hyaluronic acid into the pleural fluid and do not seem to play any resorptive role. Microvilli are more numerous on mesothelial cells of the visceral pleura as compared with the parietal pleura at a similar intrathoracic level [5]. For further reading on pleural anatomy, the interested reader is referred to an excellent review by Wang [3].

Pleural infections

Intrathoracic infections are leading causes of morbidity and mortality worldwide, and empyema (infection of the pleural space producing a fibrino-suppurative exudate) has been described since the time of Hippocrates. Infection of the pleura and pleural space is most often a result of disease arising in the ipsilateral lung, but trauma and vascular dissemination also play important roles. We have assembled a short compendium of common and rare infections seen in practice today. Pathogens have changed significantly over the past 50 years in developed countries, but the mechanisms of infection and the stereotypic responses of the pleura to them remain as relative constants.

The pleural membrane is composed of several tissue boundaries of differing degrees of strength [6]. The direct apposition of the pleura to other structures also influences susceptibility to infection. For example, the parietal pleura overlying the diaphragm and chest wall is most resistant to penetration by infection, whereas the parietal pleura overlying the medi-

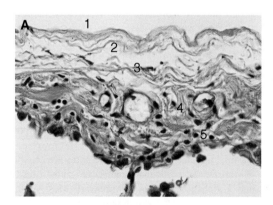
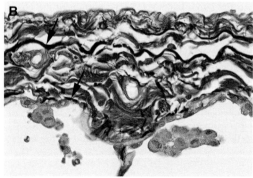

Fig. 2. Histologic findings of the pleura (routine hematoxylin-eosin stain). (*A*) The normal pleura is made up of five relatively indistinct anatomic layers (labeled 1–5 here). The elastic laminae are not easily visible on routine staining. The dilated structures located centrally in the photograph are blood vessels. (*B*) With an elastic tissue stain, the elastic laminae become undulating black lines (*arrows*). Collagen is stained in red, and macrophages in underlying alveoli (*light brown*) are unstained (Verhoeff's stain for elastic tissue).

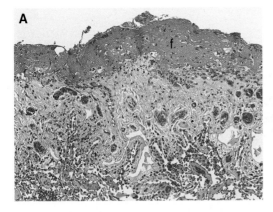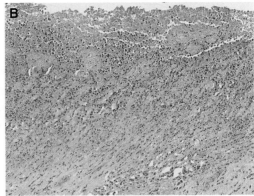

Fig. 3. Fibrinous and necroinflammatory reactions in the pleura (routine hematoxylin-eosin stain). (*A*) Fibrinous pleuritis is characterized by a variably thick surface layer of brightly eosinophilic fibrin derived from the blood (f), overlying a variable inflammatory reaction in underlying pleura. (*B*) Empyema is characterized by the presence of neutrophilic debris and necrosis, typically extending across all layers of the pleura. The pleural surface is at the top of the photograph.

astinum is most easily penetrated by invading organisms. Every class of infectious organism is capable of causing pleural infection. Because the pleura is a membranous structure in constant motion, the pathologic finding of pleural infection differs somewhat from that caused by the same organism in a different organ.

Most empyemas occur as a complication of pneumonia or lung abscess, but perhaps 15% to 30% occur after thoracic surgery and 10% occur in association with an intra-abdominal infection [7]. Two thirds of all pleural space infections arise from infection in the underlying lung or from transthoracic trauma [8]. Despite the current widespread use of antibiotics for respiratory tract infections, pleural em-

pyema still occurs as a significant complication of pneumonia (7–10 cases per 100,000 inhabitants per year) [9]. Empyema associated with lung infections tends to be polymicrobial with anaerobic bacterial organisms predominating, whereas postsurgical empyemas tend involve a single bacterial organism and the common nosocomial pathogens are overwhelmingly represented (*Staphylococcus aureus* and aerobic gram-negative bacilli) [7].

When the pleura is faced with an infectious organism, it responds with edema and exudation of protein and neutrophils. Within the pleural space, this translates to the classically observed exudative pleural effusion (Fig. 3). Mesothelial cells orchestrate inflammatory and exudative reactions through the release

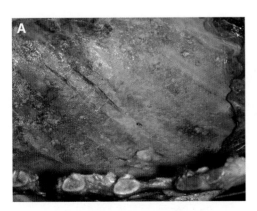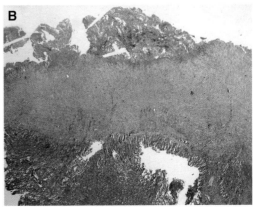

Fig. 4. Gross empyema and consequences (routine hematoxylin-eosin stain). (*A*) A coating of plaque-like yellow-gray exudate can be seen covering the surface of the lung in this case of *Nocardia* empyema; note transected ribs (*bottom*). (*B*) Unresolved empyema can lead to marked pleural fibrosis (eg, *horizontal light pink band of collagen*). Loose fibrinous adhesions are still present superficially (*top*).

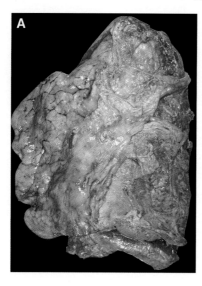

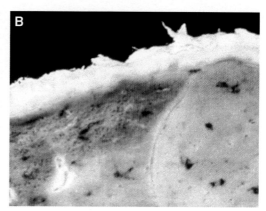

Fig. 5. Gross pleural fibrosis with adhesions. (*A*) Pleural fibrosis after infection can result in extensive pleural fibrosis with obliteration of the pleural space, causing nearly total encasement of the lung here. (*B*) A close-up view of pleural fibrosis after chronic empyema. Note the irregular "shaggy" surface (*top*). The underlying lung parenchyma has peribronchovascular anthracosis (*black pigment*).

of cytokines, chemokines, oxidants, and proteases. Mesothelial cells are also capable of phagocytosis and likely engulf infectious organisms as a direct defense mechanism [10]. As is the case with most other mammalian organs, if the infectious injury is promptly resolved, healing typically occurs with few permanent sequelae. In the case of severe or persistent necroinflammatory damage, structural integrity may be reconstituted with the addition of a fibrotic reaction produced by the submesothelial fibroblast (Fig. 4) [11]. During this fibrotic response, the pleural space may become focally or massively obliterated and be accompanied by the formation of dense fibrous adhesions (Fig. 5) [6].

Common infections

Bacterial infections

Infection of the pleura always results in empyema; as mentioned previously, bacteria are the most common etiologic agents (Box 1) [12,13]. *S aureus*, *Streptococcus* pneumonia, and enteric gram-negative bacilli are the principle bacteria involved. In a review of 193 cases of pleuropulmonary infections involving anaerobic bacteria, Bartlett [14] identified aspiration pneumonia, lung abscess, and empyema as the most common associated conditions. *Nocardia* and *Actinomycetes* are primarily implicated in the setting of immunocompromise (former) and aspiration pneumonia (latter).

Tuberculous pleuritis

Today, tuberculous pleuritis is an uncommon occurrence in Western countries. In a publication by the Centers for Disease Control and Prevention in 1978, approximately 1100 cases of tuberculous pleuritis were reported annually in the United States [15]. The disease produces a granulomatous reaction within the pleura (Fig. 6) and likely results from rupture of a focus within the lung through the visceral pleura [16]. In developed countries, pleural tuberculosis tends to occur in older individuals, with an increased

---

Box 1. Causes of empyema (pyothorax)

Infectious pneumonias [6,10, 12–14,112]
   Staphylococcus aureus
   Fusobacterium nucleatum
   Bacteroides spp
   Clostridium
   Escherichia coli
   Pseudomonas spp
Thoracic trauma [113]
Esophageal rupture [114]
Thoracotomy or thoracentesis [115]
Sepsis [116–119]
Abdominal abscess [120]

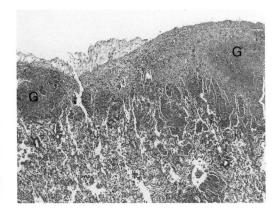

Fig. 6. Granulomatous pleuritis (routine hematoxylin-eosin stain). Tuberculous empyema likely results from rupture of granulomas (G) arising in underlying lung, with passage of organisms and granulomatous exudate into the pleural space.

incidence of reactivation disease. In a 2005 review by Ibrahim and colleagues [17], a retrospective study of 100 patients discharged from a Middle Eastern general hospital (Hamad General Hospital, Qatar) with a diagnosis of pleural tuberculosis between 1996 and 2002 revealed a younger age group, with 84% of patients younger than the age of 45 years. In this study, the disease was mostly a result of primary infection. Most of the described patients had no predisposing medical conditions. The pathologic stages of pleural tuberculosis are presented in Box 2 [16].

Uncommon infections

Fungi

Granulomatous inflammation of the pleura always requires a search for mycobacterial, fungal, and higher bacterial infections (*Actinomyces* and *Nocardia*). These infections may account for as much as 10% of all empyemas [18]. Unlike common bacterial infections, which may spread across the pleura from underlying pneumonia, mycobacterial and fungal empyemas likely require a physical event to transgress the pleura (rupture of a mycetoma in underlying lung or perforating physical trauma through the chest wall). In fact, most extremely active fungal pneumonias seem to encounter a formidable barrier in the pleura (Fig. 7). The increasing use of therapeutic agents that compromise normal host immunity and the increasing prevalence of HIV infections have resulted in a change in the epidemiology of pleural fungal infections. In hospitalized patients, ubiquitous environmental fungi, such as *Pneumocystis jiroveci* (Fig. 8), have become relatively common pathogens [19]. In certain areas of the United States, such as the desert Southwest (*Coccidioides* species) and the Mississippi and Ohio River Valleys (*Histoplasma* species), endemic fungi still play a significant role in pleural infection (Fig. 9).

Protozoa

Although parasitic infection remains relatively uncommon in the United States, parasitosis is a rea-

---

Box 2. Stages of tuberculous pleurisy

Serofibrinous pleuritis
Patchy granulation tissue with mainly nonnecrotizing granulomas
Confluent granulation tissue with necrotizing granulomas
Tuberculous ''empyema''[a] (ruptured tuberculous pulmonary cavity)
Calcification of pleural granulomas

[a] Histiocytic semiliquid exudate with necrotic material (not neutrophils).
(*Adapted from* Abrams WB, Small MJ. Current concepts of tuberculous pleurisy with effusion as derived from pleural biopsy studies. Dis Chest 1960;38:60–5.)

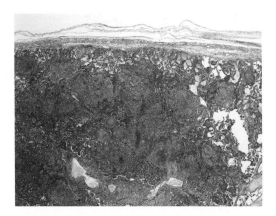

Fig. 7. The pleura is a strong barrier to infection (routine hematoxylin-eosin stain). In spite of the occurrence of empyema, under most circumstances, the pleura is an excellent barrier to infectious organisms involving underlying lung. Here, in a case of miliary parenchymal tuberculosis, the inflammatory reaction is well confined by the pleura (*top*).

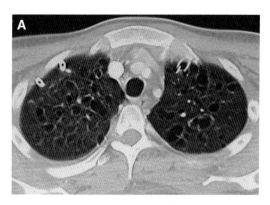
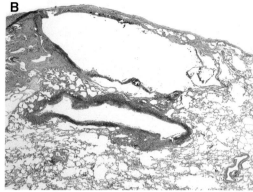

Fig. 8. Cystic *Pneumocystis* infection (routine hematoxylin-eosin stain). (*A*) Multiple cystic spaces in the lung (CT scan) in a case of *Pneumocystis* pneumonia occurring in an HIV-infected host on antiretroviral therapy. (*B*) The histopathologic finding in this patient's lung at scanning magnification was one of cysts lined by a granulomatous inflammation. At higher magnification (not shown), numerous organisms were present within patchy fibrinous exudates lining the cyst walls (pleural surface, *top*).

sonable consideration for pleural effusion of unclear cause. Parasitic infestations outside the thorax may be contributory, such as the case of hepatic amoebiasis crossing the diaphragm from a liver abscess [20]. Cysticercosis can be a primary pleural disease; however, like amebic pleuritis, the disease more often spreads from the underlying lung or liver [21]. Paragonimiasis may be confused with tuberculous pleuritis on occasion, but pleural fluid is often diagnostic [22,23]. Other less common protozoan infestations of the pleura include schistosomiasis, anisakiasis, and strongyloidiasis [23].

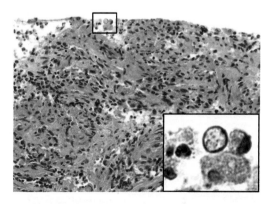

Fig. 9. Pleural empyema in coccidioidomycosis (routine hematoxylin-eosin stain). In regions where coccidioidomycosis is endemic, pleural empyema can occur after rupture of a cavitary lung parenchymal cyst. *Coccidioides* is one of the few fungi that can be readily identified on routine hematoxylin-eosin stains. (Box and inset show a spherule of *Coccidioides* spp.)

Noninfectious inflammatory and fibrotic conditions of the pleura

Nonspecific inflammation of the pleura (pleuritis) is a relatively common condition seen in pleural pulmonary pathologic conditions, with underlying etiologies that include systemic connective tissue diseases, renal disease (uremia), drug reactions, pneumoconiosis, trauma, and even transdiaphragmatic extension of intra-abdominal inflammatory processes (eg, pancreatitis). The hallmarks of pleuritis are fibrin and neutrophils in acute forms and lymphocytes and plasma cells in chronic forms. Box 3 presents some common causes of noninfectious pleuritis.

Systemic immunologic (autoimmune) diseases

Systemic immunologic diseases may produce pleural effusion with varying degrees of pleural inflammation (Fig. 10). The collagen vascular diseases figure most prominently, and these, with their described pleural findings, are presented in Box 4. Drug reactions, postcardiac injury syndrome, and sarcoidosis are also acknowledged causes. Pneumoconiosis is well known to produce pleural fibrosis, especially that occurring in association with asbestos exposure [24–27]. The pleural fluid findings are typically nondiagnostic in these conditions, although rheumatoid arthritis and systemic lupus erythematosus may be associated with characteristic abnormalities [28].

Pleural fibrosis and its mechanisms have been the subject of excellent recent reviews [29,30]. Most investigators have focused on the role of the subpleural

Box 3. Causes of pleuritis

Systemic autoimmune disease (eg, systemic lupus erythematosus, drug-induced lupus, rheumatoid arthritis, Sjogren's syndrome, Wegener's granulomatosis) [121–125]
Drug-induced (eg, nitrofurantoin, bromocriptine, methysergide, procarbazine) [31,32,126]
Trauma (eg, external, esophageal rupture, intra-abdominal abscesses) [113,124]
Pancreatitis [127,128]
Thoracic irradiation [129]
Postcardiac injury syndrome [130]
Pneumoconioses (asbestosis) [53,131]
Metabolic disease (uremia) [132,133]
Metastatic tumor [43,44]

Box 4. Systemic immune diseases that commonly affect the pleura

Rheumatoid arthritis [123,134–138]
Acute fibrinous pleuritis
Nonspecific chronic inflammation with effusion
Pyopneumothorax
Localized rheumatoid nodules
Diffuse rheumatoid nodules (necrotizing rheumatoid pleuritis)
Ruptured rheumatoid nodule with bronchopleural fistula
Systemic lupus erythematosus [122,139–141]
Acute fibrinous pleuritis
Chronic nonspecific pleuritis
Cellular effusions with ''lupus erythematosus cells''
Sjogren's syndrome [142,143]
Chronic lymphocytic pleuritis
Wegener's granulomatosis [144–146]

fibroblast; however, more recently, the potential for mesothelial cells to initiate and orchestrate the deposition of matrix proteins has gained favor [30]. Fibrosis of the pleura is most often associated with an exudative pleural effusion, because it seems that a phase of fibrinous pleuritis is required for the eventual propagation of fibrosis. The cytokines transforming growth factor (TGF)-β and TNFα have been implicated in fibrin matrix deposition. Clinically significant pleural fibrosis requires involvement of the visceral pleura [29]. Box 5 [147] presents some of the known causes of diffuse visceral and parietal pleural fibrosis.

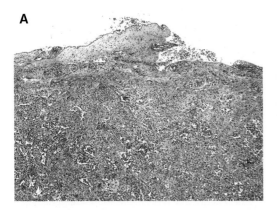
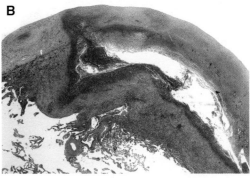

Fig. 10. Pleural manifestations of systemic connective tissue disease (routine hematoxylin-eosin stain). (*A*) Systemic lupus erythematosus can produce acute and chronic pleuritis (pleura, *top*). There is a brisk inflammatory reaction in the underlying lung as well as evidence of subacute lung injury (organizing pneumonia pattern). (*B*) Rheumatoid arthritis has a number of pleural pulmonary manifestations. Here, a rheumatoid nodule can be seen within the substance of the pleura as an irregular dark blue cyst. The dark blue is produced by dense neutrophilic debris. A rheumatoid nodule can simulate granulomatous infection as well as Wegener's granulomatosis.

Box 5. Causes of pleural fibrosis

Diffuse visceral (parietal) pleural fibrosis
  Collagen-vascular disease
  Asbestos exposure
  Drug reactions
  Any other cause of recurrent
    exudative effusions
Fibrothorax
  Organization of a hemothorax
  Organization of an empyema
  Secondary to plombage therapy for
    tuberculosis with escape of
    plombage material
  Severe asbestos-induced visceral
    pleural fibrosis adherent to
    pleural plaques
Apical caps
Pleural plaques
  Asbestos exposure
  Chest trauma
  Hemothorax
  Organized empyema
Rounded atelectasis (folded lung)
  Pleural fibrosis secondary to
    asbestos exposure
  Pleural fibrosis secondary to
    renal disease
  Pleural fibrosis secondary
    to infections
  Pleural fibrosis secondary to trauma

(*From* Churg AM. Diseases of the pleura. In: Churg AM, Myers JL, Tazelaar HD, et al, editors. Thurlbeck's pathology of the lung. New York: Thieme; 2005. p. 997; with permission.)

Drug reactions

Many medications in current clinical use are capable of producing pleural inflammation and sometimes fibrosis. The best known and most extensively studied agents are methysergide, ergotamine, ergonovine, bromocriptine, practolol, oxprenolol, amiodarone, methotrexate, bleomycin, and mitomycin. Fortunately, compared with the number of drugs known to produce parenchymal lung disease, those that produce pleural disease are relatively small in number. Several excellent reviews on drugs and the pleura are available [31–33].

Interstitial lung diseases

Many inflammatory interstitial lung diseases are associated with pathologic changes in the pleura. In fact, evaluation of the pleura can be helpful in the approach to the surgical biopsy for interstitial lung disease (Fig. 11). Every named systemic connective tissue disease has been associated with lung manifestations, ranging from diffuse alveolar damage to pulmonary fibrosis. One potentially relevant finding in this regard is the complete absence of significant pleuritis in association with usual interstitial pneumonia (UIP) in the context of clinical idiopathic pulmonary fibrosis (IPF). The reasons for this are unknown, but the exquisite peripheral localization of fibrosis in lung lobules in IPF may have a direct effect on fluid transport across the pleura. It is also said that patients with IPF do not develop pleural effusions. By contrast, patients with lung fibrosis related to underlying connective tissue disease often have evidence of pleural inflammation and may have associated effusion visible on chest imaging.

Pneumoconiosis-associated pleural disease

Asbestos exposure and asbestosis are the best-documented inorganic environmental exposures known to cause pleural fibrosis. Workers exposed to asbestos have a common occurrence of pleural fibrosis on chest imaging. The process begins as circumscribed plaques of dense hyaline fibrosis on the parietal pleural surfaces, typically involving the diaphragm and chest wall (Fig. 12) [34]. The presence of these pleural plaques is believed to be indicative of significant exposure to asbestos, although the presence of these lesions carries no direct implication regarding the presence of pulmonary asbestosis. The fibrogenic properties of the amphibole and serpentine forms of asbestos are well known. Box 6 [147a] presents an overview of the naturally occurring forms of asbestos. Potential nonmining exposures to asbestos are presented in Box 7 [148].

Other types of pneumoconiosis also may produce pleural fibrosis. For example Arakawa and coworkers [35] found pleural thickening in 58% of individuals with silicosis, and this finding was more prominent in patients with complicated silicosis. Mazziotti and colleagues [36] found that 8 of 28 patients with a history of pumice (amorphous silica) inhalation had pleural fibrosis. Finally, coal workers' pneumoconiosis may be associated with pleural fibrosis, as illustrated by a study of 98 Appalachian former coal

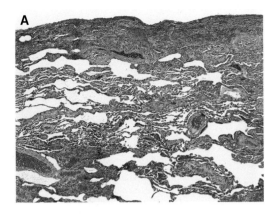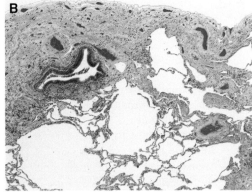

Fig. 11. The pleura in interstitial lung disease (routine hematoxylin-eosin stain). (*A*) This overtly inflammatory interstitial lung disease (cellular nonspecific pneumonia [NSIP] pattern) is associated with fibrinous pleuritis and dense lymphocytic infiltration into pleura. (*B*) UIP, conversely, has little if any inflammation in the pleura. Fibrosis accrues beneath the pleura and extends into underlying lung.

miners, in whom thickened pleura was identified in 18% of affected individuals [37].

Benign and borderline pleural lesions/neoplasms

Pulmonary hyalinizing granuloma

Pulmonary hyalinizing granuloma is a distinct nodular fibrosing pleural lesion characterized by whorled deposits of lamellar collagen (Fig. 13). Based on two large survey publications [38,39], the condition is of unknown etiology, and, in most in-

stances, the lesions are multiple and bilateral. Affected patients may be mildly symptomatic. As many as half of the patients had associated auto-immune phenomena. In the original description in 1977, 4 of the 20 patients presented also had sclerosing mediastinitis. One hypothesis for the etiology of pulmonary hyalinizing granuloma is that these lesions represent resolved foci of granulomatous infection (possibly related to *Histoplasma* species) [38]. The lesions may be mistaken for metastatic carcinoma radiologically. In the series by Yousem and Hochholzer [38], a significant association with sclerosing mediastinitis was also found.

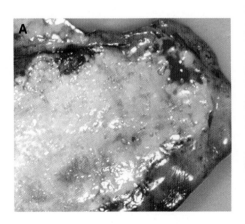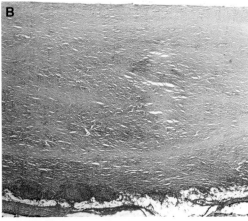

Fig. 12. Pleural plaque related to asbestos exposure. (*A*) Glistening, white, circumscribed pleural plaque can occur after asbestos exposure. This is not a marker for "asbestosis." (*B*) Under the microscope, pleural plaque consists of dense paucicellular collagen with characteristic slit-like retraction spaces oriented parallel to the pleural surface (routine hematoxylin-eosin stain).

Box 6. Six naturally-occurring fibrous silicates (asbestos)

> Serpentine asbestos (''plate-like'' and
>   serpentine forms)
>   Chrysotile (white asbestos)
> Amphibole Asbestos (long
>   slender fibers)
>   Crocidolite (blue asbestos)
>   Amosite (brown asbestos)
>   Tremolite
>   Anthophyllite
>   Actinolite

(*Adapted from* Craighead JE, Mossman BT, Bradley BJ. Comparative studies on the cytotoxicity of amphibole and serpentine asbestos. Environ Health Perspect 1980;34:37–46.)

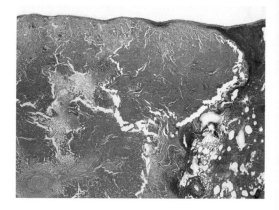

Fig. 13. Pulmonary hyalinizing granuloma (routine hematoxylin-eosin stain). Dense hyalinized collagen forms a pleural-based nodule in this example of pulmonary hyalinizing granuloma (pleural surface, *top*).

Calcifying fibrous pseudotumor

Calcifying fibrous pseudotumors were described in soft tissue before their recognition as a lesion of the pleura. In the soft tissues, these pseudotumors occur

Box 7. Potential nonmining sources for asbestos exposure

> Manufacture and processing of
>   asbestos-containing cement
> Demolition and construction industries
> Dockyard work (''ship-fitting'')
> Electricians
> Plumbers
> Boiler manufacturing
> Railway workers
> Naval servicemen
> Insulation work
> Manufacture and fitting of brake linings
> Environmental exposure near mines
> Household exposure related to asbestos worker
> City dwelling with heavy road traffic
>   (brake lining decay)

(*Adapted from* Hendry NW. The geology, occurrences and major uses of asbestos. Ann NY Acad Sci B 1965;132(1):12–22.)

most commonly on the extremities, trunk, scrotum, groin, neck, or axilla. Pinkard and coworkers [40] described three cases of pleural calcifying fibrous pseudotumor, with all three occurring in relatively young individuals (34, 28, and 23 years of age at presentation, respectively). Two of the three patients presented with chest pain. Pleural-based nodular masses were identified with central attenuation attributable to microcalcification. Histopathologically, calcifying fibrous pseudotumors are unencapsulated and consist of hyalinized and collagenized fibrotic tissue with interspersed lymphoplasmacellular infiltrates with calcification (Fig. 14). Psammomatous-type calcifications were commonly seen. The lesions did not involve the underlying lung parenchyma. We

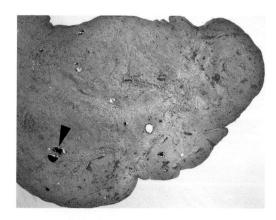

Fig. 14. Calcifying fibrous pseudotumor (routine hematoxylin-eosin stain). This nodular lesion also has dense hyalinized collagen, but admixed are numerous calcified bodies, some of which are psammomatous with lamellar rings (*arrowhead*).

have seen one recent case in consultation that was typical morphologically except for the presence of a few included benign-appearing mesothelial tubular glands.

Localized fibrous tumor of pleura (solitary fibrous tumor of pleura)

First described in 1942 by Stout as "benign localized mesothelioma" and later as "solitary fibrous tumor of the pleura," the lesion now known as "localized fibrous tumor" is neither a lesion restricted to the pleura nor is it always solitary. Localized fibrous tumors have been described at many body sites, and malignant and benign forms occur. In 1981, Briselli and coworkers [41] described 8 cases and reviewed the world's literature of 360 additional cases. Approximately three quarters of patients had symptoms at the time of diagnosis, including cough, chest pain, dyspnea, or pulmonary osteoarthropathy. Eighty percent of these tumors arose from the visceral pleura, whereas 20% are described as arising in the parietal pleura. The tumors are generally circumscribed, ranging in size from 1 to 36 cm, with a mean of approximately 6 cm. Many are pedunculated, with attachment to the pleura by a pedicle (Fig. 15). Histopathologically, these are cellular tumors in which spindle cells alternate with hyalinized connective tissue. In the benign forms, there is minimal cellular atypia and rare mitotic figures. Eighty-eight percent of the described cases behaved in a benign fashion. Patients who succumbed to tumor did so after extensive intrathoracic growth, typically in the context of late diagnosis and unresectable tumor. These original authors could identify no pathologic finding other than the presence of a pedicle that would otherwise infer a more favorable prognosis. Nuclear pleomorphism and high mitotic rates were only implicated as poor prognostic features if the tumor lacked circumscription. A further discussion of malignant localized fibrous tumor can be found later in this article. Localized fibrous tumor has no known association with asbestos exposure.

Adenomatoid tumor

Adenomatoid tumors are benign neoplasms demonstrating mesothelial differentiation [42]. They are rare in the pleura and occur most commonly along the genital tract mesothelium. When adenomatoid tumors occur in the pleura, they are nodular expansile lesions 1 to 2 cm in diameter. They are composed of epithelioid cells forming tubules and irregularly dilated glands within a fibrovascular stroma (Fig. 16). The cells typically have an eccentrically placed nucleus and generous eosinophilic cytoplasm, many times with prominent vacuolization.

Adenomatoid tumors are most important as mimickers of malignant pleural disease (metastatic adenocarcinoma to pleura or epithelial mesothelioma). Adenomatoid tumors of the pleura are rareand can be distinguished from carcinomas and mesotheliomas by their relatively bland cytology (compared with metastatic carcinomas) and their exquisite circum-

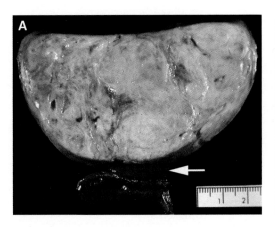
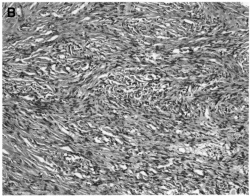

Fig. 15. Localized (solitary) fibrous tumor of pleura. (*A*) This pedunculated tumor has a narrow attachment to pleura (*arrow*). The cross-sectional appearance resembles that of leiomyoma of the uterus, with whorled and nodular subpatterns. (*B*) The microscopic appearance is distinctive, consisting of spindled cells with elongated nuclei woven into a tapestry of collagen (routine hematoxylin-eosin stain).

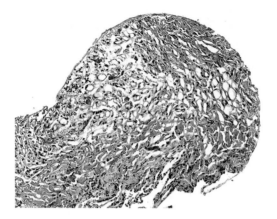

Fig. 16. Adenomatoid tumor (routine hematoxylin-eosin stain). This rare benign tumor of the pleura can be confused with a vascular neoplasm or a mesothelioma. Loose collagen bundles surround variable numbers of ring-like vascular channels and epithelial inclusions.

scription (helpful in separating this tumor from mesothelioma) [42].

Malignant pleural neoplasms

An overview of malignant pleural tumors is presented in Box 8. Mesothelioma clearly dominates any discussion of pleural tumors for many reasons, ranging from the distinctive etiologic relation with asbestos exposure to the diagnostic challenges that these tumors pose. Litigious issues related to occupational asbestos exposure also figure prominently in the landscape of mesothelioma, but these are beyond the scope of this article. It is more common for a malignant tumor of the pleura to be a metastasis from another site, so we begin with these.

Metastatic tumors

Metastatic carcinoma

Metastatic tumors to the pleura are another common cause of exudative effusions, and the risk of this process increases with age. The most common cause of malignant effusion with metastatic carcinoma to pleura is underlying lung cancer. The mechanism is most often contiguous spread and invasion of tumor into the pulmonary vasculature and lymphatics [43]. Metastatic tumor from lung, breast, ovary, stomach, or lymphoproliferative origins accounts for 80% of all malignant effusions [43]. In patients older than 50 years of age, neoplasms of the pleura are second only to congestive heart failure as a

cause of pleural effusion [44]. Adenocarcinoma is the most common form of metastatic carcinoma involving pleura [44].

A peculiar manifestation of metastatic carcinoma to pleura may grossly simulate diffuse malignant mesothelioma, so-called "pleurotropic" or "pseudomesotheliomatous" carcinomas (Fig. 17) [45,46].

Metastatic sarcoma

Most sarcomas of the pleura are metastatic to this site from known or clinically occult soft tissue tumors. Nearly every named soft tissue sarcoma has been reported to involve the pleura by direct extension or metastasis.

Lymphoproliferative diseases

Beyond the well-established association of long-standing chronic empyema and Epstein-Barr virus associated with primary pleural lymphoma [47], lymphoproliferative diseases primarily occurring in the pleura are rare. One relatively notorious form is so-called "effusion-based lymphoma," a human herpes virus type 8 (HHV8)–associated lymphoma occurring mainly in HIV-infected hosts [48]. Isolated pleural effusion as a first manifestation of disease is relatively rare [49].

When the pleura is secondarily involved by lymphoma or leukemia, the extrathoracic primary site of

---

Box 8. Malignant pleural neoplasms

Metastatic tumors
    Lung carcinoma
    Extrathoracic carcinomas
Sarcomas
    Fibromatosis
    Malignant fibrous histiocytoma
    Synovial sarcoma
    Angiosarcoma
    Liposarcoma
    Rhabdomyosarcoma
    Fibrosarcoma
Lymphoproliferative diseases
    Lymphoma
    Hodgkin's disease
    Leukemia
Mesothelioma
    Epithelial
    Sarcomatoid
    Biphasic

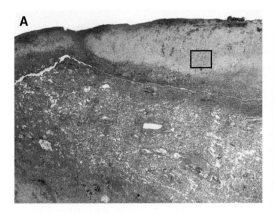
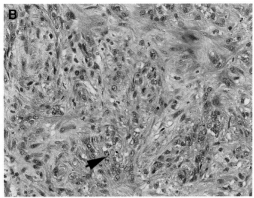

Fig. 17. Pseudomesotheliomatous carcinoma (routine hematoxylin-eosin stain). (*A*) At scanning magnification, the pleura (*top*) is markedly thickened and covered with a thin layer of bright red fibrin. Within the expanded pleura, nested cells of adenocarcinoma can be seen (box: expanded in *B*). (*B*) At higher magnification, the malignant epithelial cells can be identified within dense collagen, simulating mesothelioma (*arrow*).

involvement is generally known at the time of diagnosis (Fig. 18).

Primary malignant neoplasms

Mesothelioma

Mesothelioma is a highly lethal and therapy-resistant malignant neoplasm derived from the mesothelial cell [50]. Mesothelioma is strongly linked with certain types of asbestos exposure [51], and radiation therapy to the chest is also a well-recognized risk [50].

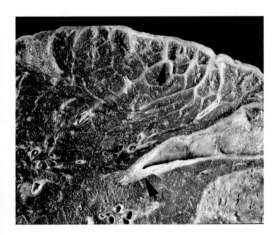

Fig. 18. Lymphoma involving pleura. When lymphoproliferative diseases involve the pleura, they do so along lymphatic routes. Here, thickened pleura and interlobular septa (*white areas*) can be seen (*arrows*).

Asbestos is a group of fibrous silicate minerals that includes two main groups known as amphiboles and serpentines (see Box 6). The tumorigenic role of amphiboles (eg, crocidolite, amosite) is well established, but the role of other asbestos particles in the causation of mesothelioma remains controversial in the scientific community [51]. Furthermore, most epidemiologic studies have focused on occupational exposure, but there is a well-recognized nonoccupational exposure risk (paraoccupational, neighborhood, and true environmental) [52].

One of the most problematic factors related to asbestos as an environmental carcinogen is the apparent minimal contact required for the eventual induction of mesothelioma, although the latency period may be 30 years or longer. The widespread use of asbestos in the shipbuilding, construction, and building maintenance trades over the past century has led to a dramatic increase in the incidence of mesothelioma [53,54]. Connelly and coworkers [55] described a doubling between the periods 1975 to 1979 and 1980 to 1984. The epidemiologic data suggest that the incidence of mesothelioma has already peaked in the United States [56,57], whereas Great Britain may not see an abatement of cases until after 2020 [58,59]. Unfortunately, the prevalence may continue to increase with the long latency period [60] between asbestos exposure and development of mesothelioma and the increasing life expectancy of the population [61].

Mesothelioma is a disease of older individuals, generally occurring between the ages of 50 and 60 years [62]. Affected individuals most commonly present with unilateral pleural effusion, chest pain,

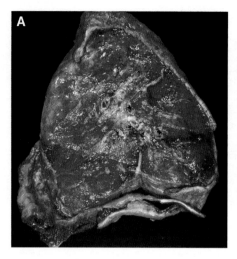
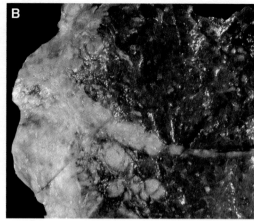

Fig. 19. Mesothelioma. (*A*) Late in mesothelioma, the lung becomes encased with a thick rind of fibrotic tumor. (*B*) Another example of advanced mesothelioma with thick tumor at the surface (*left*) and extending downward into lung parenchyma along interlobular septa; note the irregular black areas representing anthracosis of "native" pleura and interlobular septa.

and dyspnea [54,62–64]. Radiologic evidence of asbestosis is uncommon, but the pleural plaques (see Fig. 12) of asbestos exposure are frequently present [65]. The tumor grows relentlessly, finally encasing the lung, mediastinum, and chest wall in a thick sheath of tumor (Fig. 19). As listed in Box 9, mesotheliomas may present initially as (1) diffuse plaque-like and miliary nodular disease, (2) multiple distinct nodular masses, and, least commonly, (3) an isolated pleural-based tumor (localized malignant mesothelioma) [66,67]. Growth characteristics of malignant pleural mesothelioma are highly variable between individual patients, a factor that becomes important when considering surgical therapeutic options. Some tumors may be relatively well circumscribed and amenable to surgical dissection from surrounding structures; other lesions are highly infiltrative, rendering effective surgery impossible [68].

The histopathologic findings of mesothelioma take several forms, including purely epithelial types (Fig. 20), mixed epithelial and sarcomatous types (Fig. 21), and purely sarcomatous types (Fig. 22). The nuances of the histopathologic variants within each of these major groupings are beyond the scope of this article, and the interested reader is referred to several excellent reviews [66,69–76]. Suffice it to say that the diagnosis of mesothelioma can be one of the most challenging in pathology, mainly because all three forms of this tumor may have significant overlap with reactive conditions of the pleura. A particular problem for pathologists is separating the desmoplastic variant of sarcomatous mesothelioma from reactive fibrous pleurisy [72,77]. Moreover, pleural biopsies of sufficient size to guarantee a definitive diagnosis may be difficult to obtain, especially early in the disease. Even in the most experienced hands, an accurate diagnosis requires exclusion of benign and malignant imitations, often requiring the addition of a battery of immunohistochemical stains (Box 10). Even though pleural effusion is a constant (and accessible) feature, the fluid is often not entirely diagnostic. Reactive mesothelial proliferations may be more atypical cytologically than their mesothelioma counterparts [78], and no specific markers of malignancy have yet emerged as ancillary tests.

The concept of mesothelioma-in-situ, although intuitive, is still controversial in practice. Confident diagnosis by experts is only made when unequivocal invasive mesothelioma is identified in the same specimen (Fig. 23) [79]. In uncertain cases, a diagnosis of atypical mesothelial hyperplasia is appropriate.

Box 9. Gross manifestations of mesothelioma

Pleural studding and small
  plaques (discontinuous)
Pleural masses with variable confluence
Lung encasement with tumor invasion
  of chest wall and lung
Localized mass lesion (rarest)

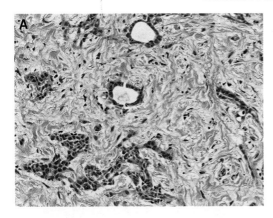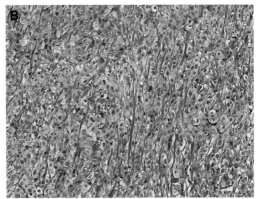

Fig. 20. Epithelial mesothelioma (routine hematoxylin-eosin stain). (*A*) The pure epithelial variant of mesothelioma closely simulates metastatic carcinoma. Note here the sparse irregular infiltration of dense collagen by nested cells, some of which form tubular structures (*upper center*) in this example of mesothelioma. (*B*) Another example of epithelial mesothelioma shows pale epithelioid mesothelial cells separated by thin strands of collagen (*dark pink*).

Primary sarcomas

Malignant localized fibrous tumor.   As discussed previously, localized fibrous tumors may behave aggressively with local recurrence and distant metastasis. England and coworkers [80] described the Armed Forces Institute of Pathology experience with localized fibrous tumor and proposed criteria for distinguishing benign from malignant forms. These authors described 223 localized fibrous tumors of pleura, 82 of which were malignant. The tumors occurred equally in the sexes and most commonly in the sixth or seventh decade of life. Twenty-five

percent of their patients had hypoglycemia, digital clubbing, or pleural effusion. Tumors occurring outside the visceral pleura or those inverted into the lung parenchyma (Fig. 24) were more often malignant in this series. Patients who were cured of malignant localized fibrous tumor had pedunculated or well-circumscribed tumors at diagnosis. Invasion into the lung parenchyma or chest wall, recurrence of disease

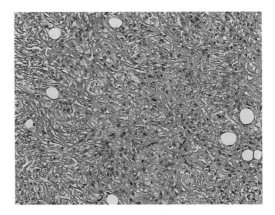

Fig. 22. Sarcomatoid mesothelioma (routine hematoxylin-eosin stain). Perhaps the most challenging of mesotheliomas, sarcomatoid mesothelioma can be quite bland on the one hand or strikingly pleomorphic on the other. Immunohistochemical stains may not be helpful in separating sarcomatoid mesothelioma from sarcomatoid carcinoma of the lung that has spread to involve the pleura. The desmoplastic variant of sarcomatoid carcinoma may be difficult to distinguish from reactive fibrous pleuritis. The white circles in this photograph represent fat invaded by tumor.

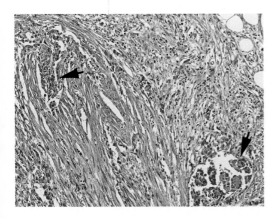

Fig. 21. Mixed epithelial and sarcomatoid (biphasic) mesothelioma (routine hematoxylin-eosin stain). Few malignant tumors of the pleura simulate biphasic mesothelioma, given the presence of distinct nested epithelioid cells (*arrows*) separated by fascicles of malignant spindle cell growth.

Box 10. Immunohistochemical stains useful in the diagnosis of mesothelioma

Positive in mesothelioma
    Pankeratin
    Cytokeratin 5/6 [149,150]
    Calretinin [151–153]
    HBME-1 [154–156]
    WT-1 [157]
    Thrombomodulin (CD141) [154]
    Vimentin [158,159]
Positive in adenocarcinomas
    (pulmonary or extrathoracic origin)
    Pankeratin
    Carcinoembryonic antigen
        [160,161]
    Thyroid transcription factor-1
        [162,163]
    BER-EP4 [164,165]
    MOC-31 [166]
    CD15 [167]
    B72.3 [168,169]

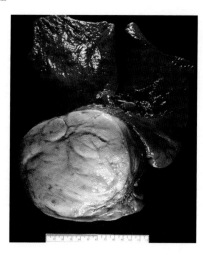

Fig. 24. Malignant localized fibrous tumor. This large fleshy tumor was almost entirely intraparenchymal. Histopathologically, sections showed pleomorphic tumor cells with many mitotic figures and areas of necrosis.

proximately 50% of localized fibrous tumors express C-KIT immunohistochemically [82].

Other sarcomas. Angiosarcoma, leiomyosarcoma, rhabdomyosarcoma, Ewing's sarcoma, primitive neurectodermal tumor, chondrosarcoma, malignant fibrous histiocytoma, osteosarcoma, synovial sarcoma, and fibrosarcoma are sarcomas described as occurring rarely as primary intrathoracic tumors. Some of these occur more often as chest wall lesions extending to involve pleura (Ewing's sarcoma, primitive

after excision, or metastases were the most common causes of mortality in those patients with malignant tumors by histopathologic criteria. Immunohistochemical stains are helpful in separating localized fibrous tumor from fibroblastic forms of mesothelioma (CD34-positive, cytokeratin-negative) [81]. Ap-

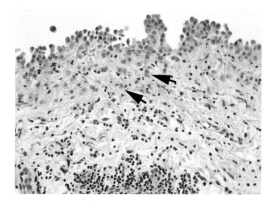

Fig. 23. Possible mesothelioma in situ (routine hematoxylin-eosin stain). Most authorities agree that purely in situ mesothelioma is impossible to diagnose with certainty. Here, superficial invasion by individual epithelioid cells (*arrows*) can be appreciated, compatible with early mesothelioma. The patient whose biopsy is illustrated here returned 6 months later with deeply invasive biphasic mesothelioma.

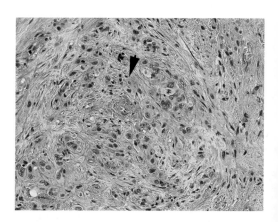

Fig. 25. Epithelioid hemangioendothelioma (routine hematoxylin-eosin stain). This malignant epithelioid vascular tumor is characterized by cells with cytoplasmic vacuoles containing red blood cells (*arrow*). Distinct vascular channels typically are not formed.

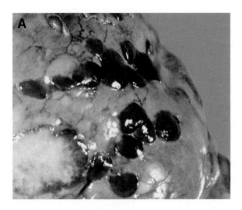 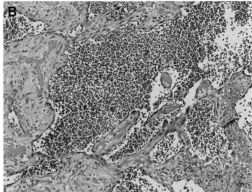

Fig. 26. Angiosarcoma. Most angiosarcomas are metastatic to pleura. (*A*) This gross example of angiosarcoma involving the pleura shows dark hemorrhagic blebs and gray-white scirrhous areas of infiltrating tumor (*lower left*). (*B*) The histopathologic finding of angiosarcoma involving the pleura is similar to the findings of angiosarcoma at other sites. Here, large irregular vascular blood lakes can be seen separated by cords of tumor-associated stromal "promontories" covered by malignant endothelial cells.

neurectodermal tumor, chondrosarcoma, malignant fibrous histiocytoma, osteosarcoma, synovial sarcoma, and fibrosarcoma) [83]. AIDS-related Kaposi's sarcoma is technically the most common sarcoma of lung, at least in large urban centers [84], and may present with pneumothorax [85], bloody pleural effusion [86], or chylothorax [87]. Epithelioid hemangioendothelioma (Fig. 25) and angiosarcoma (Fig. 26) are rare sarcomas of endothelial origin that present with serosanguineous pleural effusions [88,89] and may mimic mesothelioma grossly and microscopically [90,91]. Rare cases of pediatric pleural hemangiomas have been described [92].

Pathologic findings of pneumothorax

The potential causes of pneumothorax are presented in Box 11. Most patients with pneumothorax are not subjected to a biopsy for the purpose of diagnosing an underlying cause; however, pleura and lung samples are often submitted for histopathologic evaluation at the time of surgical intervention for repair of a persistent air leak. These samples are often nondiagnostic, much to the consternation of the surgical pathologist, who often feels obliged to render a meaningful diagnosis in this setting.

Iatrogenic pneumothorax

A well-recognized complication of invasive thoracic diagnostic procedures, iatrogenic pneumothorax, has been reported most frequently after transthoracic needle aspiration, thoracentesis, transthoracic pleural biopsy, subclavian vein catheter replacements, thoracentesis, transthoracic pleural biopsy, and barotrauma. Pneumothorax in these contexts becomes a histopathologic issue typically after transbronchial biopsy, when fragments of normal pleura may be identified in the sample. Induced pneumothorax (therapeutic pneumothorax) for the treatment of tuberculosis is rarely practiced in United States today.

Spontaneous pneumothorax

Spontaneous pneumothoraces can be divided into a primary form that occurs in patients without known underlying lung disease and a secondary form that occurs in patients with known underlying lung disease.

Box 11. Causes of pneumothorax

Trauma [170–173]
Emphysema [100,101,174,175]
Certain lung infections (*Pneumocystis*)
   [176–178]
Pulmonary Langerhans cell
   histiocytosis [179]
Lymphangioleiomyomatosis [180]
Cystic fibrosis [181]
Spontaneous [182]
Catamenial [105,107,110]
Iatrogenic and/or artificial [183,184]

Primary spontaneous pneumothorax affects men more commonly than women (7.4 versus 1.2 per 100,000 population) [93]. The etiology is unknown. The peak age for the primary form is the early third decade, and the condition rarely occurs in persons older than 40 years of age. Clinical features include acute localized chest pain with shortness of breath. The condition typically occurs when the subject is at rest [94]. There has been considerable speculation on the origin of this process, but the prevailing opinion is that the condition results from ruptured subpleural emphysematous blebs and/or bullae in the lung apices (Fig. 27). In a large series reporting the pathologic findings in spontaneous pneumothorax, Jordan and colleagues [95] found emphysema and bulla formation in 80% of their patients. Patients with primary spontaneous pneumothorax tend to be taller and thinner than age-matched controls. Larger pressure gradients from apex to base in the pleura have been postulated as producing greater distention of apical subpleural alveoli with subsequent rupture. Pneumothorax occurs more commonly in individuals with underlying airway disease (typically smoking-related airway disease) [96]. Abnormal airways are also implicated in the patient with spontaneous pneumothorax of primary type [97]. Pathologic specimens taken at the time of pneumothorax repair may cause considerable problems for pathologists. Eosinophilic pleuritis may occur [98], and there may be variable nonspecific subpleural fibrosis in resected portions of lung under these circumstances.

Secondary pneumothorax is more common in patients older than 40 years of age [99–101]. The recurrence rate for secondary pneumothorax is higher than that for primary spontaneous pneumothorax.

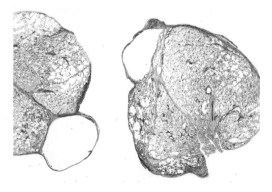

Fig. 27. Pleural blebs. Blebs are defined as cystic spaces occurring within the substance of the pleura. Here, a low-magnification image shows isolated blebs in the pleura of two lung sections.

Chronic obstructive pulmonary disease is the most commonly implicated underlying parenchymal disease, although underlying causes range from infections to malignant tumors. Patients with HIV infection may develop pneumothorax secondary to *Pneumocystis* pneumonia [102]. In these latter individuals, there may be considerable necrosis associated with the pneumothorax, making repair of persistent lesions difficult [103]. Patients with underlying cavitary infection, such as that produced by tuberculosis or coccidioidomycosis, are at risk for pneumothorax [104]. Patients with asthma are also at risk for pneumothorax presumably on the basis of mucous impaction and ball-valve hyperexpansion of peripheral lung segments.

Catamenial pneumothorax

Defined as spontaneous pneumothorax occurring within 72 hours of the onset of menstruation (often with hemoptysis), catamenial pneumothorax is believed to be a rare condition [105–107]. The lack of consistent associated intraoperative findings has led to conflicting theories as to the pathogenesis of catamenial pneumothorax [105]. Pleural or pleural parenchymal endometriosis is associated with a small subset of patients who qualify as having catamenial pneumothorax [108], but the presence of pleural parenchymal endometriosis would not adequately explain the recurrent and cyclic nature of this phenomenon [107]. A high degree of suspicion is prudent, and any ovulating woman with spontaneous pneumothorax should be evaluated for this possibility. An association with pelvic endometriosis is not required. Successful surgical management may involve plication of the diaphragmatic surface, and hormonal suppression therapy has been recommended as a helpful adjunct [105].

Regarding pneumothorax in general, there is a clear association with known malignancy, so any patient known to have primary intra- or extrathoracic malignant neoplasm and pneumothorax should be evaluated for the possibility of lung metastasis [109].

Miscellaneous rare or unusual pleural lesions

Pleural endometriosis

Thoracic endometriosis (Fig. 28) is uncommon and associated with a variety of clinical manifestations. The pathogenesis is not completely understood. An association with recurrent right-sided pneumothorax occurring within days of the onset of menstruation is

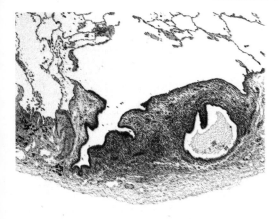

Fig. 28. Pleural endometriosis (routine hematoxylin-eosin stain). The occurrence of endometrial glands and stroma within lung parenchyma or pleura is exceptionally rare. In this example, the stippled dark blue area represents endometrial stroma, whereas the surface layer is endometrial glandular epithelium. On the lower right, a cyst lined by endometrial epithelium is formed within the pleura.

the most common presentation [110]. Patients may have known intra-abdominal endometriosis.

Pleural splenosis

Pleural splenosis is a peculiar and rare occurrence after thoracoabdominal trauma. The term refers to the presence of normal-appearing splenic tissue within the pleural cavity derived presumably by autotransplantation. Abdominal splenosis is a much more common event. Sometimes, long intervals may pass before the pleural lesion is identified as an incidental finding, possibly raising suspicion for a neoplasm radiologically [111].

References

[1] Davies J. Development of the respiratory system. In: Human developmental anatomy. New York: Ronald Press; 1963. p. 135–43.

[2] Sahn SA. State of the art. The pleura. Am Rev Respir Dis 1988;138(1):184–234.

[3] Wang NS. Anatomy of the pleura. Clin Chest Med 1998;19(2):229–40.

[4] Wang N. The preformed stomas connecting the pleural cavity and the lymphatics in the parietal pleura. Am Rev Respir Dis 1975;111:12–20.

[5] Gaudio E, Rendina EA, Pannarale L, et al. Surface morphology of the human pleura. A scanning electron microscopic study. Chest 1988;93(1):149–53.

[6] Harley RA. Pathology of pleural infections. Semin Respir Infect 1988;3(4):291–7.

[7] Hughes CE, Van Scoy RE. Antibiotic therapy of pleural empyema. Semin Respir Infect 1991;6(2): 94–102.

[8] Magovern CJ, Rusch VW. Parapneumonic and post-traumatic pleural space infections. Chest Surg Clin N Am 1994;4(3):561–82.

[9] Krasnik M, Storm HK, Frimodt-Moller N. [Pleural empyema]. Ugeskr Laeger 1996;158(15):2109–12 [in Danish].

[10] Antony VB, Mohammed KA. Pathophysiology of pleural space infections. Semin Respir Infect 1999; 14(1):9–17.

[11] Strange C, Sahn SA. Management of parapneumonic pleural effusions and empyema. Infect Dis Clin North Am 1991;5(3):539–59.

[12] Bartlett JG. Bacterial infections of the pleural space. Semin Respir Infect 1988;3(4):308–21.

[13] Everts RJ, Reller LB. Pleural space infections: microbiology and antimicrobial therapy. Semin Respir Infect 1999;14(1):18–30.

[14] Bartlett JG. Anaerobic bacterial infections of the lung and pleural space. Clin Infect Dis 1993;16(Suppl 4): S248–55.

[15] Center for Disease Control. Extrapulmonary tuberculosis in the United States. US Department of Health, Education, and Welfare, Public Health Service, Center for Disease Control, 1978 Series HEW publication no. CDC 78-8360.

[16] Abrams WB, Small MJ. Current concepts of tuberculous pleurisy with effusion as derived from pleural biopsy studies. Dis Chest 1960;38:60–5.

[17] Ibrahim WH, Ghadban W, Khinji A, et al. Does pleural tuberculosis disease pattern differ among developed and developing countries. Respir Med 2005; 99(8):1038–45.

[18] George RB, Penn RL, Kinasewitz GT. Mycobacterial, fungal, actinomycotic, and nocardial infections of the pleura. Clin Chest Med 1985;6(1):63–75.

[19] Lambert RS, George RB. Fungal diseases of the pleura: clinical manifestations, diagnosis, and treatment. Semin Respir Infect 1988;3(4):343–51.

[20] Shamsuzzaman SM, Hashiguchi Y. Thoracic amebiasis. Clin Chest Med 2002;23(2):479–92.

[21] Mayo F, Baier H. Cysticercotic cyst involving the pleura. An unusual case of an abnormal chest roentgenogram. Arch Intern Med 1979;139(1):115–6.

[22] Im JG, Whang HY, Kim WS, et al. Pleuropulmonary paragonimiasis: radiologic findings in 71 patients. AJR Am J Roentgenol 1992;159(1):39–43.

[23] Roberts PP. Parasitic infections of the pleural space. Semin Respir Infect 1988;3(4):362–82.

[24] Hillerdal G. Non-malignant asbestos pleural disease. Thorax 1981;36:669–75.

[25] Stephens M, Gibbs A, Pooley F, et al. Asbestos induced diffuse pleural fibrosis: pathology and mineralogy. Thorax 1987;42:583–8.

[26] Mintzer R, Cugell D. The association of asbestos-

induced pleural disease and rounded atelectasis. Chest 1982;81:457–60.

[27] Cugell DW, Kamp DW. Asbestos and the pleura: a review. Chest 2004;125(3):1103–17.

[28] Sahn SA. Immunologic diseases of the pleura. Clin Chest Med 1985;6(1):83–102.

[29] Huggins JT, Sahn SA. Causes and management of pleural fibrosis. Respirology 2004;9(4):441–7.

[30] Mutsaers SE, Prele CM, Brody AR, et al. Pathogenesis of pleural fibrosis. Respirology 2004;9(4):428–40.

[31] Antony VB. Drug-induced pleural disease. Clin Chest Med 1998;19(2):331–40.

[32] Huggins JT, Sahn SA. Drug-induced pleural disease. Clin Chest Med 2004;25(1):141–53.

[33] Morelock S, Sahn S. Drugs and the pleura. Chest 1999;116:212–21.

[34] Remy-Jardin M, Sobaszek A, Duhamel A, et al. Asbestos-related pleuropulmonary diseases: evaluation with low-dose four-detector row spiral CT. Radiology 2004;233(1):182–90.

[35] Arakawa H, Honma K, Saito Y, et al. Pleural disease in silicosis: pleural thickening, effusion, and invagination. Radiology 2005;236(2):685–93.

[36] Mazziotti S, Gaeta M, Costa C, et al. Computed tomography features of liparitosis: pneumoconiosis due to amorphous silica. Eur Respir J 2004;23(2):208–13.

[37] Young Jr RC, Rachal RE, Carr PG, et al. Patterns of coal workers' pneumoconiosis in Appalachian former coal miners. J Natl Med Assoc 1992;84(1):41–8.

[38] Engleman P, Liebow AA, Gmelich J, et al. Pulmonary hyalinizing granuloma. Am Rev Respir Dis 1977;115(6):997–1008.

[39] Yousem SA, Hochholzer L. Pulmonary hyalinizing granuloma. Am J Clin Pathol 1987;87(1):1–6.

[40] Pinkard NB, Wilson RW, Lawless N, et al. Calcifying fibrous pseudotumor of pleura. A report of three cases of a newly described entity involving the pleura. Am J Clin Pathol 1996;105(2):189–94.

[41] Briselli M, Mark E, Dickersin G. Solitary fibrous tumors of the pleura: eight new cases and review of 360 cases in the literature. Cancer 1981;47:2678–89.

[42] Kaplan MA, Tazelaar HD, Hayashi T, et al. Adenomatoid tumors of the pleura. Am J Surg Pathol 1996;20(10):1219–23.

[43] Sahn SA. Malignancy metastatic to the pleura. Clin Chest Med 1998;19(2):351–61.

[44] Matthay RA, Coppage L, Shaw C, et al. Malignancies metastatic to the pleura. Invest Radiol 1990;25(5):601–19.

[45] Attanoos RL, Gibbs AR. 'Pseudomesotheliomatous' carcinomas of the pleura: a 10-year analysis of cases from the Environmental Lung Disease Research Group, Cardiff. Histopathology 2003;43(5):444–52.

[46] Koss LG. Benign and malignant mesothelial proliferations. Am J Surg Pathol 2001;25(4):548–9.

[47] Molinie V, Pouchot J, Navratil E, et al. Primary Epstein-Barr virus-related non-Hodgkin's lymphoma of the pleural cavity following long-standing tuberculous empyema. Arch Pathol Lab Med 1996;120(3):288–91.

[48] Hengge UR, Ruzicka T, Tyring SK, et al. Update on Kaposi's sarcoma and other HHV8 associated diseases. Part 2: pathogenesis, Castleman's disease, and pleural effusion lymphoma. Lancet Infect Dis 2002;2(6):344–52.

[49] Vu HN, Jenkins FW, Swerdlow SH, et al. Pleural effusion as the presentation for primary effusion lymphoma. Surgery 1998;123(5):589–91.

[50] Jaurand MC, Fleury-Feith J. Pathogenesis of malignant pleural mesothelioma. Respirology 2005;10(1):2–8.

[51] Marchevsky AM, Wick MR. Current controversies regarding the role of asbestos exposure in the causation of malignant mesothelioma: the need for an evidence-based approach to develop medicolegal guidelines. Ann Diagn Pathol 2003;7(5):321–32.

[52] Bourdes V, Boffetta P, Pisani P. Environmental exposure to asbestos and risk of pleural mesothelioma: review and meta-analysis. Eur J Epidemiol 2000;16(5):411–7.

[53] Borow M, Conston A, Livornese LL, et al. Mesothelioma and its association with asbestosis. JAMA 1967;201(8):587–91.

[54] Borow M, Conston A, Livornese L, et al. Mesothelioma following exposure to asbestos: a review of 72 cases. Chest 1973;64(5):641–6.

[55] Connelly RR, Spirtas R, Myers MH, et al. Demographic patterns for mesothelioma in the United States. J Natl Cancer Inst 1987;78(6):1053–60.

[56] Nishimura SL, Broaddus VC. Asbestos-induced pleural disease. Clin Chest Med 1998;19(2):311–29.

[57] Peto J, Decarli A, La Vecchia C, et al. The European mesothelioma epidemic. Br J Cancer 1999;79(3–4):666–72.

[58] Peto J, Hodgson JT, Matthews FE, et al. Continuing increase in mesothelioma mortality in Britain. Lancet 1995;345(8949):535–9.

[59] Treasure T, Waller D, Swift S, et al. Radical surgery for mesothelioma. BMJ 2004;328(7434):237–8.

[60] Lanphear BP, Buncher CR. Latent period for malignant mesothelioma of occupational origin. J Occup Med 1992;34(7):718–21.

[61] Ohar J, Sterling DA, Bleecker E, et al. Changing patterns in asbestos-induced lung disease. Chest 2004;125(2):744–53.

[62] Legha SS, Muggia FM. Pleural mesothelioma: clinical features and therapeutic implications. Ann Intern Med 1977;87(5):613–21.

[63] Brenner J, Sardillo P, Magill G, et al. Malignant mesothelioma of the pleura. Review of 123 patients. Cancer 1982;49:2431–5.

[64] Adams V, Krishnan K, Muhm J, et al. Diffuse malignant mesothelioma of pleura: diagnosis and survival in 92 cases. Cancer 1986;58:1540–51.

[65] Elmes PC, Simpson JC. The clinical aspects of mesothelioma. Q J Med 1976;45(179):427–49.

[66] Crotty TB, Myers JL, Katzenstein AL, et al. Lo-

calized malignant mesothelioma. A clinicopathologic
and flow cytometric study. Am J Surg Pathol 1994;
18(4):357–63.

[67] Allen TC, Cagle PT, Churg AM, et al. Localized
malignant mesothelioma. Am J Surg Pathol 2005;
29(7):866–73.

[68] van Ruth S, Baas P, Zoetmulder FA. Surgical treatment of malignant pleural mesothelioma: a review.
Chest 2003;123(2):551–61.

[69] Butnor KJ, Sporn TA, Hammar SP, et al. Well-
differentiated papillary mesothelioma. Am J Surg
Pathol 2001;25(10):1304–9.

[70] Hammar S, Bolen J. Sarcomatoid pleural mesothelioma. Ultrastruct Pathol 1985;9:337–43.

[71] Klima M, Bossart M. Sarcomatous type of ma-
ligant mesothelioma. Ultrastruct Pathol 1983;4:
349–58.

[72] Mangano W, Cagle P, Churg A, et al. The diagnosis
and desmoplastic malignant mesothelioma and its
distinction from fibrous pleurisy: a histologic and
immunohistochemical analysis of 31 cases including
p53 immunostaining. Am J Clin Pathol 1998;18:
195–9.

[73] Attanoos RL, Gibbs AR. Pathology of malignant
mesothelioma. Histopathology 1997;30(5):403–18.

[74] Roggli VL, Kolbeck J, Sanfilippo F, et al. Pathology
of human mesothelioma. Etiologic and diagnostic
considerations. Pathol Annu 1987;22(Pt 2):91–131.

[75] Van Marck E. Pathology of malignant mesothelioma.
Lung Cancer 2004;45(Suppl 1):S35–6.

[76] Corson JM. Pathology of mesothelioma. Thorac Surg
Clin 2004;14(4):447–60.

[77] Churg A, Colby TV, Cagle P, et al. The separation
of benign and malignant mesothelial proliferations.
Am J Surg Pathol 2000;24(9):1183–200.

[78] Kutty CP, Remeniuk E, Varkey B. Malignant-
appearing cells in pleural effusion due to pancreatitis: case report and literature review. Acta Cytol 1981;
25(4):412–6.

[79] Henderson DW, Shilkin KB, Whitaker D. Reactive
mesothelial hyperplasia vs mesothelioma, including
mesothelioma in situ: a brief review. Am J Clin Pathol
1998;110(3):397–404.

[80] England DM, Hochholzer L, McCarthy MJ. Localized benign and malignant fibrous tumors of the
pleura. A clinicopathologic review of 223 cases. Am J
Surg Pathol 1989;13(8):640–58.

[81] Flint A, Weiss SW. CD-34 and keratin expression
distinguishes solitary fibrous tumor (fibrous mesothelioma) of pleura from desmoplastic mesothelioma.
Hum Pathol 1995;26(4):428–31.

[82] Butnor KJ, Burchette JL, Sporn TA, et al. The
spectrum of Kit (CD117) immunoreactivity in lung
and pleural tumors: a study of 96 cases using a single-
source antibody with a review of the literature. Arch
Pathol Lab Med 2004;128(5):538–43.

[83] Gladish GW, Sabloff BM, Munden RF, et al. Primary thoracic sarcomas. Radiographics 2002;22(3):
621–37.

[84] Ognibene FP, Shelhamer JH. Kaposi's sarcoma. Clin
Chest Med 1988;9(3):459–65.

[85] Floris C, Sulis ML, Bernascani M, et al. Pneumothorax in pleuropulmonary Kaposi's sarcoma related
to acquired immunodeficiency syndrome. Am J Med
1989;87(1):123–4.

[86] O'Brien RF, Cohn DL. Serosanguineous pleural effusions in AIDS-associated Kaposi's sarcoma. Chest
1989;96(3):460–6.

[87] Pandya K, Lal C, Tuchschmidt J, et al. Bilateral chylothorax with pulmonary Kaposi's sarcoma. Chest
1988;94(6):1316–7.

[88] Yousem SA. Angiosarcoma presenting in the lung.
Arch Pathol Lab Med 1986;110(2):112–5.

[89] Bocklage T, Leslie K, Yousem S, et al. Extracuta-
neous angiosarcomas metastatic to the lungs: clinical
and pathologic features of twenty-one cases. Mod
Pathol 2001;14(12):1216–25.

[90] Lin BT, Colby T, Gown AM, et al. Malignant vascular tumors of the serous membranes mimicking
mesothelioma. A report of 14 cases. Am J Surg Pathol
1996;20(12):1431–9.

[91] Falconieri G, Bussani R, Mirra M, et al. Pseudomesotheliomatous angiosarcoma: a pleuropulmonary
lesion simulating malignant pleural mesothelioma.
Histopathology 1997;30(5):419–24.

[92] Hurvitz CH, Greenberg SH, Song CH, et al. He-
mangiomatosis of the pleura with hemorrhage and
disseminated intravascular coagulation. J Pediatr Surg
1982;17(1):73–5.

[93] Melton III LJ, Hepper NG, Offord KP. Incidence
of spontaneous pneumothorax in Olmsted County,
Minnesota: 1950 to 1974. Am Rev Respir Dis 1979;
120(6):1379–82.

[94] Bense L, Wiman LG, Hedenstierna G. Onset of
symptoms in spontaneous pneumothorax: correlations
to physical activity. Eur J Respir Dis 1987;71(3):
181–6.

[95] Jordan KG, Kwong JS, Flint J, et al. Surgically
treated pneumothorax. Radiologic and pathologic
findings. Chest 1997;111(2):280–5.

[96] Bense L, Eklund G, Wiman LG. Smoking and the
increased risk of contracting spontaneous pneumothorax. Chest 1987;92(6):1009–12.

[97] Bense L. Spontaneous pneumothorax. Chest 1992;
101(4):891–2.

[98] Askin F, McCann B, Kuhn C. Reactive eosinophilic
pleuritis: a lesion to be distinguished from pulmonary
eosinophilic granuloma. Arch Pathol Lab Med 1977;
101:187–91.

[99] Shields TW, Oilschlager GA. Spontaneous pneumothorax in patients 40 years of age and older. Ann
Thorac Surg 1966;2(3):377–83.

[100] Dines DE, Clagett OT, Payne WS. Spontaneous pneumothorax in emphysema. Mayo Clin Proc 1970;
45(7):481–7.

[101] George RB, Herbert SJ, Shames JM, et al. Pneumothorax complicating pulmonary emphysema. JAMA
1975;234(4):389–93.

[102] Newsome GS, Ward DJ, Pierce PF. Spontaneous pneumothorax in patients with acquired immunodeficiency syndrome treated with prophylactic aerosolized pentamidine. Arch Intern Med 1990;150(10): 2167–8.

[103] Gerein AN, Brumwell ML, Lawson LM, et al. Surgical management of pneumothorax in patients with acquired immunodeficiency syndrome. Arch Surg 1991;126(10):1272–6 [discussion: 1276–7].

[104] Wilder RJ, Beacham EG, Ravitch MM. Spontaneous pneumothorax complicating cavitary tuberculosis. J Thorac Cardiovasc Surg 1962;43:561–73.

[105] Korom S, Canyurt H, Missbach A, et al. Catamenial pneumothorax revisited: clinical approach and systematic review of the literature. J Thorac Cardiovasc Surg 2004;128(4):502–8.

[106] Marshall MB, Ahmed Z, Kucharczuk JC, et al. Catamenial pneumothorax: optimal hormonal and surgical management. Eur J Cardiothorac Surg 2005;27(4):662–6.

[107] Peikert T, Gillespie DJ, Cassivi SD. Catamenial pneumothorax. Mayo Clin Proc 2005;80(5):677–80.

[108] Velasco OA, Hilario RE, Santamaria GJL, et al. Catamenial pneumothorax with pleural endometriosis and hemoptysis. Diagn Gynecol Obstet 1982;4(4): 295–9.

[109] Srinivas S, Varadhachary G. Spontaneous pneumothorax in malignancy: a case report and review of the literature. Ann Oncol 2000;11(7):887–9.

[110] Johnson MM. Catamenial pneumothorax and other thoracic manifestations of endometriosis. Clin Chest Med 2004;25(2):311–9.

[111] Yammine JN, Yatim A, Barbari A. Radionuclide imaging in thoracic splenosis and a review of the literature. Clin Nucl Med 2003;28(2):121–3.

[112] Hage CA, Abdul-Mohammed K, Antony VB. Pathogenesis of pleural infection. Respirology 2004;9(1): 12–5.

[113] Mandal AK, Thadepalli H, Chettipalli U. Posttraumatic empyema thoracis: a 24-year experience at a major trauma center. J Trauma 1997;43(5):764–71.

[114] Oba S, Akuma M. [Localized bilateral empyema caused by spontaneous esophageal rupture]. Rinsho Hoshasen 1985;30(3):395–6 [in Japanese].

[115] Sees DW, Obney JA, Tripp HF. Empyema complicating muscle-sparing thoracotomy: the role of wound management. Am Surg 2002;68(4):390–1.

[116] Irving AD, Turner MA. Pleural empyema in association with renal sepsis. Br J Surg 1976;63(1):70–2.

[117] Clarridge J, Roberts C, Peters J, et al. Sepsis and empyema caused by Yersinia enterocolitica. J Clin Microbiol 1983;17(5):936–8.

[118] Ballantyne KC, Sethia B, Reece IJ, et al. Empyema following intra-abdominal sepsis. Br J Surg 1984; 71(9):723–5.

[119] Iscovich AL, Salvucci AA. Streptococcal sepsis and death caused by empyema. Am J Emerg Med 1986; 4(1):28–30.

[120] Samelson SL, Ferguson MK. Empyema following percutaneous catheter drainage of upper abdominal abscess. Chest 1992;102(5):1612–4.

[121] Smith PR, Nacht RI. Drug-induced lupus pleuritis mimicking pleural space infection. Chest 1992; 101(1):268–9.

[122] Good Jr JT, King TE, Antony VB, et al. Lupus pleuritis. Clinical features and pleural fluid characteristics with special reference to pleural fluid antinuclear antibodies. Chest 1983;84(6):714–8.

[123] Graham WR. Rheumatoid pleuritis. South Med J 1990;83(8):973–5.

[124] Owens MW, Milligan SA. Pleuritis and pleural effusions. Curr Opin Pulm Med 1995;1(4):318–23.

[125] Chou CW, Chang SC. Pleuritis as a presenting manifestation of rheumatoid arthritis: diagnostic clues in pleural fluid cytology. Am J Med Sci 2002;323(3): 158–61.

[126] Morelock SY, Sahn SA. Drugs and the pleura. Chest 1999;116(1):212–21.

[127] Kaye M. Pleuropulmonary complications of pancreatitis. Thorax 1968;23:297–306.

[128] Saugier B, Emonot A, Berard P, et al. [Pleuresies in chronic pancreatitis and in pancreatic pseudocysts. A study apropos of 20 cases]. Poumon Coeur 1976; 32(5):233–40 [in French].

[129] Fentanes de Torres E, Guevara E. Pleuritis by radiation: reports of two cases. Acta Cytol 1981;25(4): 427–9.

[130] Shrivastava R, Venkatesh S, Pavlovich BB, et al. Immunological analysis of pleural fluid in postcardiac injury syndrome. Postgrad Med J 2002; 78(920):362–3.

[131] Vallyathan NV, Green FH, Craighead JE. Recent advances in the study of mineral pneumoconiosis. Pathol Annu 1980;15(Pt 2):77–104.

[132] Maher JF. Uremic pleuritis. Am J Kidney Dis 1987; 10(1):19–22.

[133] Yoshii C, Morita S, Tokunaga M, et al. Bilateral massive pleural effusions caused by uremic pleuritis. Intern Med 2001;40(7):646–9.

[134] Ellman P, Cudkowicz L, Elwood J. Widespread serous membrane involvement by rheumatoid nodules. J Clin Pathol 1954;7:239–44.

[135] Jurik AG, Graudal H. Pleurisy in rheumatoid arthritis. Scand J Rheumatol 1983;12(2):75–80.

[136] Robinson AC, Power J, Clancy L, et al. Recurrent pneumothorax in rheumatoid arthritis. Ir J Med Sci 1984;153(12):437–8.

[137] Engel U, Aru A, Francis D. Rheumatoid pleurisy. Acta Pathol Microbiol Immunol Scand 1986;94: 53–6.

[138] Anaya JM, Diethelm L, Ortiz LA, et al. Pulmonary involvement in rheumatoid arthritis. Semin Arthritis Rheum 1995;24(4):242–54.

[139] Pines A, Kaplinsky N, Olchovsky D, et al. Pleuropulmonary manifestations of systemic lupus erythematosus: clinical features of its subgroups. Prognostic and therapeutic implications. Chest 1985;88(1): 129–35.

[140] Wang DY, Chang DB, Kuo SH, et al. Systemic lupus erythematosus presenting as pleural effusion: report of a case. J Formos Med Assoc 1995;94(12): 746–9.

[141] Wang DY. Diagnosis and management of lupus pleuritis. Curr Opin Pulm Med 2002;8(4):312–6.

[142] Quismorio Jr FP. Pulmonary involvement in primary Sjogren's syndrome. Curr Opin Pulm Med 1996; 2(5):424–8.

[143] Kawamata K, Haraoka H, Hirohata S, et al. Pleurisy in primary Sjogren's syndrome: T cell receptor beta-chain variable region gene bias and local autoantibody production in the pleural effusion. Clin Exp Rheumatol 1997;15(2):193–6.

[144] Weir IH, Muller NL, Chiles C, et al. Wegener's granulomatosis: findings from computed tomography of the chest in 10 patients. Can Assoc Radiol J 1992;43(1):31–4.

[145] Kuhlman JE, Hruban RH, Fishman EK. Wegener granulomatosis: CT features of parenchymal lung disease. J Comput Assist Tomogr 1991;15(6): 948–52.

[146] Maguire R, Fauci AS, Doppman JL, et al. Unusual radiographic features of Wegener's granulomatosis. AJR Am J Roentgenol 1978;130(2):233–8.

[147] Churg AM. Disease of the pleura. In: Churg AM, Myers JL, Tazelaar HD, et al, editors. Thurlbeck's pathology of the lung. New York: Thieme; 2005. p. 997.

[147a] Craighead JE, Mossman BT, Bradley BJ. Comparative studies on the cytotoxicity of amphibole and serpentine asbestos. Environ Health Perspect 1980; 34:37–46.

[148] Hendry NW. The geology, occurrences and major uses of asbestos. Ann N Y Acad Sci B 1965;132(1): 12–22.

[149] Clover J, Oates J, Edwards C. Anti-cytokeratin 5/6: a positive marker for epithelioid mesothelioma. Histopathology 1997;31(2):140–3.

[150] Ordonez NG. Value of cytokeratin 5/6 immunostaining in distinguishing epithelial mesothelioma of the pleura from lung adenocarcinoma. Am J Surg Pathol 1998;22(10):1215–21.

[151] Tos AP, Doglioni C. Calretinin: a novel tool for diagnostic immunohistochemistry. Adv Anat Pathol 1998;5(1):61–6.

[152] Ordonez NG. Value of calretinin immunostaining in differentiating epithelial mesothelioma from lung adenocarcinoma. Mod Pathol 1998;11(10):929–33.

[153] Ordonez NG. The immunohistochemical diagnosis of mesothelioma: a comparative study of epithelioid mesothelioma and lung adenocarcinoma. Am J Surg Pathol 2003;27(8):1031–51.

[154] Ordonez NG. The value of antibodies 44–3A6, SM3, HBME-1, and thrombomodulin in differentiating epithelial pleural mesothelioma from lung adenocarcinoma: a comparative study with other commonly used antibodies. Am J Surg Pathol 1997; 21(12):1399–408.

[155] Gonzalez-Lois C, Ballestin C, Sotelo MT, et al. Combined use of novel epithelial (MOC-31) and mesothelial (HBME-1) immunohistochemical markers for optimal first line diagnostic distinction between mesothelioma and metastatic carcinoma in pleura. Histopathology 2001;38(6):528–34.

[156] Gumurdulu D, Zeren EH, Cagle PT, et al. Specificity of MOC-31 and HBME-1 immunohistochemistry in the differential diagnosis of adenocarcinoma and malignant mesothelioma: a study on environmental malignant mesothelioma cases from Turkish villages. Pathol Oncol Res 2002;8(3):188–93.

[157] Foster MR, Johnson JE, Olson SJ, et al. Immunohistochemical analysis of nuclear versus cytoplasmic staining of WT1 in malignant mesotheliomas and primary pulmonary adenocarcinomas. Arch Pathol Lab Med 2001;125(10):1316–20.

[158] al-Saffar N, Hasleton PS. Vimentin, carcinoembryonic antigen and keratin in the diagnosis of mesothelioma, adenocarcinoma and reactive pleural lesions. Eur Respir J 1990;3(9):997–1001.

[159] Duggan MA, Masters CB, Alexander F. Immunohistochemical differentiation of malignant mesothelioma, mesothelial hyperplasia and metastatic adenocarcinoma in serous effusions, utilizing staining for carcinoembryonic antigen, keratin and vimentin. Acta Cytol 1987;31(6):807–14.

[160] Wang NS, Huang SN, Gold P. Absence of carcinoembryonic antigen-like material in mesothelioma: an immunohistochemical differentiation from other lung cancers. Cancer 1979;44(3):937–43.

[161] Riera JR, Astengo-Osuna C, Longmate JA, et al. The immunohistochemical diagnostic panel for epithelial mesothelioma: a reevaluation after heat-induced epitope retrieval. Am J Surg Pathol 1997;21(12): 1409–19.

[162] Khoor A, Whitsett JA, Stahlman MT, et al. Utility of surfactant protein B precursor and thyroid transcription factor 1 in differentiating adenocarcinoma of the lung from malignant mesothelioma. Hum Pathol 1999;30(6):695–700.

[163] Ordonez NG. Value of thyroid transcription factor-1, E-cadherin, BG8, WT1, and CD44S immunostaining in distinguishing epithelial pleural mesothelioma from pulmonary and nonpulmonary adenocarcinoma. Am J Surg Pathol 2000;24(4):598–606.

[164] Gaffey MJ, Mills SE, Swanson PE, et al. Immunoreactivity for BER-EP4 in adenocarcinomas, adenomatoid tumors, and malignant mesotheliomas. Am J Surg Pathol 1992;16(6):593–9.

[165] Ordonez NG. Value of the Ber-EP4 antibody in differentiating epithelial pleural mesothelioma from adenocarcinoma. The M.D. Anderson experience and a critical review of the literature. Am J Clin Pathol 1998;109(1):85–9.

[166] Ordonez NG. Value of the MOC-31 monoclonal antibody in differentiating epithelial pleural mesothelioma from lung adenocarcinoma. Hum Pathol 1998; 29(2):166–9.

[167] Comin CE, Novelli L, Boddi V, et al. Calretinin, thrombomodulin, CEA, and CD15: a useful combination of immunohistochemical markers for differentiating pleural epithelial mesothelioma from peripheral pulmonary adenocarcinoma. Hum Pathol 2001;32(5):529–36.

[168] Szpak CA, Johnston WW, Roggli V, et al. The diagnostic distinction between malignant mesothelioma of the pleura and adenocarcinoma of the lung as defined by a monoclonal antibody (B72.3). Am J Pathol 1986;122(2):252–60.

[169] Warnock ML, Stoloff A, Thor A. Differentiation of adenocarcinoma of the lung from mesothelioma. Periodic acid-Schiff, monoclonal antibodies B72.3, and Leu M1. Am J Pathol 1988;133(1):30–8.

[170] Bridges KG, Welch G, Silver M, et al. CT detection of occult pneumothorax in multiple trauma patients. J Emerg Med 1993;11(2):179–86.

[171] Hill SL, Edmisten T, Holtzman G, et al. The occult pneumothorax: an increasing diagnostic entity in trauma. Am Surg 1999;65(3):254–8.

[172] Henderson SO, Shoenberger JM. Anterior pneumothorax and a negative chest X-ray in trauma. J Emerg Med 2004;26(2):231–2.

[173] Misthos P, Kakaris S, Sepsas E, et al. A prospective analysis of occult pneumothorax, delayed pneumothorax and delayed hemothorax after minor blunt thoracic trauma. Eur J Cardiothorac Surg 2004;25(5):859–64.

[174] Peguero FA, Netzman A. Bullous emphysema and pneumothorax. J Med Soc NJ 1985;82(9):743–5.

[175] DeVries WC, Wolfe WG. The management of spontaneous pneumothorax and bullous emphysema. Surg Clin North Am 1980;60(4):851–66.

[176] Beers MF, Sohn M, Swartz M. Recurrent pneumothorax in AIDS patients with Pneumocystis pneumonia. A clinicopathologic report of three cases and review of the literature. Chest 1990;98(2):266–70.

[177] Pastores SM, Garay SM, Naidich DP, et al. Review: pneumothorax in patients with AIDS-related Pneumocystis carinii pneumonia. Am J Med Sci 1996;312(5):229–34.

[178] Tumbarello M, Tacconelli E, Pirronti T, et al. Pneumothorax in HIV-infected patients: role of Pneumocystis carinii pneumonia and pulmonary tuberculosis. Eur Respir J 1997;10(6):1332–5.

[179] Mendez JL, Nadrous HF, Vassallo R, et al. Pneumothorax in pulmonary Langerhans cell histiocytosis. Chest 2004;125(3):1028–32.

[180] Bearz A, Rupolo M, Canzonieri V, et al. Lymphangioleiomyomatosis: a case report and review of the literature. Tumori 2004;90(5):528–31.

[181] Flume PA. Pneumothorax in cystic fibrosis. Chest 2003;123(1):217–21.

[182] Noppen M, Baumann MH. Pathogenesis and treatment of primary spontaneous pneumothorax: an overview. Respiration (Herrlisheim) 2003;70(4):431–8.

[183] Sassoon CS, Light RW, O'Hara VS, et al. Iatrogenic pneumothorax: etiology and morbidity. Results of a Department of Veterans Affairs Cooperative Study. Respiration (Herrlisheim) 1992;59(4):215–20.

[184] Despars JA, Sassoon CS, Light RW. Significance of iatrogenic pneumothoraces. Chest 1994;105(4):1147–50.

ELSEVIER
SAUNDERS

Clin Chest Med 27 (2006) 181 – 191

CLINICS
IN CHEST
MEDICINE

Pleural Fibrosis

Michael A. Jantz, MD, FCCP*, Veena B. Antony, MD

*Division of Pulmonary and Critical Care Medicine, University of Florida, 1600 SW Archer Road, Room M352,
PO Box 100225, Gainesville, FL 32610–0225, USA*

Pleural fibrosis can result from a variety of inflammatory processes that include immunologic diseases like rheumatoid pleurisy, infections like bacterial empyema and tuberculous pleurisy, asbestos exposure, malignancy, improperly drained hemothorax, post–coronary artery bypass graft (CABG) surgery, uremic pleurisy, and medications. The pathogenesis of pleural fibrosis is related to inflammation of the pleura. The response of the pleural mesothelial cell to injury and the ability to maintain its integrity are crucial in determining whether normal healing or pleural fibrosis occurs. Although pleural fibrosis may resolve over a period of several months, persistence of pleural fibrosis may result in impaired pleural and pulmonary function with increased morbidity for the patient.

Pathogenesis

The lungs and inner surface of the thoracic wall are covered by an elastic serous membrane to form the pleural cavity. The pleura provides protection and allows for a smooth lubricating surface for movement of the lungs during inspiration and expiration. In addition to a protective barrier, the pleura serves as an immunologically and metabolically active membrane that is involved in maintaining homeostasis as well as in responding to pleural inflammation [1]. The pleura is lined by a monolayer of mesothelial cells that rest on a thin basement membrane supported by connective tissue, blood vessels, and lymphatics. The

pleural mesothelial cell is a functionally dynamic cell that has an apical surface covered with microvilli and a defined basilar surface. The mesothelial cells secrete glycosaminoglycans and other surfactant-like molecules to lubricate the pleural surface. In addition, the mesothelial cells also have other important functions, including (1) movement of fluid, particulates, and cells across the pleural cavity; (2) release of proinflammatory and anti-inflammatory mediators; (3) antigen presentation; (4) secretion of factors that promote fibrin deposition and fibrin clearance; (5) and synthesis of growth factors and extracellular matrix proteins to assist in pleural membrane repair [2].

The primary or earliest events during pleural inflammation are mediated via the response of the mesothelial cell and secondarily by inflammatory cells recruited by cytokines that are activated by the primary mesothelial responses. Mesothelial cells phagocytize foreign substances, such as bacteria, talc particles, and asbestos fibers, with subsequent cell activation and release of cytokines, such as interleukin (IL)-8 [3–6]. Activated macrophages release mediators that also stimulate mesothelial cells to release inducers of neutrophil and monocyte chemokines including IL-8, interferon-inducible protein (IP)-10, monocyte chemoattractant protein (MCP)-1, and regulated-on-activation normal T-cell expressed and secreted (RANTES) protein [3,7,8]. Secretion of these chemokines is polarized toward the apical cell surface, creating a chemotactant gradient from the basilar surface of the mesothelium that is covered by a capillary network toward the apical surface of the mesothelium [7,9,10].

Movement of leukocytes from the circulation to the site of inflammation is facilitated by expression of integrins and adhesion molecules. Pleural mesothe-

* Corresponding author.

E-mail address: jantzma@medicine.ufl.edu
(M.A. Jantz).

lial cells express several cell adhesion molecules, including intercellular adhesion molecule (ICAM)-1, vascular cellular adhesion molecule (VCAM)-1, E-cadherin, N-cadherin, L-selectin, P-selectin, and E-selectin [11–13]. After exposure to tumor necrosis factor (TNF)-α, interferon-γ, and IL-1β, these adhesion molecules are expressed on the cell surface of the mesothelial cell and allow for adherence of the neutrophils or monocytes to the mesothelial cell via the CD11/CD18 integrin on the leukocyte [11,14,15].

As noted, the mesothelial cell plays a critical role in the initiation of inflammatory responses in the pleural space because it is the first cell to recognize a perturbation in the pleural space. Pleural inflammation is not only associated with an influx of a large number of inflammatory cells but with a transfer of proteins and a change in the permeability of the pleura. The pleural mesothelial cells release cytokines in a polar fashion, with a high concentration being released on the apical surface, which leads to directed migration of leukocytes into the pleural space. In addition to release from mesothelial cells, a number of cytokines are released from the inflammatory cells recruited to the pleural space (Fig. 1). We examine some of these cytokines that may play a part in the

pathogenesis of pleural fibrosis and discuss the role of disordered fibrin turnover in the development of pleural fibrosis.

Transforming growth factor–β

Transforming growth factor (TGF)-β is a family of multifunctional growth-modulating cytokines. Virtually all cells, including mesothelial cells, can produce and have receptors for TGFβ. Overproduction of TGFβ is the principal abnormality in most fibrotic diseases, and elevated levels of TGFβ have been found in pleural effusions [16]. TGFβ regulates a number of cellular processes, including cell proliferation, cell migration, cell differentiation, and extracellular matrix production. It is a potent chemoattractant for fibroblasts, which are important in collagen synthesis and pleural fibrosis [17]. Mesothelial cells also participate in extracellular matrix turnover. After stimulation by TGFβ, mesothelial cells can synthesize collagen, matrix proteins, matrix metalloproteinase (MMP)-1, MMP-9, and tissue inhibitor of matrix metalloproteinases (TIMP)-2 [18,19]. TGFβ suppresses fibrinolysis by reducing tissue plasminogen activators as well as increasing the meso-

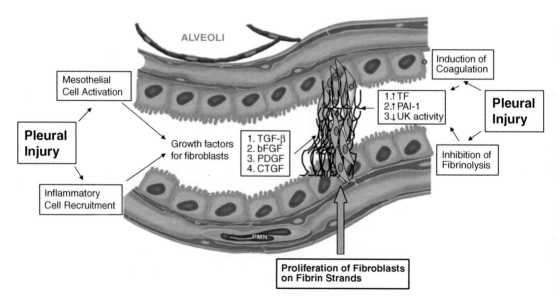

Fig. 1. Mechanisms of pleural fibrosis. Pleural injury leads to activation of mesothelial cells and recruitment of inflammatory cells into the pleural space. The activated pleural mesothelial cells and recruited inflammatory cells release growth factors for fibroblasts such as TGF-ß, bFGF, PDGF, and CTGF. In addition, pleural injury induces induction of the coagulation pathway and inhibition of fibrinolysis resulting in increased levels of tissue factor and plasminogen activator inhibitor-1 and decreased urokinase activity. Together, these processes produce fibrin strand formation, fibroblast proliferation, and generation of extracellular matrix with subsequent pleural fibrosis. bFGF, basic fibroblast growth factor; CTGF, connective tissue growth factor; PAI-1, plasminogen activator inhibitor-1; PDGF, platelet-derived growth factor; TF, tissue factor; TGF-ß, transforming growth factor-beta; UK, urokinase.

thelial cell production of plasminogen activator inhibitor (PAI)-1 and PAI-2 [20,21]. TGFβ has been demonstrated to be present at high levels in empyema, tuberculous pleuritis, and asbestos-related pleural effusions, suggesting a role in the pleural fibrosis associated with these conditions [22–24]. In addition, intrapleural administration of TGFβ has been demonstrated to induce pleurodesis (ie, pleural fibrosis) in animal models [25,26].

Basic fibroblast growth factor

Basic fibroblast growth factor (bFGF), also known as fibroblast growth factor-2, is one of the fibroblast growth factor families. bFGF is known to stimulate mesothelial cell proliferation in vitro and in vivo [27]. bFGF is mitogenic for fibroblasts, smooth muscle cells, and endothelial cells; in addition, it is a known angiogenic factor [28–30]. bFGF is present in pleural effusions due to various etiologies [31,32]. In a recent study, pleural fluid levels of bFGF were higher in patients who underwent successful talc pleurodesis compared with those who failed treatment with talc pleurodesis or had thoracoscopy alone without talc pleurodesis [33]. In this study, the addition of bFGF antibody to the pleural fluids obtained from these patients caused a significant decrease in fibroblast growth activity. Mesothelial cells stimulated with talc were noted to release higher amounts of bFGF compared with controls [33].

Platelet-derived growth factor

Platelet-derived growth factor (PDGF) is a mitogenic cytokine for mesothelial cells [34]. Mesothelial cells are known to produce PDGF [35]. PDGF can also promote the growth of fibroblasts and stimulates hyaluronan production in fibroblasts and mesothelial cells [36,37]. In addition, PDGF can stimulate collagen production by mesothelial cells. PDGF has been demonstrated to be an important mediator of fibroblast proliferation in the pleura in response to inhaled crocidolite asbestos fibers in rodent models. Antibodies against PDGF inhibit fibroblast proliferation in these models [38]. Finally, PDGF also induces the expression of TGFβ, further potentiating the fibrotic response [39].

Disordered fibrin turnover

During the process of wound healing, formation of a transitional fibrin neomatrix contributes to tissue organization and fibrotic repair. It has been proposed that disordered fibrin turnover plays a central role in the pathogenesis of pleural fibrosis (see Fig. 1) [40]. The extravascular deposition of fibrin that occurs along the parietal and visceral pleural surfaces is a marker of early pleural injury. As a result of pleural injury and increased microvascular permeability, plasma is extravasated into the tissue or body compartment. Coagulation at the site of injury is initiated by tissue factor forming a complex with activated factor VII and resultant formation of transitional fibrin. Remodeling of the transitional fibrin occurs through the release of proteases from inflammatory cells that invade the neomatrix. Continued formation and resorption of extravascular fibrin are facilitated by cytokines, such as TNFα and TGFβ. The mesothelial cells and recruited inflammatory cells can produce components of the fibrinolytic system and inhibitors of the fibrinolytic system, including tissue plasminogen activator, urokinase, urokinase receptor, and PAI-1. The relative expression of urokinase, which is thought to be the major plasminogen activator of extravascular fibrin in the lung, versus that of PAIs and antiplasmins, is a key determinant of local fibrinolytic activity. With ongoing remodeling rather than clearance of transitional fibrin, collagen deposition occurs, which ultimately leads to progressive scarring and fibrotic repair [40,41].

Tissue factor is locally secreted in the pleural compartment and is detectable in pleural fluid [42]. In addition, tissue factor is expressed by cells in the pleural compartment, including mesothelial cells, macrophages, and fibroblasts [20,43,44]. The process of coagulation in the pleural space is regulated by concurrent expression of tissue factor pathway inhibitor (TFPI) [42]. Pleural mesothelial cells elaborate tissue factor as well as TFPI [45]. In the setting of pleural injury, the intrapleural elaboration of tissue factor seems to exceed that of TFPI, given the intrapleural fibrin deposition that is observed with pleural inflammation. Intrapleural coagulation has been demonstrated to be upregulated in patients with exudative effusions compared with patients with effusions caused by congestive heart failure [42].

Urokinase, urokinase receptor, and PAI-1 are also hypothesized to be involved in the pathogenesis of pleural injury and fibrosis. These components of the fibrinolysis system have been identified in pleural fluid [42]. Plasminogen is present in pleural fluids and can be activated by urokinase or tissue plasminogen activator, with the subsequent generation of plasmin. Urokinase and tissue plasminogen activator are secreted by cultured human pleural mesothelial cells, and both of these molecules are detectable in pleural effusions in a free form and complexed to PAI-1 and

PAI-2 [20,42]. Tissue plasminogen activator is mainly responsible for intravascular thrombolysis, whereas urokinase is mainly involved in extravascular proteolysis and tissue remodeling [46]. Localized generation of plasmin by urokinase, in free form or via interaction with urokinase receptors on the cell surface, allows mesothelial cells and other cells to degrade extracellular matrix [46]. Urokinase receptors are expressed on the surface of pleural mesothelial cells, macrophages, and lung fibroblasts [47–49]. Urokinase and urokinase receptors are involved in regulation of cytokine-mediated cellular signaling and cell trafficking [50]. In addition, urokinase is a chemotaxin and a mitogen for mesothelial cells and lung fibroblasts [47,51]. PAI-1 and PAI-2 are the major inhibitors of urokinase. PAI-1 and PAI-2 are produced by mesothelial cells and lung fibroblasts [20]. The expression of urokinase-mediated fibrinolytic activity in pleural fluids is inhibited by PAI-1 as well as by antiplasmins [42]. Levels of PAI-1 have been noted to be markedly increased in exudative effusions compared with transudative effusions attributable to congestive heart failure. By inhibiting intrapleural fibrin clearance, these PAIs produce a fibrinolytic defect that leads to accelerated pleural connective tissue matrix organization and pleural fibrosis. Thus, the interplay of urokinase, urokinase receptor, and PAI responses seems to influence the processes of pleural inflammation and repair versus the development of pleural fibrosis.

Causes of pleural fibrosis

Asbestos-related pleural fibrosis

There are two distinct forms of asbestos-related pleural fibrosis: parietal pleural plaques and diffuse pleural thickening. Parietal pleural plaques are the most common manifestation of asbestos exposure. When bilateral and partially calcified, they are virtually pathognomonic of past asbestos exposure. The latency period from first exposure to development of radiographically identifiable plaques averages 20 to 30 years [52]. Parietal pleural plaques are most commonly found on the posterior and lateral walls of the lower half of the thorax and follow the course of the ribs. The costophrenic angles and apices are usually spared. Plaques can also form on the domes of the diaphragm, mediastinal pleura, and pericardium. Simple asbestos-related pleural plaques typically do not cause respiratory symptoms. They are often discovered incidentally during radiographic evaluation for another process. Pulmonary function in patients with parietal pleural plaques is often normal, but a reduced forced vital capacity has been observed in some patients [53,54].

The mechanism of pleural plaque formation is not known for certain. It has been suggested that asbestos fibers protrude out of the visceral pleura and scratch the parietal pleural surface during respiration, with the generation of an inflammatory tissue reaction. This theory has not been generally accepted, however. Another hypothesis is that asbestos fibers that have reached the visceral pleural surface penetrate through the pleura to enter the pleural space and are then transported to the parietal pleural surface [55]. Another possibility is that asbestos fibers reach the parietal pleura via retrograde lymphatic drainage from the mediastinal lymph nodes to the intercostal lymphatics. When the mesothelial cells are exposed to asbestos fibers, an inflammatory reaction that leads to fibrosis is initiated [56,57].

In contrast to parietal pleural plaques, diffuse pleural thickening involves the visceral pleura. The costophrenic angles are often involved. Diffuse pleural thickening may be the sequela of an asbestos-related benign pleural effusion [58]. Alternatively, diffuse pleural thickening may be secondary to repeated bouts of asbestos-related pleurisy, with subsequent development of pleural fibrosis. In some studies, the incidence of diffuse pleural thickening is less than that of parietal pleural plaques [59]; in other studies, diffuse pleural thickening was noted more often than parietal pleural plaques [60].

Diffuse pleural thickening is often associated with respiratory symptoms, with dyspnea on exertion being the most common complaint [61]. A small number of patients may have pleuritic chest pain [62,63]. Studies evaluating pulmonary function in patients with diffuse pleural thickening have noted a decrease in forced vital capacity, total lung capacity, and diffusing capacity, although the reported diffusing capacities were not corrected for lung volume [64,65].

Treatment options for patients with diffuse pleural thickening and pulmonary impairment are limited. Decortication can be attempted when clinically significant pulmonary parenchymal fibrosis is not present, although results are mixed [66]. Supportive care is usually the best option. Oxygen therapy may be required for patients with hypoxemia at rest or with exertion.

Tuberculous pleurisy

Tuberculous pleurisy is the most frequent extrapulmonary manifestation of tuberculosis [67]. The frequency of tuberculous pleurisy varies among countries, with 4% of patients in the United States having pleurisy as their manifestation of tuberculosis [68]. Residual pleural thickening of 2 to 10 mm has been reported in 20% to 50% of cases [69,70]. No apparent relations have been noted between the development of pleural fibrosis and clinical symptoms, size of effusion, and microbiologic or biochemical characteristics of the pleural fluid [69,70]. Pleural fibrosis related to tuberculous pleurisy typically does not significantly affect lung function, although patients with more extensive fibrosis may have restrictive physiology and dyspnea on exertion.

Steroids have been proposed in the treatment of pleural tuberculosis to limit the degree of pleural inflammation and subsequent fibrosis [71–73]. A review by Matchaba and Volmink [74] analyzing the results of randomized, double-blind, placebo-controlled trials of corticosteroids for tuberculous pleurisy concluded that there was insufficient evidence to support the use of corticosteroids for the prevention of pleural fibrosis. Treatment with corticosteroids, however, can result in more rapid resolution of the effusion and improvement in symptoms.

Rheumatoid pleurisy

Pleural pathologic findings in rheumatoid pleurisy vary from small fibrous plaques to extensive reactive fibrosis of the pleura [75]. Pathologic studies have demonstrated that pleural effusion and pleural fibrosis occur in up to 50% of patients [76]. Interstitial lung disease and other parenchymal abnormalities are noted in approximately 30% of patients with rheumatoid pleurisy [77]. Those patients with recurrent or protracted rheumatoid pleurisy may develop significant pleural fibrosis and subsequent trapped lung. Treatment with systemic and intrapleural corticosteroids has been used with variable success [78–80]. The effect of disease-modifying antirheumatic drugs on rheumatoid pleurisy and pleural fibrosis is unknown. In symptomatic patients with pleural fibrosis, decortication may be considered, although surgery may be problematic in rheumatoid disease [81,82].

Uremic pleuritis

Fibrinous pleuritis has been observed in 20% of uremic patients at autopsy [83]. Uremic pleuritis generally responds to hemodialysis with residual pleural thickening that is not clinically important. In a small number of patients, the pleural fluid becomes gelatinous and a thick fibrous pleural peel develops. Fibrosing uremic pleuritis can result in restrictive physiology and significant dyspnea [84–86]. Fibrosing uremic pleuritis may occur in patients with end-stage renal disease several years into hemodialysis therapy. The use of corticosteroids in preventing pleural fibrosis and trapped lung from uremic pleuritis has not been well studied. With severe fibrosing pleuritis and disabling symptoms, surgical decortication can be considered [85,86].

Coronary artery bypass graft surgery

Exudative left-sided pleural effusions after CABG surgery are common [87,88]. The incidence of pleural effusions has been noted to be higher with internal mammary artery grafting than with saphenous vein grafting alone in some studies [89,90] but not in others [87]. Studies have demonstrated mixed results in assessing whether receiving a pleurotomy during internal mammary artery grafting is associated with an increase in the incidence of pleural effusion [89,90]. Usually, these effusions gradually resolve. In a small number of patients, the effusion may persist for months after CABG surgery. Pleural biopsy specimens from patients undergoing thoracoscopy for persistent pleural effusions after CABG surgery demonstrate an intense lymphocytic pleuritis [91]. Over time, there is a decline in cellular inflammation with a concurrent increase in pleural fibrosis and subsequent development of a trapped lung. No controlled studies are available to assess the efficacy of corticosteroids or nonsteroidal anti-inflammatory agents in treating this group of patients. In patients with significant dyspnea and restrictive physiology, decortication has been performed successfully [92].

Hemothorax

Hemothoraces are usually caused by trauma or are iatrogenic after procedures but may also be attributable to causes like primary and metastatic pleural tumors, anticoagulation and bleeding diatheses, pleural endometriosis, and arteriovenous malformations. Diffuse pleural thickening producing a fibrothorax is a potential late complication of a residual clotted hemothorax. Fibrothorax, however, seems to be an uncommon complication of a hemothorax, even if the residual blood is not removed from the pleural space [93]. Nevertheless, early drainage of every hemothorax by a chest tube is indicated to reduce the incidence of fibrothorax as well as empyema. Controversy exists as to whether a residual clotted hemothorax should be treated by thoracotomy or by more conservative methods. Intrapleural fibrinolytic therapy seems to be an effective therapy when applied within 10 days of the development of a clotted hemothorax [94,95]. When a fibrothorax or trapped lung does develop, decortication can be performed with good results.

Medication-induced pleural fibrosis

Many medications have been associated with the development of pleural effusions, but drug-induced pleural thickening and pleural fibrosis are less commonly observed. Ergoline or ergot derivatives have been associated with pleural fibrosis, alone or in combination with fibrosis of the pericardium, mediastinum, retroperitoneum, and cardiac valves [96]. Methysergide was the first ergot recognized to cause pleural fibrosis in patients who were receiving the drug for migraine headaches [97]. Bromocriptine, used for the treatment of Parkinson's disease, has also been reported to cause pleural fibrosis [98]. Newer ergolines being used in the treatment of Parkinson's disease, such as pergolide, cabergoline, lisuride, and nicergoline, have also been associated with the development of pleural fibrosis [96,99]. The incidence has been estimated at 2% to 4% of the treated population and may be greater in patients exposed to asbestos [100]. Involvement is usually bilateral and more often along the lateral and basilar aspects of the thorax. Associated loculated pleural effusions may be present. Mild to severe restriction may be noted on pulmonary function testing. Most patients improve after stopping the medication, with gradual improvement in pleural thickening over months to years. The pleural thickening may not completely resolve in those patients with marked pleural involvement. Corticosteroids do not seem to accelerate recovery of the pleural abnormalities or hasten improvement in symptoms [101]. In general, decortication is not required in these patients. Rechallenge with another ergoline drug should be discouraged, because recurrences may develop.

Other medications have also been associated with pleural thickening and fibrosis. Cyclophosphamide, in addition to causing pulmonary fibrosis, can produce pleural fibrosis that involves the upper and lateral aspects of the pleura bilaterally [102]. In patients with amiodarone pneumonitis, smooth-edged pleural thickening may be noted on imaging studies [103,104]; pleural effusion in the absence of parenchymal involvement may also occur [104,105]. On drug discontinuation, some degree of pleural thickening may persist.

Cryptogenic fibrosing pleuritis

Buchanan and colleagues [106] have described four patients who developed progressive bilateral pleural fibrosis after the occurrence of exudative pleural effusions. Histologic examination revealed thickened fibrous tissue affecting the parietal and visceral pleurae with obliteration of the pleural space. Extensive evaluation of the patients failed to reveal an attributable cause. The term *cryptogenic fibrosing pleuritis* was used by the authors to describe these cases. Decortication was successful in three patients. Corticosteroids seemed to control contralateral disease in one patient, whereas progressive pleural fibrosis occurred in another patient despite corticosteroid therapy. Since that report, other case reports and case series of cryptogenic fibrosing pleuritis have been published [107–109]. We have also encountered a case similar to those in these reports.

Fibrothorax and trapped lung

The clinical entities of fibrothorax and trapped lung are two unique and uncommon consequences of pleural fibrosis. Fibrothorax represents the most severe form of pleural fibrosis. With a fibrothorax, there is dense fibrosis of the visceral and parietal pleural surfaces, leading to fusion of these membranes. Contracture of the involved hemithorax and reduced mobility of the lung and thoracic cage occur because of the symphysis of the pleural membranes and progressive pleural fibrosis. Over time, the size of the ipsilateral hemithorax decreases, the intercostal spaces narrow, and the mediastinum is shifted ipsilaterally [110]. Decortication is the only potentially effective treatment for fibrothorax in patients with severe respiratory compromise. The timing of decortication is important, because the degree of pleural thickening and symptoms may improve over several months. When pleural fibrosis has been stable or is progressive over a 6-month period, decortication should be considered in the symptomatic patient.

A trapped lung is characterized by the inability of the lung to expand and fill the thoracic cavity because of a restrictive, fibrous, visceral pleural peel and is the result of a remote inflammatory process [111]. A trapped lung presents as a chronic unilateral pleural effusion that develops from filling of the pleural space with low-protein pleural fluid because of restriction of lung parenchyma expansion and subsequent negative pressure and hydrostatic disequilibrium in the pleural space. Any of the aforementioned causes of pleural fibrosis may produce a trapped lung if the associated pleural effusion persists long enough to allow fibrous tissue to develop on the visceral pleural surface of the lung while the visceral and parietal pleural surfaces remain separated. The diagnosis of a trapped lung implies chronicity, stability over time, and a purely mechanical cause for the persistence of a fluid-filled pleural space [111]. In contrast, lung entrapment is the result of an active inflammatory process or malignancy in the pleural space, leading to a restricted pleural space. Pleural fluid from lung entrapment is an exudate, whereas pleural fluid from a trapped lung is usually a transudate.

The diagnosis of a trapped lung requires documentation of chronicity and the absence of pleural inflammation, pleural malignancy, or endobronchial obstruction. Pleural fluid analysis demonstrates protein and lactate dehydrogenase (LDH) values in the transudative range or, on occasion, borderline exudative values. The pleural fluid nucleated cell count is usually less than 1000 cells/mm^3, with a differential consisting predominantly of lymphocytes. The pathognomonic radiographic sign of a trapped lung is the pneumothorax ex vacuo, a small to moderate-sized air collection in the pleural space after evacuation of the effusion, often in association with visible thickening of the visceral pleural surface. Measurements of pleural liquid pressure are negative initially and substantially decrease with fluid removal [112–114]. Negative initial pleural liquid pressures, however, may also be observed in patients with lung entrapment from malignancy and in occasional transudative and exudative effusions without entrapment. Increased pleural elastance, defined as a change of greater than 25 cm H$_2$O after removing 1 L of pleural fluid, is suggestive of a trapped lung or lung entrapment [114,115]. Reaccumulation after fluid removal to prethoracentesis levels usually occurs rapidly.

Patients with a trapped lung usually do not experience improvement in dyspnea after thoracentesis [111]. In contrast, thoracentesis typically improves symptoms in patients with lung entrapment; however, they develop chest pain after a critical volume of fluid is removed. Management of the patient with a trapped lung should take into consideration that a trapped lung produces a benign chronic effusion. An asymptomatic patient obviously does not benefit from a decortication procedure. In symptomatic patients, decortication should be considered. The underlying lung parenchyma should be assessed before decortication. If the trapped lung is severely diseased and fibrotic, decortication is unlikely to result in lung re-expansion and the procedure does not provide symptomatic benefit. For patients with lung entrapment associated with malignancy, the use of chronic indwelling pleural catheters can be helpful in alleviating dyspnea [116].

Decortication is the only effective therapy for symptomatic patients with a trapped lung.

Summary

Pleural fibrosis can result from a variety of inflammatory conditions. The development of pleural fibrosis follows severe pleural inflammation, which is usually associated with an exudative pleural effusion. Interactions among resident and inflammatory cells, cytokines, growth factors, and blood-derived products are important in the pathogenesis of pleural fibrosis. Pleural injury and repair are characterized by disordered fibrin turnover, which contributes to the pathogenesis of pleural fibrosis. Cytokines, such as TGFβ, bFGF, and PDGF, likely play key roles in the development of pleural fibrosis. Other cytokines, such as TNFα, IL-1, IL-6, IL-8, and vascular endothelial growth factor (VEGF), may also be involved in pleural fibrosis. The pathogenesis of pleural fibrosis remains incompletely understood; it is also unclear why the same injury causes pleural fibrosis in some individuals and complete resolution without sequelae in others.

A spectrum of derangements is observed in pleural fibrosis, ranging from radiographic abnormalities alone without symptoms to severe restrictive physiology and disabling dyspnea. In general, corticosteroid therapy does not seem to prevent or lessen the development of pleural fibrosis or its progression, with the possible exception of some patients with rheumatoid pleurisy. Decortication can be considered for patients with a trapped lung who are symptomatic and have normal underlying lung parenchyma. Decortication should be entertained only after stability or progression of pleural fibrosis has been demonstrated over a 6-month period, however.

References

[1] Antony VB. Immunological mechanisms in pleural disease. Eur Respir J 2003;21:539–44.
[2] Mutsaers SE. Mesothelial cells: their structure, function, and role in serosal repair. Respirology 2002;7:171–91.
[3] Antony VB, Hott JW, Kunkel SL, et al. Pleural mesothelial cell expression of C-C (monocyte chemotactic peptide) and C-X-C (interleukin 8) chemokines. Am J Respir Cell Mol Biol 1995;12:581–8.
[4] Nasreen N, Hartman DL, Mohammed KA, et al. Talc-induced expression of C-C and C-X-C chemokines and intercellular adhesion molecule-1 in mesothelial cells. Am J Respir Crit Care Med 1998;158:971–8.

[5] Visser CE, Steenbergen JJ, Betges MG, et al. Interleukin-8 production by human mesothelial cells after direct stimulation with staphylococci. Infect Immun 1995;63:4206–9.

[6] Tanaka S, Choe N, Iwagaki A, et al. Asbestos exposure induces MCP-1 secretion by pleural mesothelial cells. Exp Lung Res 2000;26:241–55.

[7] Nasreen N, Mohammed KA, Hardwick J, et al. Polar production of interleukin-8 by mesothelial cells promotes the transmesothelial migration of neutrophils: role of intercellular adhesion molecule-1. J Infect Dis 2001;183:1638–45.

[8] Betjes MG, Tuk CW, Struijk DG, et al. Interleukin-8 production by human peritoneal mesothelial cells in response to tumor necrosis factor-alpha, interleukin-1, and medium conditioned by macrophages cocultured with Staphylococcus epidermidis. J Infect Dis 1993; 168:1202–10.

[9] Li FK, Davenport A, Robson RL, et al. Leukocyte migration across human peritoneal mesothelial cells is dependent on directed chemokine secretion and ICAM-1 expression. Kidney Int 1998;54:2170–83.

[10] Zeillemaker AM, Mul FP, Hoynck van Papendrecht AA, et al. Polarized secretion of interleukin-8 by human mesothelial cells: a role in neutrophil migration. Immunology 1995;84:227–32.

[11] Liberek T, Topley N, Luttmann W, et al. Adherence of neutrophils to human peritoneal mesothelial cells; role of intercellular adhesion molecule-1. J Am Soc Nephrol 1996;7:208–17.

[12] Cannistra SA, Ottensmeier C, Tidy J, et al. Vascular cell adhesion molecule-1 expressed by peritoneal mesothelium partly mediates the binding of activated T lymphocytes. Exp Hematol 1994;22:996–1002.

[13] Jonjic N, Peri G, Bernasconni S, et al. Expression of adhesion molecules and chemotactic cytokines in cultured human mesothelial cells. J Exp Med 1992; 176:1165–75.

[14] Goodman RB, Wood RG, Martin TR, et al. Cytokine-stimulated human mesothelial cells produce chemotactic activity for neutrophils including Nap-1/IL-8. J Immunol 1992;148:457–65.

[15] Antony VB, Godbey SW, Kunkel SL, et al. Recruitment of inflammatory cells to the pleural space. Chemotactic cytokines, IL-8, and monocyte chemotactic peptide-1 in human pleural fluids. J Immunol 1993;151:7216–23.

[16] Lee YC, Lane KB. The many faces of transforming growth factor-beta in pleural diseases. Curr Opin Pulm Med 2001;7:173–9.

[17] Antony VB, Sahn SA, Mossman B, et al. Pleural cell biology in health and disease. Am Rev Respir Dis 1992;145:1236–9.

[18] Harvey W, Amlot PL. Collagen production by human mesothelial cells in vitro. J Pathol 1993;19: 445–52.

[19] Ma C, Tarnuzzer RW, Chegini N. Expression of matrix metalloproteinases and tissue inhibitors of matrix metalloproteinases in mesothelial cells and their regulation by transforming growth factor-beta 1. Wound Repair Regen 1999;7:477–85.

[20] Idell S, Zweib C, Kumar A, et al. Pathways of fibrin turnover of human pleural mesothelial cells in vitro. Am J Respir Cell Mol Biol 1992;7: 414–26.

[21] Falk P, Ma C, Chegini N, et al. Differential regulation of mesothelial cell fibrinolysis by transforming growth factor beta 1. Scan J Clin Lab Invest 2000; 60:439–47.

[22] Sasse SA, Jadus MR, Kukes GD. Pleural fluid transforming growth factor-beta1 correlates with pleural fibrosis in experimental empyema. Am J Respir Crit Care Med 2003;168:700–5.

[23] Maeda J, Ueki N, Oshkawa T, et al. Local production and localization of transforming growth factor-beta in tuberculous pleurisy. Clin Exp Immunol 1993;92:32–8.

[24] Jagirdar J, Lee TC, Reibman J, et al. Immunohistochemical localization of transforming growth factor beta isoforms in asbestos-related diseases. Environ Health Perspect 1997;105(Suppl 5):1197–203.

[25] Light RW, Cheng DS, Lee YCG, et al. A single intrapleural injection of transforming growth factor beta-2 produces an excellent pleurodesis in rabbits. Am J Respir Crit Care Med 2000;162:98–104.

[26] Lee YCG, Lane KB, Parker RE, et al. Transforming growth factor beta-2 (TGF-β2) produces effective pleurodesis in sheep with no systemic complications. Thorax 2000;55:1058–62.

[27] Mutsaers SE, McAnulty RJ, Laurent GJ, et al. Cytokine regulation of mesothelial cell proliferation in vitro. Eur J Cell Biol 1997;72:24–9.

[28] Bikfalvi A, Klein S, Pintucci G, et al. Biologic roles of fibroblast growth factor-2. Endocr Rev 1997;18: 26–45.

[29] Folkman J, Klagsbrun M, Sasse J, et al. A heparin-binding angiogenic protein-basic fibroblast growth factor-is stored within basement membrane. Am J Pathol 1988;130:393–400.

[30] Friesel RE, Maciag T. Molecular mechanisms of angiogenesis: fibroblast growth factor signal transduction. FASEB J 1995;9:919–25.

[31] Abramov Y, Anteby SO, Fasouliotis SJ, et al. Markedly elevated levels of vascular endothelial growth factor, fibroblast growth factor, and interleukin 6 in Meigs syndrome. Am J Obstet Gynecol 2001;184:354–5.

[32] Strizzi L, Vianale G, Catalano A, et al. Basic fibroblast growth factor in mesothelioma pleural effusions: correlation with patient survival and angiogenesis. Int J Oncol 2001;18:1093–8.

[33] Antony VB, Nasreen N, Mohammed KA, et al. Talc pleurodesis: basic fibroblast growth factor mediates pleural fibrosis. Chest 2004;126:1522–8.

[34] Owens MW, Milligan SA. Growth factor modulation of rat pleural mesothelial cell mitogenesis and collagen synthesis. Effects of epidermal growth factor

and platelet-derived factor. Inflammation 1994;18: 77–87.

[35] Waters CM, Chang JY, Glucksberg MR, et al. Mechanical forces alter growth factor release by pleural mesothelial cells. Am J Physiol 1997; 272(3 Part 1):L552.

[36] Safi A, Sadmi M, Martinet N, et al. Presence of elevated levels of platelet-derived growth factor (PDGF) in lung adenocarcinoma pleural effusions. Chest 1992;102:204–7.

[37] Heldin P, Asplund T, Ytterberg D, et al. Characterization of the molecular mechanism involved in the activation of hyaluronan synthetase by platelet-derived growth factor in human mesothelial cells. Biochem J 1992;283:165–70.

[38] Adamson IYR, Prieditis H, Young L. Lung mesothelial cell and fibroblast responses to pleural and alveolar macrophage supernatants and to lavage fluids from crocidolite-exposed rats. Am J Respir Cell Mol Biol 1997;16:650–6.

[39] Pierce GF, Mustoe TA, Lingelbach J, et al. Platelet-derived growth factor and transforming growth factor-beta enhance tissue repair activities by unique mechanisms. J Cell Biol 1989;109:429–40.

[40] Idell S. Pleural fibrosis. In: Light RW, Lee YCG, editors. Textbook of pleural diseases. London: Arnold Publishing; 2003. p. 96–108.

[41] Mutsaers SE, Prele CM, Brody AR, et al. Pathogenesis of pleural fibrosis. Respirology 2004;9:428–40.

[42] Idell S, Girard W, Koenig KB, et al. Abnormalities of fibrin turnover in the human pleural space. Am Rev Respir Dis 1991;144:187–94.

[43] McGee M, Rothberger H. Tissue factor in bronchoalveolar lavage fluids. Evidence for an alveolar macrophage source. Am Rev Respir Dis 1985;131: 331–6.

[44] Idell S, Zwieb C, Boggaram J, et al. Mechanisms of fibrin formation and lysis by human lung fibroblasts: influence of TGF-β and TNF-α. Am J Physiol 1992; 263(4 Part 1):L487.

[45] Bajaj MS, Pendurthi U, Koenig K, et al. Tissue factor pathway inhibitor expression by human pleural mesothelial and mesothelioma cells and lung fibroblasts. Eur Respir J 2000;15:1069–78.

[46] Vassalli JD, Sappino AP, Berlin D. The plasminogen activator/plasmin system. J Clin Invest 1991;88: 1067–72.

[47] Shetty S, Kumar A, Johnson AR, et al. Regulation of mesothelial cell mitogenesis by antisense oligonucleotides for the urokinase receptor. Antisense Res Dev 1995;5:307–14.

[48] Sitrin RG, Todd III RF, Albrecht E, et al. The urokinase receptor (CD87) facilitates CD11b/CD18-mediated adhesion of human monocytes. J Clin Invest 1996;97:1942–51.

[49] Shetty S, Idell S. A urokinase receptor mRNA binding protein from rabbit lung fibroblasts and mesothelial cells. Am J Physiol 1998;274(Part 1):L871.

[50] Chapman HA. Plasminogen activators, integrins, and the coordinated regulation of cell adhesion and migration. Curr Opin Cell Biol 1997;9:714–24.

[51] Shetty S, Kumar A, Johnson AR, et al. Differential expression of the urokinase receptor in fibroblasts from normal and fibrotic human lungs. Am J Respir Cell Mol Biol 1996;15:78–87.

[52] Hillerdal G. Pleural plaques in a health survey material. Frequency, development and exposure to asbestos. Scand J Respir Dis 1978;59:257–63.

[53] Bourbeau J, Ernst P, Chrome J, et al. The relationship between respiratory impairment and asbestos-related pleural abnormality in an active work force. Am Rev Respir Dis 1990;142:837–42.

[54] Oliver LC, Eisen EA, Greene R, et al. Asbestos-related pleural plaques and lung function. Am J Ind Med 1988;14:649–56.

[55] Hillerdal G. The pathogenesis of pleural plaques and pulmonary asbestosis: possibilities and impossibilities. Eur J Respir Dis 1980;61:129–38.

[56] Robledo R, Mossman B. Cellular and molecular mechanisms of asbestos-induced fibrosis. J Cell Physiol 1999;180:158–66.

[57] Kawahara M, Kagan E. The mesothelial cell and its role in asbestos-induced pleural injury. Int J Exp Pathol 1995;76:163–70.

[58] Lilis R, Lerman Y, Selikoff IJ. Symptomatic benign pleural effusions among asbestos insulation workers: residual radiographic abnormalities. Br J Ind Med 1988;45:443–9.

[59] Hillerdal G. Non-malignant asbestos pleural disease. Thorax 1981;36:669–75.

[60] de Klerk NH, Cookson WO, Musk AW, et al. Natural history of pleural thickening after exposure to crocidolite. Br J Ind Med 1989;46:461–7.

[61] Yates DH, Browne K, Stidolph PN, et al. Asbestos-related bilateral diffuse pleural thickening: natural history of radiographic and lung function abnormalities. Am J Respir Crit Care Med 1996;153:301–6.

[62] Miller A. Chronic pleuritic pain in four patients with asbestos induced pleural fibrosis. Br J Ind Med 1990;7:147–53.

[63] Mukherjee S, de Klerk N, Palmer LJ, et al. Chest pain in asbestos-exposed individuals with benign pleural and parenchymal disease. Am J Respir Crit Care Med 2000;162:1807–11.

[64] Yates DH, Browne K, Stidolph PN, et al. Asbestos-related bilateral diffuse pleural thickening: natural history of radiographic and lung function abnormalities. Am J Respir Crit Care Med 1996;153:301–6.

[65] Kee ST, Gamsu G, Blanc P. Causes of pulmonary impairment in asbestos-exposed individuals with diffuse pleural thickening. Am J Respir Crit Care Med 1996;154:789–93.

[66] Wright PH, Hanson A, Kreel L, et al. Respiratory function changes after asbestos pleurisy. Thorax 1980;35:31–6.

[67] Seibert AF, Haynes J, Middleton R, et al. Tuberculous

pleural effusion. Twenty years experience. Chest 1991;99:883–6.

[68] Mehta JB, Dutt A, Havill L, et al. Epidemiology of extrapulmonary tuberculosis. A comparative analysis with pre-AIDS era. Chest 1991;99(5): 1134–8.

[69] de Pablo A, Villena V, Eschave Sustaeta J, et al. Are pleural fluid parameters related to the development of residual pleural thickening in tuberculosis. Chest 1997;112:1293–7.

[70] Barbas CS, Cukier A, de Varhalho CR, et al. The relationship between pleural fluid findings and the development of pleural thickening in patients with pleural tuberculosis. Chest 1991;100:1264–7.

[71] Wyser C, Walzl G, Smedema J, et al. Corticosteroids in the treatment of tuberculous pleurisy. A double-blind, placebo-controlled, randomized study. Chest 1996;110:333–8.

[72] Lee CH, Wang WJ, Lan RS, et al. Corticosteroids in the treatment of tuberculous pleurisy: a double-blind, placebo-controlled randomized study. Chest 1988; 94:1256–9.

[73] Galarza I, Cafiete C, Granados A, et al. Randomized trial of corticosteroids in the treatment of tuberculous pleurisy. Thorax 1995;50:1305–7.

[74] Matchaba PT, Volmink J. Steroids for treating tuberculous pleurisy. Cochrane Database Syst Rev 2000;2:CD001876.

[75] Brunk JR, Drash EC, Swineford O. Rheumatoid pleuritis successfully treated with decortication. Report of a case and review of the literature. Am J Med Sci 1966;251:545–51.

[76] Joseph J, Sahn SA. Connective tissue diseases and the pleura. Chest 1993;104:262–70.

[77] Stanford RE. Rheumatoid and other collagen lung disease. Semin Respir Med 1982;4:107–12.

[78] Jurik AG, Grudal H. Pleurisy in rheumatoid arthritis. Scand J Rheumatol 1983;12:75–80.

[79] Chapman PT, O'Donnell JL, Moller PW. Rheumatoid pleural effusion: response to intrapleural corticosteroids. J Rheumatol 1992;19:478–80.

[80] Russell ML, Gladman DD, Mintz S. Rheumatoid pleural effusion: lack of response to intrapleural corticosteroids. J Rheumatol 1986;13:412–5.

[81] Brunk JR, Drash EC, Swineford O. Rheumatoid pleuritis successfully treated with decortication. Report of a case and review of the literature. Am J Med Sci 1966;251:545–51.

[82] Yarbrough JW, Sealy WC, Miller JA. Thoracic surgical problems associated with rheumatoid arthritis. J Thorac Cardiovasc Surg 1975;69:347–54.

[83] Hopps HC, Wissler RW. Uremic pneumonitis. Am J Pathol 1955;31:261–73.

[84] Maher JF. Uremic pleuritis. Am J Kidney Dis 1987; 10:19–22.

[85] Gilbert L, Ribot S, Frankel H, Jacobs M, et al. Fibrinous uremic pleuritis: a surgical entity. Chest 1976;67:53–6.

[86] Rodelas R, Rakowski TA, Argy WP, et al. Fibrosing uremic pleuritis during hemodialysis. JAMA 1980; 243:2424–5.

[87] Peng MJ, Vargas FS, Cukier A, et al. Postoperative pleural changes after coronary revascularization. Chest 1992;101:327–30.

[88] Light RW, Rogers JT, Cheng DS, et al. Large pleural effusions occurring after coronary bypass grafting. Ann Intern Med 1999;130:891–6.

[89] Hurlbut D, Myers ML, Lefcoe M, et al. Pleuropulmonary morbidity: internal thoracic artery versus saphenous vein graft. Ann Thorac Surg 1990;50: 959–64.

[90] Landymore RW, Howell F. Pulmonary complications following myocardial revascularization with the internal mammary artery graft. Eur J Cardiothorac Surg 1990;4:156–62.

[91] Lee YCG, Vaz MAC, Ely KA, et al. Symptomatic persistent post-coronary artery bypass graft pleural effusions requiring operative treatment: clinical and histologic features. Chest 2001;119:795–800.

[92] Lee YCG, Vaz MAC, Ely KA, et al. Symptomatic persistent post-coronary artery bypass graft pleural effusions requiring operative treatment: clinical and histologic features. Chest 2001;119:795–800.

[93] Wilson JM, Boren CH, Peterson SR, et al. Traumatic hemothorax: is decortication necessary? J Thorac Cardiovasc Surg 1979;77:489–95.

[94] Inci I, Ozcelik C, Ulku R, et al. Intrapleural fibrinolytic treatment of traumatic clotted hemothorax. Chest 1998;114:160–5.

[95] Jerjes-Sanchez C, Ramirez-Rivera A, Elizalde JJ, et al. Intrapleural fibrinolysis with streptokinase as an adjunctive treatment in hemothorax and empyema: a multicenter trial. Chest 1996;109:1514–9.

[96] Pfitzenmeyer P, Foucher P, Dennewald G, et al. Pleuropulmonary changes induced by ergoline drugs. Eur Respir J 1996;9:1013–9.

[97] Graham JR, Suby HI, LeCompte PR, et al. Fibrotic disorders associated with methysergide therapy for headache. N Engl J Med 1966;274:350–68.

[98] McElvaney NG, Wilcox PG, Churg A, et al. Pleuropulmonary disease during bromocriptine treatment of Parkinson's disease. Arch Intern Med 1988;148: 2231–6.

[99] Bhatt MH, Keenan SP, Fleetham JA, et al. Pleuropulmonary disease associated with dopamine agonist therapy. Ann Neurol 1991;30:613–6.

[100] De Vuyst P, Pfitzenmeyer P, Camus P. Asbestos, ergot drugs, and the pleura. Eur Respir J 1997;10: 2695–8.

[101] Robert M, Derbaudrenghien JP, Blampain JP, et al. Fibrotic processes associated with long-term ergotamine therapy. N Engl J Med 1984;311:601–2.

[102] Malik SW, Myers JL, DeRemee RA, et al. Lung toxicity associated with cyclophosphamide use. Two distinct patterns. Am J Respir Crit Care Med 1996; 154:1851–6.

[103] Standerskjold-Nordenstam CG, Wandtke JC, Hood WJJ, et al. Amiodarone pulmonary toxicity. Chest

radiography and CT in asymptomatic patients. Chest 1985;88:143–5.

[104] Gonzalez-Rothi RJ, Hannan SE, Hood I, et al. Amiodarone pulmonary toxicity presenting as bilateral exudative effusions. Chest 1987;92:179–82.

[105] Stein B, Zaatari GS, Pine JR. Amiodarone pulmonary toxicity. Clinical, cytological, and ultrastructural findings. Acta Cytol 1987;31:357–61.

[106] Buchanan DR, Johnston IDA, Kerr IH, et al. Cryptogenic bilateral fibrosing pleuritis. Br J Dis Chest 1988;82:186–93.

[107] Hayes JP, Wiggins J, Ward K, et al. Familial cryptogenic fibrosing pleuritis with Fanconi's syndrome (renal tubular acidosis). A new syndrome. Chest 1995;107:576–8.

[108] Lee-Chiong Jr TL, Hilbert J. Extensive idiopathic benign bilateral asynchronous pleural fibrosis. Chest 1996;109:564–5.

[109] Azoulay E, Paugam B, Heymann MF, et al. Familial extensive idiopathic bilateral pleural fibrosis. Eur Respir J 1999;14:971–3.

[110] Morton JR, Boushy SF, Guinn GA. Physiological evaluation of results of pulmonary decortication. Ann Thorac Surg 1970;9:321–6.

[111] Doelken P, Sahn SA. Trapped lung. Semin Respir Crit Care Med 2001;22:631–5.

[112] Light RW, Stansbury DW, Brown SE. Observations on pleural fluid pressures as fluid is withdrawn during thoracentesis. Am Rev Respir Dis 1980;121: 799–804.

[113] Light RW, Stansbury DW, Brown SE. The relationship between pleural pressures and changes in pulmonary function after therapeutic thoracentesis. Am Rev Respir Dis 1986;133:658–61.

[114] Villena V, Lopez-Encuentra A, Pozo F, et al. Measurement of pleural pressures during therapeutic thoracentesis. Am J Respir Crit Care Med 2000;162: 1534–8.

[115] Lan R, Singh KL, Chuang M, et al. Elastance of the pleural space: a predictor for the outcome of pleurodesis in patients with malignant effusions. Ann Intern Med 1997;126:768–74.

[116] Pien GW, Gant MJ, Washam CL, et al. Use of an implantable pleural catheter for trapped lung syndrome in patients with malignant pleural effusion. Chest 2001;119:1641–6.

ELSEVIER SAUNDERS

CLINICS
IN CHEST
MEDICINE

Clin Chest Med 27 (2006) 193 – 213

Imaging of Pleural Disease

Nagmi R. Qureshi, MRCP, FRCR*, Fergus V. Gleeson, FRCP, FRCR

Department of Radiology, Churchill Hospital, Headington, Oxford OX3 7LJ, UK

Imaging plays an important role in the diagnosis and subsequent management of patients with pleural disease. The presence of a pleural abnormality is usually suggested following a routine chest x-ray, with a number of imaging modalities available for further characterization. This article describes the radiographic and cross-sectional appearances of pleural diseases, which are commonly encountered in every day practice. The conditions covered include benign and malignant pleural thickening, pleural effusions, empyema and pneumothoraces. The relative merits of CT, MRI and PET in the assessment of these conditions and the role of image-guided intervention are discussed.

Normal pleural anatomy

Understanding the appearances of the normal pleura on a CXR and CT scan allows its differentiation from pathologic changes, such as pleural plaque and thickening. The normal parietal pleura is never visualized on posteroanterior (PA) CXRs. The visceral pleura is only seen on CXRs when it invaginates the lung parenchyma to form the fissures or junctional lines or if a pneumothorax is present. The fissures are only seen when they are imaged tangentially to the x-ray beam and thus often appear incomplete [1].

On CT, the appearance of the fissures is dependent on the slice thickness and the plane of the fissures relative to the CT beam. On conventional single-slice spiral CT, the fissures appear as curvilinear, avascular, ill-defined areas of low attenuation extending from the hilum to the chest wall [2]. The oblique fissure, which is oblique to the CT beam, is more readily visualized than the horizontal fissure, which is imaged tangential to the beam.

High-resolution CT (HRCT), which is performed with a 1- to 2-mm slice thickness and a high spatial resolution algorithm, and volumetric thin-section multislice CT allow better visualization not only of the fissures, which are seen as well-defined high-attenuation bands, but of the costal pleura (Fig. 1). Classically, the costal pleura appears as a 1- to 2-mm thick line, the "intercostal stripe," representing the visceral pleura, normal physiologic pleural fluid, parietal pleura, endothoracic fascia, and innermost intercostal muscles. The stripe extends to the lateral margins of the adjacent ribs and also along the paravertebral margins (Fig. 2).

The transversus thoracic muscle is often seen arising anteriorly from the back of the sternum and inserting into the second through sixth ribs and costal cartilages (Fig. 3). At the same level, the subcostalis muscle can be seen posteriorly. These muscles are symmetric and uniform, unlike pleural plaques [3].

Normal pleura, parietal and visceral, is never visualized on MRI.

Pleural thickening

As the pleura becomes thickened in disease, it is more readily seen on all forms of imaging. It is of importance to differentiate benign from malignant disease and to determine an etiologic cause. To help in this differentiation, it is easiest to separate pleural thickening into focal and diffuse categories.

* Corresponding author.
   E-mail address: nagmiqureshi@doctors.org.uk
(N.R. Qureshi).

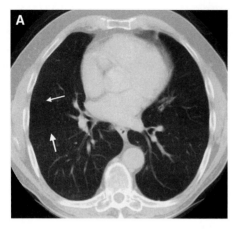

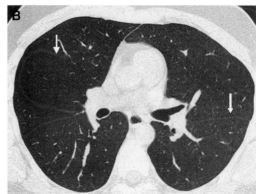

Fig. 1. Typical appearance of the oblique fissures (*bold arrow*) and horizontal fissure (*arrow*) on (*A*) conventional spiral CT and (*B*) HRCT.

Focal pleural thickening

Pleural plaques

Pleural plaques are the most common manifestation of asbestos exposure, with a latency period of 20 to 30 years. The plaques represent areas of dense hyaline collagen within the mesothelial layers of the pleura and predominantly involve the parietal pleura. Visceral plaques can occur but are relatively rare; when present as fissural plaques, they may simulate a parenchymal nodule or mass [4].

Pleural plaques are usually bilateral, although unilateral plaques are seen in 25% of cases on CXRs and are more common and usually more extensive on the left, with a posterolateral predominance [5].

The CXR has reported sensitivities ranging from 30% to 80% in the detection of pleural plaques [6]. Detection is dependent on a number of factors, including plaque thickness, size, and position; radiographic technical factors; and the presence of calcification. In certain patients, detection of plaques can be problematic because prominent extrapleural

fat or composite shadows from the adjacent chest wall can mimic plaque formation, accounting for a false-positive rate of 20% on a PA CXR. On occasion, oblique and lateral views may be useful; however, they are rarely performed because they offer limited additional information. In a retrospective study of 2018 patients, a lateral view demonstrated an additional 18% of plaques [7], whereas a right anterior oblique view was found to increase sensitivities by 13% to 26% [8]. A significant false-positive rate was noted in both of these studies compared with the PA CXR, attributable to composite shadowing.

On a CXR, plaques typically appear as smooth opacities less than 1 cm in thickness parallel to the

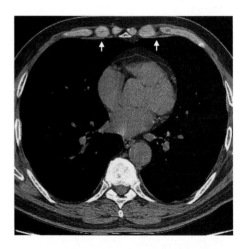

Fig. 3. Transversus thoracic muscle is seen anteriorly and arises from the posterior aspect of the sternum and inserts into the costal cartilage or adjacent 2–6 ribs (*arrows*). This muscle should not be confused with pleural plaques, which are typically asymmetrical.

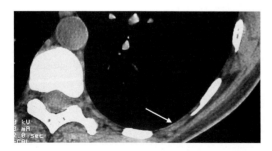

Fig. 2. HRCT of the normal pleura demonstrating the normal intercostal stripe.

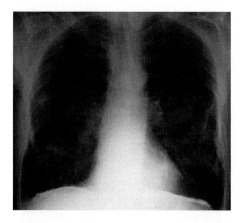

Fig. 4. CXR demonstrating bilateral calcified pleural plaques and diaphragmatic calcification.

chest wall and involving the posterolateral aspects of the seventh through 10th ribs and the lateral aspect of the sixth through ninth ribs [9]. Plaque calcification, however small, can increase the conspicuity of a plaque. Calcification is seen in 15% to 25% [6] of patients after a latency period of 30 to 40 years. Diaphragmatic calcification is virtually pathognomonic of previous exposure to asbestos, with relative sparing of the apices and costophrenic angles being common (Fig. 4).

HRCT is superior to CXRs and conventional spiral CT for demonstrating and delineating the extent of pleural plaque formation and readily differentiates plaques from extrapleural fat and adjacent composite shadows [10]. Sensitivities for depicting plaques are 95% on CT compared with 59% on CXRs [11]. Recently, low-dose multislice CT has been shown to be as sensitive and specific as HRCT in the detection of plaques (Fig. 5) [12].

Patients should be scanned in the prone position to overcome problems in differentiating dependent basal changes from coexisting asbestos-related lung disease. On CT, plaques appear as well-circumscribed areas of pleural thickening separated from the underlying rib and extrapleural fat by a thin layer of fat. Plaques typically have edges that are thicker than the central portion and can progress in size, extent, and calcification with time. Associated adjacent parenchymal changes characterized by fine interstitial lines radiating from the plaque, a "hairy plaque," may be seen in approximately half of the cases (Fig. 6) [13]. These hairy plaques are not associated with respiratory impairment, and their significance remains unclear. In the paravertebral region, plaques need to be differentiated from segments of intercostal vein and hairy plaques need to be differentiated from parenchymal changes associated with degenerative bony osteophytosis.

On MRI, pleural plaques return low signal on T1-, T2-, and proton density–weighted sequences. In a recent case series of 24 patients, high-resolution MRI was compared with CT in the diagnosis of asbestos-related pleural disease. Similar interobserver agreement in detecting pleural plaques was seen between MRI and CT. MRI was superior at demonstrating diffuse pleural thickening, extrapleural fat, and pleural effusions, whereas CT was considered superior to MRI in detecting pleural calcification [14].

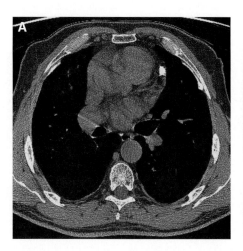
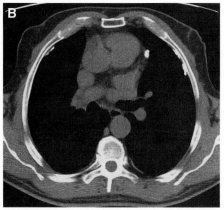

Fig. 5. Bilateral pleural plaques which are readily visualized on both (A) HRCT slice thickness 0.625mm and (B) low dose CT slice thickness 1.25mm.

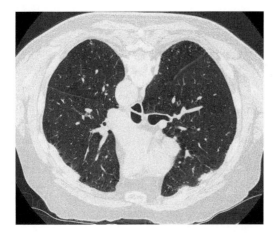

Fig. 6. CT scan performed prone, demonstrating bilateral calcified pleural plaques associated with short interstitial lines radiating perpendicularly from the plaques—"hairy plaques".

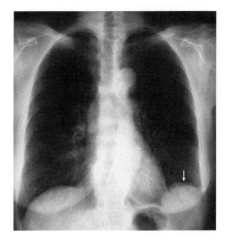

Fig. 7. CXR demonstrating a smooth soft tissue opacity in the left costophrenic angle in keeping with a pleural fibroma (arrowed).

Localized fibrous tumor of the pleura

These tumors are rare and account for less than 5% of all pleural tumors [15]. They arise from the submesenchymal cells of the pleura, with 80% arising from the visceral pleura. The mean age at presentation is 50 years, with a slight female predominance. Their cause is unknown. Cases occurring in patients with asbestos exposure and after radiation treatment for a keloid scar have been described [16]. These tumors are typically solitary and slow growing. A correlation between tumor size and patient symptoms has been elicited, with masses measuring less than 10 cm in size tending to be asymptomatic and masses greater than 16 cm in size associated with local symptoms [17].

Radiologic features are also dependent on tumor size. Typically, the fibromas appear as smooth or lobulated masses within the lower thorax. Masses abutting the hemidiaphragm may mimic diaphragmatic eventration (Fig. 7). In 40% of cases, a vascular pedicle attaches the tumor to the pleural surface, accounting for its mobility on sequential radiographs and with respiration [18].

On CT, small tumors are characteristically of homogeneous intermediate attenuation, similar to muscle, which is attributable to their high collagen density and vascular nature. They are well defined and have a smooth tapering margin that forms an obtuse angle to the pleural surface. Visualization of a pedicle is rare. Larger tumors are usually more lobulated, form an acute angle, are heterogeneous in character, and tend to displace adjacent structures (Fig. 8). Calcification is uncommon, occurring in less than 10% of cases, is usually punctate, and is most frequently seen in large tumors [19]. Contrast en-

hancement is intense and generally homogeneous. Heterogeneous enhancement may be seen in larger tumors as a result of areas of necrosis, hemorrhage, and myxoid degeneration [20].

Associated pleural effusions are seen in up to 20% of cases. Involvement of associated lymph nodes has not been described, however [16].

There are no pathognomonic radiologic features on CT to differentiate malignant from benign disease. The presence of compressive atelectasis, mediastinal mass effect, heterogeneity, and pleural effusions is more common in malignant masses, however [16].

MRI appearances conform to the expected MRI characteristics of fibrous tissue. They typically return low to intermediate signal on T1-, T2- and proton density–weighted sequences. High signal on T2-weighted sequences is seen in areas of necrosis and myxoid degeneration (Fig. 9). After administration of

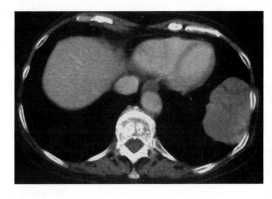

Fig. 8. Contrast-enhanced CT of the pleural fibroma. Note the pleural less tumor forms an acute angle with the pleural surface, whereas smaller fibromas typically form an obtuse angle.

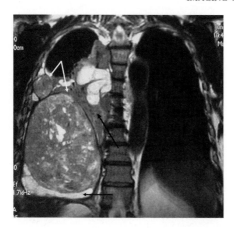

Fig. 9. Coronal T2W images showing multiple pleural fibromas (*white arrows*) and a septated pleural effusion (*black arrow*). The largest fibroma causing compression of the adjacent lung (*bold arrow*).

gadolinium, intense homogeneous enhancement is typical, reflecting the vascularity of the tumor [21]. A rim of low signal surrounding the tumor on T2-weighted images may also be present.

Lipomas and liposarcomas

Lipomas are rare, asymptomatic, benign pleural tumors. The pleural origin and fat density of these tumors are not always evident on CXRs. On CT, benign lipomas have a uniform density and measure less than 50 Hounsfield units (HU), which is indicative of fat density (Fig. 10) [22]. Linear soft tissue strands may be present. MRI appearances are of a well-defined homogeneous mass, hyperintense on T1-weighted images and moderately intense on T2-weighted images [23]. Fat suppression sequences are also useful if diagnostic doubt persists.

Liposarcomas are typically large, infiltrative, and symptomatic. There is no evidence to suggest that they arise from preexisting lipomas. They appear as heterogeneous masses on CT with soft tissue and fat components, and they measure less than 50 HU on pre- and postintravenous contrast enhancement. On MRI, they return high signal on T2-weighted sequences because of myxoid degeneration and low signal on T1-weighted sequences.

Diffuse pleural thickening

Diffuse pleural thickening primarily involves the visceral pleura and is usually preceded by a pleural effusion with subsequent visceral pleural fibrosis, which then adheres to the parietal pleura. Prior tuberculosis (TB) empyema, trauma, drugs, and asbestos

exposure may result in diffuse pleural thickening. Unlike pleural plaques, asbestos-related diffuse pleural thickening is uncommon, occurring in less than 10% of patients exposed to asbestos.

Asbestos-related diffuse pleural thickening

The International Labor Organization (ILO) has established a classification that allows epidemiologic comparison of radiographic pleural abnormalities by means of comparison with a standard set of radiographs. The classification describes findings on a PA CXR but does not define pathologic entities.

The refined 2000 criteria for defining diffuse pleural thickening on a PA CXR include the following:

- Bilateral thickening involving at least 25% of the chest or 50% if unilateral
- Pleural thickness greater than 5 mm at any site
- Obliteration of the costophrenic angle

On a CXR, diffuse pleural thickening is characterized by a smooth uninterrupted pleural density, with obliteration of the costophrenic angle (Fig. 11). In a study of 287 patients, Ameille and colleagues [24] suggested that obliteration of the costophrenic angle was a more reliable sign than the dimensional criteria used by the ILO classification. Changes to the ILO classification in 2000 have supported this finding.

As with pleural plaques, bilateral involvement can be confused with prominent extrapleural fat. Generally, bilateral asymmetric thickening is more suggestive of diffuse pleural thickening than overlying composite shadowing.

HRCT and low-dose multislice CT are more sensitive than CXRs and conventional single-slice spiral

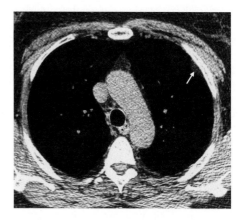

Fig. 10. Within the left upper zone there is a pleurally based low attenuation mass. Note the attenuation is similar to the subcutaneous fat in keeping with a lipoma (*arrow*).

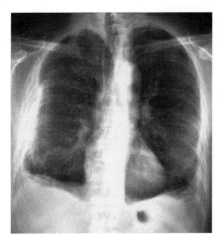

Fig. 11. Frontal chest radiograph showing smooth bilateral pleural thickening with blunting of the costophrenic angles and volume loss in keeping with longstanding pleural thickening.

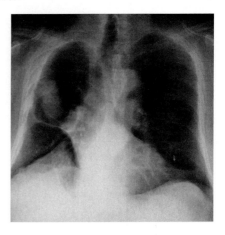

Fig. 12. Frontal radiograph showing right-sided pleural thickening with adjacent volume loss and a parenchymal mass with vessels pulled into it, in keeping with an area of rounded atelectasis.

CT in determining the extent of diffuse thickening and in assessing associated parenchymal changes, which may occur in up to 90% of cases. The value of CT is in the confirmation of diffuse pleural thickening when there is doubt from the CXR, exclusion of malignant disease, and detection of additional associated parenchymal disease. In 20% of patients with known asbestos-related disease, the CXR is normal.

On CT, diffuse pleural thickening is defined as a continuous sheet of thickening at least 5 cm in lateral extent, 8 to 10 cm in craniocaudal extent, and with a 3-mm thickness [25]. Proliferation of the overlying extrapleural fat is commonly demonstrated and thought to represent an inflammatory reaction to the pleural retraction.

Unlike pleural plaques, diffuse pleural thickening rarely calcifies. It is also, unlike plaque disease, associated with a restrictive pattern on pulmonary function tests [26].

Rounded atelectasis

Rounded atelectasis is commonly associated with asbestos-related pleural disease. Any benign pleural effusion that subsequently results in pleural thickening can cause rounded atelectasis, however. Two theories regarding the pathogenesis of rounded atelectasis have been postulated: it develops from entrapment and infolding of an area of compressive atelectasis adjacent to a resolving pleural effusion or from an area of maturing fibrous pleural tissue that contracts and distorts the adjacent parenchyma.

Radiographically, appearances are of a rounded peripheral mass 3 to 5 cm in size abutting the pleural

surface. Curvilinear densities radiating from the mass to the hilum may be visible (Fig. 12). CT features are characteristically of a rounded mass with adjacent pleural thickening, with swirling of bronchi and vessels extending from the hilum and converging on the mass producing a "comet tail" appearance (Fig. 13) [27]. Air bronchograms within the mass are common. These masses typically arise posteriorly within the lower lobe but can occur in the middle lobe and lingula. Contrast enhancement is homogeneous.

MRI is not usually necessary for diagnosis, although findings similar to CT are seen and include low signal on T1-weighted sequences, high signal on T2-weighted sequences, and hypointense lines that converge toward the center of the mass in a kidney-like pattern [28].

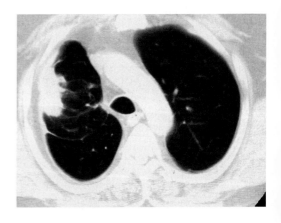

Fig. 13. CT scan section on lung windows demonstrating "comet-tail" vessels passing into the area of rounded atelectasis.

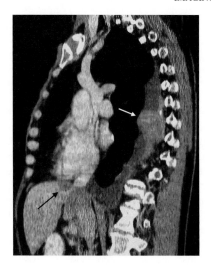

Fig. 14. Sagittal three-dimensional CT reconstruction demonstrating a malignant pleural effusion with a 2cm paravertebral pleural nodule (*white arrows*) and low attenuation liver metastasis (*black arrow*) in a patient with metastatic adenocarcinoma.

Areas of rounded atelectasis typically remain stable in size; however, complete regression can occur. An increase in size or the development of a pleural effusion should raise the possibility of malignancy and requires a biopsy.

Non−asbestos-related pleural thickening

The appearances on CXRs and CT usually reflect the underlying etiology, and frequently allow a specific etiologic diagnosis to be made.

In patients with previous TB empyema, CT features include unilateral sheet-like calcification with marked volume loss and thickening of the extrapleural fat and ribs. Pulmonary parenchymal TB changes may also be evident.

In posttraumatic hemothoraces, imaging shows pleural thickening associated with multiple healed rib fractures, with an otherwise normal underlying lung.

Pleural thickening after talc pleurodesis demonstrates a characteristic "talc sandwich" on CT, with soft tissue parietal pleural thickening, high-attenuation talc, and increased soft tissue visceral pleural thickening [29].

Diffuse malignant pleural thickening

Pleural metastatic disease

Metastatic pleural disease is the most common cause of malignant pleural thickening; bronchogenic carcinoma accounts for 40% of cases, breast carci-

noma for 20% of cases, lymphoma for 10%, and ovarian and gastric carcinoma for 5% [30]. Invasive thymoma, although rare, can also involve the pleura in a contiguous or multifocal manner. It can be impossible to differentiate pleural metastasis from mesothelioma radiologically in cases of unilateral malignant pleural thickening.

CXR appearances include circumferential lobulated pleural thickening, pleural effusion, rib crowding, and elevation of the hemidiaphragm consistent with volume loss. If large, the pleural effusion may obscure underlying pleural and parenchymal pathologic changes.

Contrast-enhanced CT is the imaging modality of choice for demonstrating and differentiating between benign and malignant pleural thickening. Ideally, this should be performed before any pleural effusion is drained. CT to include the upper abdomen should be performed routinely because it allows visualization of possible adrenal and hepatic metastasis (Fig. 14). Several studies have shown that on CT, the diagnosis of malignant disease is favored by the presence of parietal pleural thickening greater than 1 cm, circumferential pleural thickening, nodular pleural thickening (Fig. 15), and mediastinal pleural thickening. In a series by Leung and coworkers [31], the specificities of these findings were 94%, 100%, 94%, and 98%, respectively. Traill and colleagues [32] found that in the presence of a pleural effusion, circumferential pleural thickening was a less reliable indicator of malignant disease.

CT may also demonstrate the origin of the primary tumor. A spiculated pulmonary mass, enhancing breast nodule, or prominent anterior mediastinal mass would suggest a possible lung, breast, or thymic primary, respectively. With lymphoma, extensive medias-

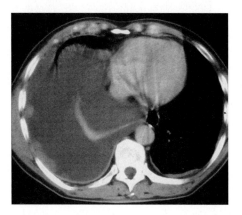

Fig. 15. Contrast-enhanced CT showing a malignant right pleural effusion with nodular pleural thickening.

tinal lymphadenopathy and parenchymal infiltrates may be present. Primary pleural lymphomatous involvement is rare and usually presents as recurrence or extension of disease from the mediastinum [33].

CT findings may therefore suggest a diagnosis of malignant disease, but histologic diagnosis is necessary for a definitive diagnosis. Scott and coworkers [34] found that the combination of CT findings and biopsy increased the sensitivity of differentiating malignant from benign disease from 83% to 100%.

MRI is usually only performed in problematic cases in which contrast-enhanced CT is contraindicated or where extrapleural infiltration has not been clearly demonstrated on CT. MRI allows excellent soft tissue contrast and multiplanar image acquisition, permitting ready assessment of chest wall and diaphragmatic invasion [35]. Typical sequences involve T1-weighted, T2-weighted, and T1-weighted postgadolinium acquisitions. Cardiac and respiratory triggering is necessary to reduce motion artifact. T1-weighted images return an intermediate signal in malignant and benign disease, whereas on T2-weighted and T1-weighted postgadolinium sequences, malignant pleural thickening shows increased signal intensity compared with intercostal muscle [36,37]. Contrast-enhanced, T1-weighted, fat-saturated sequences have been found to be particularly sensitive at demonstrating focal thickening and enhancement of the interlobar fissures, which may be seen in the absence of extensive disease as well as in mesothelioma (Fig. 16) [38]. These appearances are

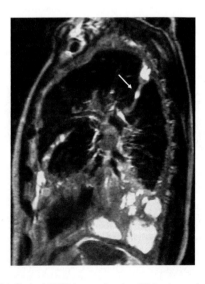

Fig. 16. Sagittal STIR image showing thickening and nodularity of the oblique fissure (*arrowed*) and pleural surfaces in a patient with mesothelioma.

sensitive but not specific for metastatic malignant pleural thickening.

A number of studies have assessed the role of MRI in distinguishing malignant from benign disease. Using the CT criteria for malignant pleural thickening described previously as well as signal intensity characteristics, sensitivities and specificities equivalent to those found with CT were demonstrated [39–41]. In two case series, pleural thickening greater than 1 cm was demonstrated in malignant and benign disease. When morphologic features and signal intensity characteristics were combined, MRI was superior to CT, with a sensitivity of 98% to 100% and a specificity of 87% to 92%, for detecting malignant pleural thickening [40–42]. Additionally, in one study, Falaschi and coworkers [43] found that pleural signal hypointensity relative to the intercostal muscles on sequences with a long repetition time (TR) was a reliable predictor of benign disease.

PET may be a useful noninvasive imaging and staging modality, although because of its scarcity and expense, it currently has a limited role in investigating pleural thickening. A few studies have examined the value of PET in distinguishing benign from malignant pleural thickening. They have demonstrated sensitivities of greater than 96% and a negative predictive value of less than 92% for identifying and differentiating malignant from benign disease [44–47]. False-positive scans after infectious and uremic pleuritis and talc pleurodesis can occur. Similarly, false-negative scans have occurred with slow-growing fibrous tumors, such as low-grade lymphoma or prostate metastasis [45]. These tumors exhibit low glycolytic and mitotic activity, accounting for the false-negative result. In view of this, patients with pleural thickening and a negative PET scan do not routinely require histologic verification but do require radiologic follow-up.

Malignant mesothelioma

Mesothelioma is the most common primary tumor of the pleura. Most cases are associated with previous asbestos exposure, developing after a latent period of 30 to 45 years. Only 5% to 7% of individuals exposed to asbestos actually develop mesothelioma, however. The incidence has been slowly increasing in industrialized countries and is expected to peak around 2020.

Mesothelioma carries a poor prognosis because most patients present with advanced disease, with a median survival of 12 months. The presence of intrathoracic lymphadenopathy, distant metastasis, and extensive pleural disease is associated with decreased survival [48].

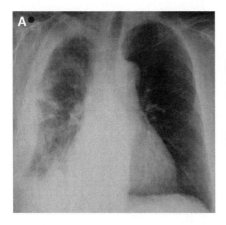
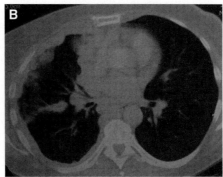

Fig. 17. (*A, B*) Frontal chest x-ray and axial CT shows right-sided lobulated pleural thickening with fissural extension in a patient with malignant pleural thickening.

Imaging plays a pivotal role in demonstrating the extent of disease and determining treatment options. On CXRs, the features are indistinguishable from diffuse metastatic malignant pleural thickening. Unilateral pleural thickening and pleural effusion are the most common manifestations of mesothelioma. Depending on the degree of pleural encasement, an associated large pleural effusion may not result in contralateral mediastinal shift. Isolated pleural thickening without an effusion is relatively uncommon, occurring in 10% to 20% of cases; extension into the fissures is frequent, occurring in 40% to 90% of cases (Fig. 17) [49].

CT is the imaging modality of choice for assessing mesothelioma. CT findings include nodular pleural thickening in 94% of cases, which involves the lower zones in 50% of cases and involves the upper zones in only a few cases. Diaphragmatic thickening and fissural involvement occur in up to 80% of patients, with pleural effusions in 80% and pleural calcification in 20%. Features suggestive of chest wall invasion include bone destruction (uncommon in mesothelioma), intercostal muscle invasion, and loss of the extrapleural fat planes (Fig. 18) [50].

MRI is not routinely used in investigating patients with mesothelioma because most patients present with advanced inoperable T4 disease, which is clearly delineated on CT. Advances in multidetector CT with multiplanar reconstructions may further reduce the need for MRI.

Currently, MRI is performed in patients under consideration for radical surgery because it allows the detection of diaphragmatic and endothoracic fascia invasion or solitary foci of chest wall invasion, enabling differentiation of T3 from T4 disease. Recently, Stewart and colleagues [51] assessed the value of contrast-enhanced MRI (CEMRI) in patients with epithelioid mesothelioma referred for surgery. They found that 17 of 49 patients had unexpected unresectable disease on CEMRI that precluded surgery.

Neither CT nor MRI can distinguish between T1a, T1b, and T2 disease because neither modality can accurately differentiate parietal from visceral involvement or detect invasion of diaphragmatic muscle or pericardium. Similarly, assessment of metastatic nodal involvement is limited, irrespective of nodal size, with sensitivities of 50% to 60% [52,53].

The role of PET in the staging of mesothelioma is poorly defined. This is primarily attributable to the fact that unlike most other malignancies, which spread systemically, mesothelioma typically spreads locally along tissue planes, with nodal and extra-

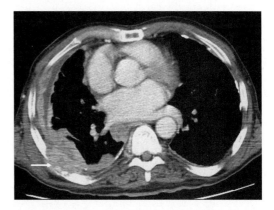

Fig. 18. Axial contrast-enhanced CT showing circumferential nodular pleural thickening with adjacent rib erosion and chest wall invasion (*arrow*) in an 80-year-old patient with mesothelioma. There are also bilateral calcified pleural plaques in keeping with previous asbestos exposure.

thoracic spread occurring late. On PET, sensitivities of greater than 90% for detecting primary tumor have been reported [54]. Extrathoracic metastasis can also be reliably detected [55]. Furthermore, when a thoracoscopic or percutaneous biopsy has been negative, PET can help to demonstrate a focal area of increased uptake and a more appropriate site for biopsy.

A recent study assessed the prognostic value of PET. The authors found that a high standardized uptake value (SUV >4) positively correlated with decreased survival ($P = .001$) and duration of survival ($P < .05$). This information may be useful clinically in determining the most appropriate treatment [56].

Pleural effusions

The normal pleural space contains 1 to 5 mL of pleural fluid. Pleural effusions occur when there is an imbalance of the normal physiologic processes that are necessary for the maintenance of equilibrium. Pleural exudates occur because of an increase in capillary permeability, most commonly attributable to malignancy, infection, or thromboembolic disease. Pleural transudates result from an increase in the capillary hydrostatic pressures or a decrease in the colloid osmotic pressures [57].

Free pleural fluid collects in the most dependent part of the pleural space on an erect CXR—normally, the posterior costophrenic recess or, less often, the

lateral recess. Approximately 50 mL of fluid causes blunting of the posterior costophrenic recess on a lateral CXR. By contrast, at least 200 mL is necessary to blunt the lateral recess on a PA CXR, and up to 500 mL of fluid can be present in some cases with no appreciable blunting [58]. A lateral decubitus film is the most sensitive view and can detect as little as 5 to 10 mL of free fluid [59].

As effusions increase in size, they produce a characteristic meniscus sign [1]. This represents fluid tracking superiorly along the pleural surface after filling of the costophrenic recess. Large effusions result in opacification of the hemithorax, with mediastinal shift. Absence of shift is suggestive of underlying lobar collapse or mediastinal fixation [60]. Massive effusions are most commonly (90%) secondary to malignancy. The most common primary malignancy is lung cancer, with breast, ovary, and gastric cancer and lymphoma accounting for 80% of all large effusions, although large pleural effusions are present in only 10% of patients with these malignancies on presentation [61].

Inversion of the hemidiaphragm can occur with massive effusions, occurring more frequently on the left side because of the protective nature of the liver on the right side [62]. After thoracocentesis, the hemidiaphragm can revert back to its normal position, with any remaining pleural fluid resulting in a slightly confusing CXR appearance of persistent pleural effusion despite thoracocentesis.

Free pleural fluid can collect in a variety of locations, such as within the fissures, abutting the mediastinum, or in a subpulmonic distribution. This

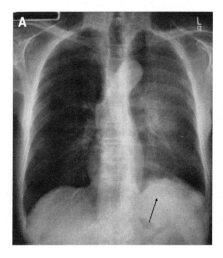 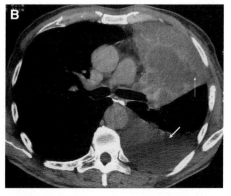

Fig. 19. (*A, B*) Frontal chest x-ray shows a veil like opacification of the left hemithorax in keeping with left upper lobe collapse. Below the left hemidiaphragm there is a paucity of lung markings and displacement of the gastric air bubble, inferiorly suggestive of a subpulmonic effusion (*arrow*). These findings were confirmed on CT (*A*).

distribution can lead to an appearance simulating a pulmonary or paramediastinal mass [63]. The fissural location of fluid is clearly evident on a lateral view, and movement of fluid from a paramediastinal or subpulmonic region laterally along the chest wall is seen on a lateral decubitus film.

Because subpulmonic effusions conform to the shape of the hemidiaphragm, they are frequently overlooked on a PA CXR, especially if they are small. Elevation and lateral displacement of the peak of the hemidiaphragm, paucity of vessels below the hemidiaphragm, and widening of the distance between the gastric bubble and hemidiaphragm should raise the suspicion of a subpulmonic effusion (Fig. 19) [64].

On a supine CXR, the presence of a large amount of fluid can be easily missed, because fluid layers posteriorly. An apical cap may suggest the diagnosis. Other features include hazy opacification of the hemithorax, blunting of the costophrenic recesses, elevation of the hemidiaphragm, and reduced lower zone vascularity (Fig. 20) [65].

CT is usually performed in patients with pleural effusions of unknown etiology and suspected malignant or complicated parapneumonic effusions and empyema. These scans should be performed after administration of intravenous contrast with a 60-second delay, enabling optimal pleural and soft tissue enhancement. This allows differentiation of pleural thickening from pleural fluid; characterization of the pleural thickening as benign or malignant; and differentiation of an exudate from a transudate, with enhancement almost always indicating an exudate (Fig. 21) [66,67]. Occasionally, it may be difficult to distinguish between pleural fluid and ascites in

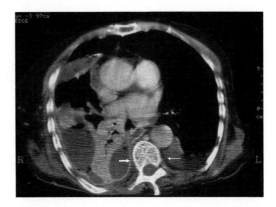

Fig. 21. The right multiloculated effusion shows pleural enhancement indicative of an exudate (*bold arrow*), whereas there is no enhancement on the left, suggesting a transudative effusion (*arrow*).

supine patients on CT. Four signs can be helpful in such cases:

1. Displaced crus sign: pleural fluid lies between the crus of the diaphragm and the vertebral bodies, causing anterior displacement of the crus. This only occurs with pleural effusions [68].
2. Interface sign: attributable to interposition of the hemidiaphragm; a hazy interface between the liver or spleen is seen with pleural fluid, compared with a sharp interface in patients with ascites [69].
3. Diaphragm sign: pleural fluid always lies peripheral to the diaphragm. With ascites, the upper abdominal viscera lie medially [70,71].
4. Bare area: the posterior aspect of the right lobe of the liver is not covered by peritoneum and is directly attached to the posterior abdominal wall; thus, peritoneal fluid cannot extend into this area.

MRI seems to be superior to CT in the characterization of pleural fluid, although it is rarely necessary for diagnosis. Triple echo (TE) pulse sequences have been shown to differentiate between an exudate and transudate, with complex exudates having greater signal intensity than simple exudates, which are still brighter than transudates [72]. Preliminary studies have suggested that single-shot diffusion-weighted imaging may also be helpful in this regard, with high diffusion seen with transudates and low diffusion seen with exudates [73]. Three-plane scanning seems to be helpful, with the sagittal and axial T2-weighted sequences being most valuable in detecting nodular pleural thickening and fat-saturated T1-weighted

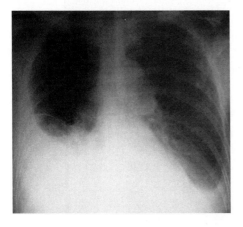

Fig. 20. Semi-supine CXR demonstrates a right loculated pleural effusion and layering of fluid posteriorly on the left. Note the bronchovascular markings are still visible.

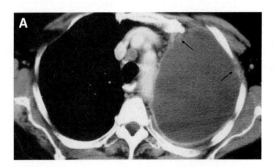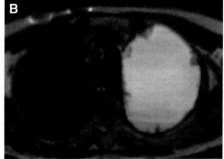

Fig. 22. (*A, B*) On contrast-enhanced CT, there is the suggestion of nodular pleural enhancement (*arrows*). T2W MR sequence shows multiple low signal pleural nodules against the pleural efussion which returns a high signal.

sequences after administration of gadolinium being useful for detecting subtle malignant thickening.

Pleural effusions are typically demonstrated as low signal on T1-weighted sequences and as high signal on T2-weighted sequences. When attempting to detect pleural nodularity, intravenous contrast is not usually necessary. On T2-weighted images, the high-signal pleural effusion and extrapleural fat act as inherent contrast, outlining the low-signal parietal pleura and clearly demonstrating pleural nodularity (Fig. 22) as well as allowing easy detection of septations, in direct comparison to their difficult detection on CT (Fig. 23). A heterogeneous appearance can also be seen on T2-weighted images because of flow artifact created by the effusion (Fig. 24).

Chylothoraces are bright on T1-weighted images and show T2 shortening with a signal intensity similar to that of subcutaneous fat.

Subacute and/or chronic hematomas demonstrate high signal on T1- and T2-weighted images. A rim of low signal attributable to hemosiderin may be seen on the T2-weighted image [74].

Parapneumonic effusions and empyema

Up to 60% of patients with pneumonia develop an associated parapneumonic effusion, and approximately 10% of these patients develop secondary infections and progress to a complicated parapneumonic effusion or empyema [71,75]. The radiographic appearances are dependent on the developmental stage of the effusion.

In most cases, a PA CXR and ultrasound scan are adequate for diagnosis and guiding drainage. The typical appearance of a parapneumonic effusion is

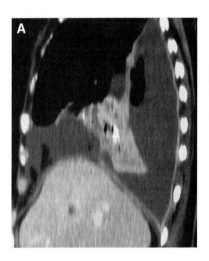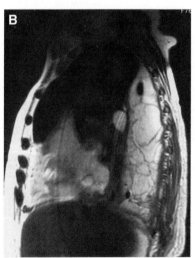

Fig. 23. (*A, B*) Sagittal CT reconstruction demonstrating an apparent non-septated pleural effusion. Sagittal T2W MR sequence clearly shows a multiseptated effusion in the same patient.

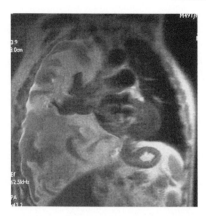

Fig. 24. The normal heterogeneous appearance of a pleural effusion due to flow artifact on MR (T2W image).

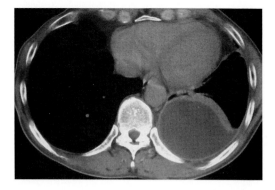

Fig. 26. Contrast-enhanced CT demonstrating separation of the left posterior-visceral and parietal pleura—the "split pleura" sign.

that of a unilateral pleural effusion associated with an area of consolidation. If bilateral effusions are present, the infected side is usually larger [76]. When patients with a pneumonic illness present late, the development of adhesions may have resulted in a loculated pleural collection. When peripheral, this may resemble a pleural mass; similarly, a fissural effusion may have the appearance of a pseudotumor (Fig. 25).

Contrast-enhanced CT is often helpful in complicated cases in which conventional treatment with antibiotics and tube drainage has failed. Complicated parapneumonic effusions and empyemas characteristically demonstrate the "split pleura" sign, which refers to the presence of thickened enhancing parietal and visceral pleura separated by pleural fluid (Fig. 26). Pleural thickening and enhancement are seen in 80% to 100% of empyemas compared with 60% of parapneumonic effusions [66,67]. There is also a tendency for increased pleural thickness to be seen with an advanced stage of pleural effu-

sion infection, although, interestingly, there is no apparent relation between the likelihood of patient response to conventional treatment and pleural thickness [77].

Other features seen on CT include thickening of the extrapleural tissues and increased attenuation of the extrapleural fat, defined as an increase of greater than 50 HU when compared with the fat posterior to the spine [77], which is thought to be attributable to inflammation and edema (Fig. 27). These features may persist for an extended period after successful treatment and have a variable likelihood of returning to normal [78–80].

Loculations are seen in 20% of cases on CT and are most commonly found with larger effusions, multiple chest drain insertions, and prolonged hospitalization. Variation in pleural fluid pH and lactate dehydrogenase (LDH) between adjacent locules can occur and may be associated with failure of patients to respond to conservative treatment [80a]. Septations are less

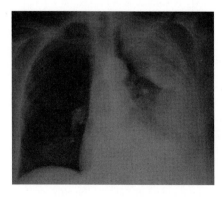

Fig. 25. Left-sided empyema mimicking a pleurally based mass.

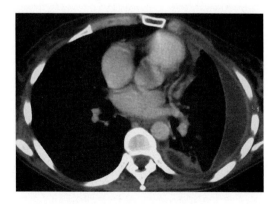

Fig. 27. Contrast-enhanced CT shows a left-sided loculated empyema with increased attenuation of the extrapleural fat (CT region of interest 1 laterally on the left).

clearly seen on CT, although they can be inferred by the presence of gas within separate locules (Fig. 28).

Moderate mediastinal lymph node enlargement, less than 2 cm, is frequently seen in community-acquired parapneumonic effusions and empyemas. This is usually ipsilateral, commonly involves the subcarinal and paratracheal nodal stations, and is more frequent on the right side. There is no apparent correlation between stage and degree of nodal enlargement [81].

Pneumothorax

Most pneumothoraces are demonstrated on a fully inspired erect PA CXR. They appear as an absence of lung markings distal to the visceral pleural line because of the presence of air between the visceral pleura and the parietal pleura. Free air tends to accumulate in the least dependent part of the pleural space, the apical portion of the lung, on an erect CXR. A 2.5-cm margin of free air between the chest wall and visceral pleura equates to a pneumothorax of approximately 30% of hemithorax volume (Fig. 29).

If there is diagnostic doubt as to the presence of a pneumothorax, an expiratory or lateral decubitus film should be taken. With expiration, reduction in the lung volume accentuates the constant volume of the pneumothorax. In the lateral decubitus position, because of the lack of composite shadows, small volumes of free air are readily demonstrated parallel to the chest wall, with sensitivities similar to those of CT [82].

The signs of a pneumothorax can be subtle on a supine film, with a false-negative rate of 30%. Air can collect in the subpulmonic, lateral, and juxtacardiac regions. Findings suggestive of a pneumothorax

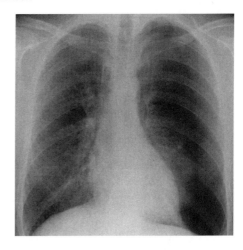

Fig. 29. Frontal chest radiograph showing an approximately 40% left pneumothorax.

on a supine film include increased radiolucency and deepening of the costophrenic angle (the deep sulcus sign), depression of the ipsilateral hemidiaphragm, and increased sharpness of the pericardial fat pad and cardiomediastinal border. In a right-sided pneumothorax, a band of air may collect in the horizontal fissure [83,84].

Skin folds and underlying clothing can mimic a pneumothorax in the supine patient. Unlike pneumothoraces, these lines are wider and continue beyond the chest wall and lung markings can be seen distal to the apparent line.

Although a tension pneumothorax is considered a medical emergency, interestingly, radiologic evidence of tension does not always correlate with the severity of clinical symptoms [85]. The radiographic signs of tension are depression of the hemidiaphragm and contralateral mediastinal shift.

CT scanning is more sensitive than a CXR at detecting pneumothoraces, with 25% to 40% of postbiopsy pneumothoraces noted on CT not detectable on a CXR [86]. After trauma and in the intensive care unit (ICU) setting, 30% to 50% of pneumothoraces can be missed on a supine film. In such patients, CT can readily demonstrate an occult or loculated pneumothorax and guide subsequent drainage (Fig. 30). Additionally, CT allows associated parenchymal abnormalities and positioning of drains and lines to be confirmed [87,88].

Differentiating between large emphysematous bullae and a pneumothorax on a CXR can be problematic. Typically, a bulla demonstrates a concave medial wall. CT may help in differentiation because air can be seen outlining both sides of the bulla wall parallel to the chest wall, the double-wall sign. Two adjacent

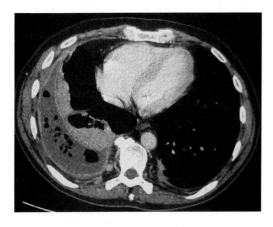

Fig. 28. Contrast-enhanced CT demonstrating a multiloculated empyema demonstrating mutiple pockets of gas.

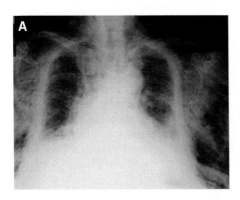
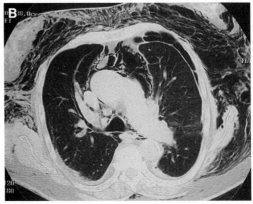

Fig. 30. (*A, B*) Frontal chest x-ray shows surgical empyema, pneumomediastinum and a pleural effusion in a patient following trauma. CT showed the injuries to be more extensive and demonstrated a left-sided pneumothorax. This finding was not evident on the plain film.

bullae can cause difficulty; however, using three-dimensional reformatting of the CT image can readily resolve this issue.

Bronchopleural fistula

Bronchopleural fistulas may occur secondary to thoracic surgery, infection, malignancy, or medical intervention. On a CXR, the presence of a persistent pneumothorax or hydropneumothorax is suggestive of an airway fistula. After pneumonectomy, the pneumonectomy space should gradually fill with fluid, with 80% to 90% opacification of the operated hemithorax by 2 weeks and complete opacification commonly by 6 months. Bronchopleural fistulas are seen in 2% to 3% of cases after pneumonectomy, with most occurring within 2 weeks [89]. The development of a fistula on sequential CXRs is suggested by the presence of increasing air, decreasing fluid, and shift of the mediastinum back to the midline (Fig. 31). CT is excellent at demonstrating a bronchopleural fistula because lung window views frequently allow direct communication between the bronchus and pleural cavity to be demonstrated, along with the underlying cause [90]. If doubt still exists, ventilation studies using xenon-133 can demonstrate the presence of a fistula during the washout phase [91].

Intervention

Thoracocentesis

In some cases, such as congestive heart failure, the cause of a pleural effusion is evident from the clinical history alone. When it is required, thoracocentesis may be performed without image guidance based on the CXR appearance and clinical signs. In the presence of a large pleural effusion, this is a relatively safe procedure. Image guidance, which is usually ultrasound, is frequently requested after a dry tap or if the effusion is small and difficult to differentiate from thickening or loculated fluid. Image-guided thoracocentesis can reduce complications and increase diagnostic yield significantly [92].

Chest tube drainage

Non–image-guided chest tube insertion, predominantly in the treatment of pneumothoraces and large

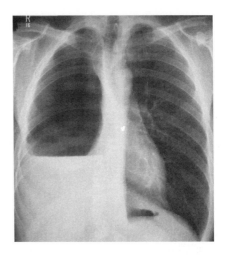

Fig. 31. Previous right pneumonectomy with a persistant air-fluid level and minor mediastinal deviation to the left should raise the possibility of a bronchopleural fistula.

effusions, is conventionally by insertion immediately cranial to the sixth rib in the midaxillary line. In case of effusion, the tip of the chest drain should ideally be positioned in the most dependent part of the effusion to maximize drainage. Practically, this may not be possible to do safely without image guidance because the effusion may be loculated, small in volume, or positioned posteriorly or medially away from the conventional site of drain insertion. Complications associated with image guidance are low, with a pneumothorax rate of less than 5% [93].

The choice of imaging modality to guide chest tube drainage is dependent on the operator as well as on the site, size, and nature of the effusion. Most guided drain insertions are placed under ultrasound, with CT usually reserved for complicated cases. CT allows visualization of pockets of fluid that are positioned behind bony structures and noncommunicating loculations that may not visible on ultrasound. Furthermore, CT may identify possible causes of failure of the lung to re-expand in patients with persistent pleural effusions and chest tubes in situ, such as underlying visceral pleural thickening, an endobronchial lesion causing pulmonary collapse, or malpositioning of the chest tube.

Traditionally, large-bore drains have been advocated to optimize effusion drainage. An increasing number of case series using small-bore catheters (8–14 French) have shown these to be as effective as large-bore drains, however, with success rates ranging from 60% to 90% [94]. There are no randomized controlled trials comparing the efficacy of large-caliber and small-caliber chest drains in patients with effusions and pneumothoraces. Three nonrandomized studies have directly compared large- and small-bore catheter drains and found no significant difference in success rates measured clinically and radiologically. Patients found placement of a small-bore drain to be more comfortable and comparable to thoracentesis [94–97]. In complicated parapneumonic effusions and empyema, indications for chest tube drainage are pus within the pleural cavity, pH less than 7.20, and a positive pleural culture. Published data, mainly observational case series, suggest that success rates of 70% to 90% can be achieved with small-bore catheters when used primarily or after failure of large-bore drains [98].

Long-term indwelling catheters are increasingly being used as an alternative to standard 8- to 14-French catheters in patients with recurrent malignant effusions. These have been shown to achieve acceptable symptomatic relief and effective pleurodesis in approximately 50% of patients in 2 to 3 months. Furthermore, they allow patients to be managed on an outpatient basis and do not require hospitalization [99,100].

Similarly, there is evidence to suggest that small-bore catheters are equally efficacious in the treatment of pneumothorax [101,102]. Indeed, success rates of 85% to 95% have been demonstrated with 5.5- to 9.4-French catheters [103–105]. Most pneumothoraces resolve by 48 hours, with failure to resolve usually attributable to a malpositioned drain or persistent air leak. In the latter situation, placement of a larger drain may be necessary. Image guidance is not usually necessary, except in cases of occult or loculated pneumothoraces.

Pleural biopsy

Pleural biopsies in patients with pleural effusions were first reported in the 1950s. Most were performed without radiologic guidance by respiratory physicians at the bedside using reverse-bevel Abrams and Cope needles. In experienced hands, diagnostic sensitivities of 50% are achievable for malignant disease, including mesothelioma, although in patients with negative pleural fluid cytology, more typical sensitivities range from 7% to 27% [106–108].

Image-guided biopsy in patients with cytology-negative effusions significantly increases the diagnostic yield when compared with an unguided Abrams biopsy. Maskell and coworkers [109] achieved a sensitivity of 87% and specificity of 100% for CT-guided biopsy in patients with pleural malignancy compared with a sensitivity of 47% and specificity of 100% for an Abrams biopsy.

Pleural biopsies are usually performed with ultrasound or CT guidance. The choice of modality depends on the operator's personal preference and competence. No studies have directly compared the clinical utility of ultrasound with that of CT, although higher sensitivities have been reported with CT guidance than with ultrasound. This is primarily because CT allows visualization and biopsy of pleural pathologic findings inaccessible to ultrasound, such as lesions internal to the rib in a paramediastinal region and deep to the scapula. Furthermore, by biopsying along the pleural plane under CT guidance, histologic cores of tissue can be attained even in patients with pleural thickening of less than 5 mm, with one study reporting a sensitivity of 75% for pleural thickness less than 5 mm and 100% for thickening greater than 5 mm (Fig. 32) [110].

Ultrasound-guided biopsy has some advantages over CT, with its lack of radiation, its ready availability, and its real-time visualization of the needle during biopsy, thereby reducing potential complica-

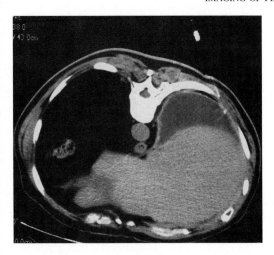

Fig. 32. There is a right-sided pleural effusion with irregular pleural thickening measuring less than 1cm. CT-guided biopsy performed prone was diagnostic for mesothelioma.

tions. Biopsies under ultrasound or CT can be performed in the absence or presence of a pleural effusion, although minimal pleural thickening is poorly demonstrated under ultrasound. The presence of an effusion reduces the risk of complications, particularly a pneumothorax.

There are no absolute contraindications to biopsy; however, as with any interventional procedure, abnormal coagulation parameters should be corrected before biopsy and severe respiratory symptoms that prevent the patient from following breath-holding instructions need to be considered.

After obtaining informed consent, biopsies can be performed with the patient in the supine or prone position. Diaphragmatic and posterobasal pleural thickening is best biopsied prone. Adequate local anesthetic infiltration of the pleura is essential to minimize patient discomfort, and core needle biopsies using an 18-gauge cutting needle should be performed. Core needle biopsy is more sensitive than fine needle aspiration biopsy at diagnosing malignant disease, especially lymphoma and mesothelioma. Adams and Gleeson [110] demonstrated sensitivities of 88% and 78% in malignant disease and 93% and 50% for mesothelioma for core biopsy and aspiration biopsy, respectively. These findings are similar to those of previous studies of malignant disease but are higher than previously reported for mesothelioma, which more typically has a sensitivity of 77% to 86% [111,112]. The diagnostic accuracy of 93% for mesothelioma is similar to that achievable with thoracoscopy. The combination of core needle and aspiration biopsy has been shown to increase the

diagnostic yield for malignant disease (88%–97%) further; however, it was unhelpful in accurately diagnosing benign disease [34].

Complications associated with percutaneous pleural biopsy occur in less than 1% of cases and include pneumothorax, hemothorax, subcutaneous hematoma, and laceration of the underlying upper abdominal viscera. Complication rates are also generally low for biopsies with Abrams needles; however, complications requiring postprocedural intervention and occasionally resulting in death have been described with an Abrams biopsy. Complication rates as high as 15% have been reported with thoracoscopy [113].

Tumour seeding along the needle track is relatively common with mesothelioma but rare with pleural metastasis from carcinoma. In mesothelioma, this occurs in 20% of patients undergoing image-guided biopsy [114]. Early radiotherapy to the biopsy track has been shown to prevent tumor seeding [115].

Summary

Imaging and image-guided intervention play a pivotal role in the diagnosis and characterization of pleural disease. The CXR remains the initial investigation for demonstrating the presence of pleural disease. In patients with an unexplained pleural effusion or pleural thickening, contrast-enhanced CT is usually indicated to differentiate benign from malignant disease and can also subsequently guide intervention. Ultrasound plays an increasingly important role in the investigation and management of patients with pleural disease, as discussed elsewhere. MRI is rarely necessary. Its superior soft tissue contrast and multiplanar capabilities may help in solving problematic cases, however, usually where the local extent of disease has been poorly defined on CT. The role of PET is still under investigation, although the advent of PET-CT may increase its clinical utility in the investigation of pleural disease.

References

[1] Wilson AG. Pleura and pleural disorders. In: Armstrong P, Wilson AG, Dee P, et al, editors. Imaging of diseases of the chest. London: Mosby; 1995. p. 641–716.
[2] Proto AV, Ball Jr JB. Computed tomography of the major and minor fissures. AJR Am J Roentgenol 1983;140:439–48.
[3] Im JG, Webb WR, Rosen A, et al. Costal pleura: appearances at high-resolution CT. Radiology 1989; 171:125–31.

[4] Rockoff SD, Kagan E, Schwartz A, et al. Visceral pleural thickening in asbestos exposure: the occurrence and implications of thickened interlobar fissures. J Thorac Imaging 1987;2:58–66.

[5] Proto AV. Conventional chest radiographs: anatomic understanding of newer observations. Radiology 1992;183:593–603.

[6] Peacock C, Copley SJ, Hansell DM. Asbestos-related benign pleural disease. Clin Radiol 2000;55:422–32.

[7] Hillerdal G. Value of the lateral view in diagnosing pleural plaques. Arch Environ Health 1986;41: 391–2.

[8] Ameille J, Brochard P, Brechot JM, et al. Pleural thickening: a comparison of oblique chest radiographs and high-resolution computed tomography in subjects exposed to low levels of asbestos pollution. Int Arch Occup Environ Health 1993;64:545–8.

[9] Muller NL. Imaging of the pleura. Radiology 1993; 186:297–309.

[10] Staples CA. Computed tomography in the evaluation of benign asbestos-related disorders. Radiol Clin North Am 1992;30:1191–207.

[11] al Jarad N, Poulakis N, Pearson MC, et al. Assessment of asbestos-induced pleural disease by computed tomography—correlation with chest radiograph and lung function. Respir Med 1991;85:203–8.

[12] Remy-Jardin M, Sobaszek A, Duhamel A, et al. Asbestos-related pleuropulmonary diseases: evaluation with low-dose four-detector row spiral CT. Radiology 2004;233:182–90.

[13] Roach HD, Davies GJ, Attanoos R, et al. Asbestos: when the dust settles, an imaging review of asbestos-related disease. Radiographics 2002;22(Suppl):S167.

[14] Weber MA, Bock M, Plathow C, et al. Asbestos-related pleural disease: value of dedicated magnetic resonance imaging techniques. Invest Radiol 2004; 39:554–64.

[15] Theros EG, Feigin DS. Pleural tumours and pulmonary tumours: differential diagnosis. Semin Roentgenol 1977;12:239–47.

[16] Bilbey JH, Muller NL, Miller RR, et al. Localized fibrous mesothelioma of pleura following external ionizing radiation therapy. Chest 1988;94:1291–2.

[17] Rosado-de-Christenson ML, Abbott GF, McAdams HP, et al. Localised fibrous tumors of the pleura. Archives of the AFIP. Radiographics 2003;23: 759–83.

[18] England DM, Hochholzer L, McCarthy MJ, et al. Localised benign and malignant fibrous tumors of the pleura. Am J Surg Pathol 1988;13:640–8.

[19] Ferretti GR, Chiles C, Choplin RH, et al. Localized benign fibrous tumors of the pleura. AJR Am J Roentgenol 1997;169:683–6.

[20] England DM, Hochholzer L, McCarthy MJ. Localised benign and malignant fibrous tumors of the pleura: a clinicopathologic review of 223 cases. Am J Surg Pathol 1989;13:640–8.

[21] Tateishi U, Nishihara H, Morikawa T, et al. Solitary fibrous tumors of the pleura: MR appearance and enhancement pattern. J Comput Assist Tomogr 2002; 26:174–9.

[22] Epler GR, McLoud TC, Munn CS, et al. Pleural lipoma. Diagnosis by computed tomography. Chest 1986;90:265–8.

[23] Davies C, Gleeson FV. Diagnostic radiology. In: Light RW, Lee YC, editors. Textbook of pleural diseases. London: Arnold; 2003. p. 210–37.

[24] Ameille J, Matrat M, Paris C, et al. Asbestos-related pleural diseases: dimensional criteria are not appropriate to differentiate diffuse pleural thickening from pleural plaques. Am J Ind Med 2004;45:289–96.

[25] Lynch DA, Gamsu G, Ray CS, et al. Asbestos-related focal lung masses: manifestations on conventional and high-resolution CT scans. Radiology 1988;169: 603–7.

[26] Copley SJ, Wells AU, Rubens MB, et al. Functional consequences of pleural disease evaluated with chest radiography and CT. Radiology 2001;220:237–43.

[27] McHugh K, Blaquiere RM. CT features of rounded atelectasis. AJR Am J Roentgenol 1989;153:257–60.

[28] Munden RF, Libshitz HI. Rounded atelectasis and mesothelioma. AJR Am J Roentgenol 1998;170: 1519–22.

[29] Murray JG, Patz Jr EF, Erasmus JJ, et al. CT appearance of the pleural space after talc pleurodesis. AJR Am J Roentgenol 1997;169:89–91.

[30] Henschke CI, Yankelevitz DF, Davis SD. Pleural diseases: multimodality imaging and clinical management. Curr Probl Diagn Radiol 1991;20:155–81.

[31] Leung AN, Muller NL, Miller RR. CT in differential diagnosis of diffuse pleural disease. AJR Am J Roentgenol 1990;154:487–92.

[32] Traill ZC, Davies RJ, Gleeson FV. Thoracic computed tomography in patients with suspected malignant pleural effusions. Clin Radiol 2001;56:193–6.

[33] Shuman LS, Libshitz HI. Solid pleural manifestations of lymphoma. AJR Am J Roentgenol 1984;142: 269–73.

[34] Scott EM, Marshall TJ, Flower CD, et al. Diffuse pleural thickening: percutaneous CT-guided cutting needle biopsy. Radiology 1995;194:867–70.

[35] Lorigan JG, Libshitz HI. MR imaging of malignant pleural mesothelioma. J Comput Assist Tomogr 1989; 13:617–20.

[36] Hierholzer J, Luo L, Bittner RC, et al. MRI and CT in the differential diagnosis of pleural disease. Chest 2000;118:604–9.

[37] Falaschi F, Battolla L, Mascalchi M, et al. Usefulness of MR signal intensity in distinguishing benign from malignant pleural disease. AJR Am J Roentgenol 1996;166:963–8.

[38] Knuuttila A, Kivisaari L, Kivisaari A, et al. Evaluation of pleural disease using MR and CT. With special reference to malignant pleural mesothelioma. Acta Radiol 2001;42:502–7.

[39] Falaschi F, Battolla L, Zampa V, et al. [Comparison of computerized tomography and magnetic resonance in the assessment of benign and malignant pleu-

ral diseases]. Radiol Med (Torino) 1996;92:713–8 [in Italian].

[40] Hierholzer J, Luo L, Bittner RC, et al. MRI and CT in the differential diagnosis of pleural disease. Chest 2000;118:604–9.

[41] Luo L, Hierholzer J, Bittner RC, et al. Magnetic resonance imaging in distinguishing malignant from benign pleural disease. Chin Med J (Engl) 2001;114: 645–9.

[42] Falaschi F, Battolla L, Zampa V, et al. Comparison of computerized tomography and magnetic resonance in the assessment of benign and malignant pleural diseases. Radiol Med (Torino) 1996;92:713–8.

[43] Falaschi F, Battolla L, Mascalchi M, et al. Usefulness of MR signal intensity in distinguishing benign from malignant pleural disease. AJR Am J Roentgenol 1996;166:963–8.

[44] Kramer H, Pieterman RM, Slebos DJ, et al. PET for the evaluation of pleural thickening observed on CT. J Nucl Med 2004;45:995–8.

[45] Duysinx B, Nguyen D, Louis R, et al. Evaluation of pleural disease with 18-fluorodeoxyglucose positron emission tomography imaging. Chest 2004;125: 489–93.

[46] Carretta A, Landoni C, Melloni G, et al. 18-FDG positron emission tomography in the evaluation of malignant pleural diseases—a pilot study. Eur J Cardiothorac Surg 2000;17:377–83.

[47] Bury T, Daenen F, Duysinx B, et al. [18FDG-PET applications in thoracic oncology]. Rev Mal Respir 2001;18:623–30 [in French].

[48] Rusch VW. A proposed new international TNM staging system for malignant pleural mesothelioma from the International Mesothelioma Interest Group. Lung Cancer 1996;14:1–12.

[49] Kawashima A, Libshitz HI. Malignant pleural mesothelioma: CT manifestations in 50 cases. AJR Am J Roentgenol 1990;155:965–9.

[50] Ng CS, Munden RF, Libshitz HI. Malignant pleural mesothelioma: the spectrum of manifestations on CT in 70 cases. Clin Radiol 1999;54:415–21.

[51] Stewart D, Waller D, Edwards J, et al. Is there a role for pre-operative contrast-enhanced magnetic resonance imaging for radical surgery in malignant pleural mesothelioma? Eur J Cardiothorac Surg 2003;24:1019–24.

[52] Bonomo L, Feragalli B, Sacco R, et al. Malignant pleural disease. Eur J Radiol 2000;34:98–118.

[53] Patz Jr EF, Rusch VW, Heelan R. The proposed new international TNM staging system for malignant pleural mesothelioma: application to imaging. AJR Am J Roentgenol 1996;166:323–7.

[54] Flores RM, Akhurst T, Gonen M, et al. Positron emission tomography defines metastatic disease but not locoregional disease in patients with malignant pleural mesothelioma. J Thorac Cardiovasc Surg 2003;126:11–6.

[55] Scheider DB, Clary-Macy C, Challa S, et al. Positron emission tomography with 18-flurodeoxyglucose in the staging and preoperative evaluation of malignant pleural mesothelioma. J Thorac Cardiovasc Surg 2000;120:128–33.

[56] Benard F, Sterman D, Smith RJ, et al. Prognostic value of FDG PET imaging in malignant pleural mesothelioma. J Nucl Med 1999;40:1241–5.

[57] Maskell NA, Butland RJ. BTS guidelines for the investigation of a unilateral pleural effusion in adults. Thorax 2003;58(Suppl 2):ii8–17.

[58] Blackmore CC, Black WC, Dallas RV, et al. Pleural fluid volume estimation: a chest radiograph prediction rule. Acad Radiol 1996;3:103–9.

[59] Moskowitz H, Platt RT, Schachar R, et al. Roentgen visualization of minute pleural effusion. An experimental study to determine the minimum amount of pleural fluid visible on a radiograph. Radiology 1973; 109:33–5.

[60] Liberson M. Diagnostic significance of the mediastinal profile in massive unilateral pleural effusions. Am Rev Respir Dis 1963;88:176–80.

[61] Sahn SA. Pleural diseases related to metastatic malignancies. Eur Respir J 1997;10:1907–13.

[62] Mulvey RB. The effect of pleural fluid on the diaphragm. Radiology 1965;84:1080–6.

[63] Raasch BN, Carsky EW, Lane EJ, et al. Pleural effusion: explanation of some typical appearances. AJR Am J Roentgenol 1982;139:899–904.

[64] Petersen JA. Recognition of infrapulmonary pleural effusion. Radiology 1960;74:34–41.

[65] Ruskin JA, Gurney JW, Thorsen MK, et al. Detection of pleural effusions on supine chest radiographs. AJR Am J Roentgenol 1987;148:681–3.

[66] Waite RJ, Carbonneau RJ, Balikian JP, et al. Parietal pleural changes in empyema: appearances at CT. Radiology 1990;175:145–50.

[67] Aquino SL, Webb WR, Gushiken BJ. Pleural exudates and transudates: diagnosis with contrast-enhanced CT. Radiology 1994;192:803–8.

[68] Dwyer A. The displaced crus: a sign for distinguishing between pleural fluid and ascites on computed tomography. J Comput Assist Tomogr 1978;2: 598–9.

[69] Teplick JG, Teplick SK, Goodman L, et al. The interface sign: a computed tomographic sign for distinguishing pleural and intra-abdominal fluid. Radiology 1982;144:359–62.

[70] Naidich DP, Megibow AJ, Hilton S, et al. Computed tomography of the diaphragm: peridiaphragmatic fluid localization. J Comput Assist Tomogr 1983;7: 641–9.

[71] Light RW, Girard WM, Jenkinson SG, et al. Parapneumonic effusions. Am J Med 1980;69:507–12.

[72] Davis SD, Henschke CI, Yankelevitz DF, et al. MR imaging of pleural effusions. J Comput Assist Tomogr 1990;14:192–8.

[73] Baysal T, Bulut T, Gokirmak M, et al. Diffusion-weighted MR imaging of pleural fluid: differentiation of transudative vs exudative pleural effusions. Eur Radiol 2004;14:890–6.

[74] McLoud TC. CT and MR in pleural disease. Clin Chest Med 1998;19:261–76.

[75] Taryle DA, Potts DE, Sahn SA. The incidence and clinical correlates of parapneumonic effusions in pneumococcal pneumonia. Chest 1978;74:170–3.

[76] Hanna JW, Reed JC, Choplin RH. Pleural infections: a clinical-radiologic review. J Thorac Imaging 1991; 6:68–79.

[77] Kearney SE, Davies CW, Davies RJ, et al. Computed tomography and ultrasound in parapneumonic effusions and empyema. Clin Radiol 2000;55:542–7.

[78] Jimenez CD, Diaz G, Perez-Rodriguez E, et al. Prognostic features of residual pleural thickening in parapneumonic pleural effusions. Eur Respir J 2003;21:952–5.

[79] Martinez MA, Cordero PJ, Cases E, et al. Prognostic features of residual pleural thickening in metapneumonic pleural effusion. Arch Bronconeumol 1999;35: 108–12.

[80] Neff CC, van Sonnenberg E, Lawson DW, et al. CT follow-up of empyemas: pleural peels resolve after percutaneous catheter drainage. Radiology 1990;176: 195–7.

[80a] Maskell NA, Gleeson FV, Darby M, et al. Diagnostically significant variations in pleural fluid pH in loculated parapneumonic effusions. Chest 2004;126: 2022–4.

[81] Kearney SE, Davies CW, Tattersall DJ, et al. The characteristics and significance of thoracic lymphadenopathy in parapneumonic effusion and empyema. Br J Radiol 2000;73:583–7.

[82] Carr JJ, Reed JC, Choplin RH, et al. Plain and computed radiography for detecting experimentally induced pneumothorax in cadavers: implications for detection in patients. Radiology 1992;183:193–9.

[83] Tocino IM, Miller MH, Fairfax WR. Distribution of pneumothorax in the supine and semirecumbent critically ill adult. AJR Am J Roentgenol 1985;144:901–5.

[84] Gordon R. The deep sulcus sign. Radiology 1980; 136:25–7.

[85] Clark S, Ragg M, Stella J. Is mediastinal shift on chest X-ray of pneumothorax always an emergency? Emerg Med (Fremantle) 2003;15:429–33.

[86] Bungay HK, Berger J, Traill ZC, et al. Pneumothorax post CT-guided lung biopsy: a comparison between detection on chest radiographs and CT. Br J Radiol 1999;72:1160–3.

[87] Tocino IM, Miller MH, Frederick PR, et al. CT detection of occult pneumothorax in head trauma. AJR Am J Roentgenol 1984;143:987–90.

[88] Gross BH, Spizarny DL. Computed tomography of the chest in the intensive care unit. Crit Care Clin 1994;10:267–75.

[89] Malave G, Foster ED, Wilson JA, et al. Bronchopleural fistula—present-day study of an old problem. A review of 52 cases. Ann Thorac Surg 1971;11:1–10.

[90] Westcott JL, Volpe JP. Peripheral bronchopleural fistula: CT evaluation in 20 patients with pneumonia, empyema, or postoperative air leak. Radiology 1995; 196:175–81.

[91] Lowe RE, Siddiqui AR. Scintimaging of bronchopleural fistula. A simple method of diagnosis. Clin Nucl Med 1984;9:10–2.

[92] Diacon AH, Brutsche MH, Soler M. Accuracy of pleural puncture sites: a prospective comparison of clinical examination with ultrasound. Chest 2003; 123:436–41.

[93] Jones PW, Moyers JP, Rogers JT, et al. Ultrasound-guided thoracentesis: is it a safer method? Chest 2003;123:418–23.

[94] Tattersall DJ, Traill ZC, Gleeson FV. Chest drains: does size matter? Clin Radiol 2000;55:415–21.

[95] Clementsen P, Evald T, Grode G, et al. Treatment of malignant pleural effusion: pleurodesis using a small percutaneous catheter. A prospective randomized study. Respir Med 1998;92:593–6.

[96] Parker LA, Charnock GC, Delany DJ. Small bore catheter drainage and sclerotherapy for malignant pleural effusions. Cancer 1989;64:1218–21.

[97] Maskell NA, Davies CWH, Nunn AJ, et al. UK Controlled Trial of Intrapleural Streptokinase for Pleural Infection. N Engl J Med 2005;352:865–74.

[98] Patz Jr EF, Goodman PC, Erasmus JJ. Percutaneous drainage of pleural collections. J Thorac Imaging 1998;13:83–92.

[99] Pollak JS, Burdge CM, Rosenblatt M, et al. Treatment of malignant pleural effusions with tunneled long-term drainage catheters. J Vasc Interv Radiol 2001;12: 201–8.

[100] Smart JM, Tung KT. Initial experiences with a long-term indwelling tunnelled pleural catheter for the management of malignant pleural effusion: technical report. Clin Radiol 2000;55:882–4.

[101] Ulmer JL, Choplin RH, Reed JC. Image-guided catheter drainage of the infected pleural space. J Thorac Imaging 1991;6:65–73.

[102] Henry M, Arnold T, Harvey J. BTS guidelines for the management of spontaneous pneumothorax. Thorax 2003;58(Suppl 2):ii39–52.

[103] Conces Jr DJ, Tarver RD, Gray WC, et al. Treatment of pneumothoraces utilizing small caliber chest tubes. Chest 1988;94:55–7.

[104] Casola G, van Sonnenberg E, Keightley A, et al. Pneumothorax: radiologic treatment with small catheters. Radiology 1988;166:89–91.

[105] Perlmutt LM, Braun SD, Newman GE, et al. Transthoracic needle aspiration: use of a small chest tube to treat pneumothorax. AJR Am J Roentgenol 1987;148: 849–51.

[106] Escudero BC, Garcia CM, Cuesta CB, et al. Cytologic and bacteriologic analysis of fluid and pleural biopsy specimens with Cope's needle. Study of 414 patients. Arch Intern Med 1990;150:1190–4.

[107] Salyer WR, Eggleston JC, Erozan YS. Efficacy of pleural needle biopsy and pleural fluid cytopathology in the diagnosis of malignant neoplasm involving the pleura. Chest 1975;67:536–9.

[108] Prakash UB, Reiman HM. Comparison of needle biopsy with cytologic analysis for the evaluation of

pleural effusion: analysis of 414 cases. Mayo Clin Proc 1985;60:158–64.

[109] Maskell NA, Gleeson FV, Davies RJ. Standard pleural biopsy versus CT-guided cutting-needle biopsy for diagnosis of malignant disease in pleural effusions: a randomised controlled trial. Lancet 2003;361: 1326–30.

[110] Adams RF, Gleeson FV. Percutaneous image-guided cutting-needle biopsy of the pleura in the presence of a suspected malignant effusion. Radiology 2001;219: 510–4.

[111] Heilo A, Stenwig AE, Solheim OP. Malignant pleural mesothelioma: US-guided histologic core-needle biopsy. Radiology 1999;211:657–9.

[112] Adams RF, Gray W, Davies RJ, et al. Percutaneous image-guided cutting needle biopsy of the pleura in the diagnosis of malignant mesothelioma. Chest 2001;120:1798–802.

[113] Harris RJ, Kavuru MS, Mehta AC, et al. The impact of thoracoscopy on the management of pleural disease. Chest 1995;107:845–52.

[114] Screaton NJ, Flower CD. Percutaneous needle biopsy of the pleura. Radiol Clin North Am 2000;38: 293–301.

[115] Boutin C, Rey F, Viallat JR. Prevention of malignant seeding after invasive diagnostic procedures in patients with pleural mesothelioma. A randomized trial of local radiotherapy. Chest 1995;108:754–8.

ELSEVIER
SAUNDERS

Clin Chest Med 27 (2006) 215 – 227

CLINICS
IN CHEST
MEDICINE

Pleural Ultrasonography

Paul H. Mayo, MD[a],*, Peter Doelken, MD[b]

[a]Albert Einstein College of Medicine, Bronx, NY, USA
[b]Division of Pulmonary, Critical Care, Allergy, and Sleep Medicine, Medical University of South Carolina, Charleston, SC, USA

Ultrasonography is a useful tool for physicians managing pleural diseases. It permits imaging of pleural effusion and other pleural pathology. In addition, ultrasonography has utility in the guidance of thoracentesis and various pleural interventions. This article reviews the field of pleural ultrasonography with emphasis on clinical applications.

Pleural ultrasonography physics

Medical ultrasonography uses ultrasound waves to create images of the body for diagnostic purposes and to guide procedures. Whether imaging the abdomen, heart, vascular structures, or pleura, the physical principles of ultrasonography are the same. The transducer sends out a brief pulse of high-frequency sound that penetrates the tissue. The sound waves are reflected back to the transducer, which serves as the sensor and the source of signal. Ultrasound is reflected at tissue boundaries and interfaces. The degree of reflection is determined by the acoustic impedance of the adjacent tissue. Acoustic impedance is related largely to tissue density, although the propagation velocity of sound through different tissues also is a factor. Another factor that influences the detection of an acoustic interface is the angle at which the sound beam strikes the interface of interest. Ultrasound undergoes refraction, scattering, and attenuation as it

passes through tissue, all of which degrade image quality on examining deeper structures.

Ultrasound examination of the pleura is particularly influenced by the presence of ribs and aerated lung. In bone, there is nearly complete absorption of sound waves; this yields a shadowing artifact. Ribs completely stop transmission of ultrasound and block any view of structures deep to the rib in question. Air is a powerful ultrasound reflector. As a result, most of the ultrasound wave is reflected back from the lung surface if the lung is filled with air. It is impossible to view normally aerated lung with ultrasound. This point of reflection of air from the lung surface corresponds to the pleural surface. If the lung is not normally aerated, as in consolidation or atelectasis, it can be readily visualized [1].

Image artifacts are common in ultrasonography. Bone shadowing and lung air reflection artifacts are predictable problems with thoracic ultrasonography. Artifacts related to the beam itself, such as reverberation, mirroring, marginal, and scatter artifacts, may confuse the examiner. Enhancement, resolution, and beam-thickness artifacts are problematic. Translational artifacts that occur when the patient is breathing at a high respiratory rate may make it difficult to discern dynamic pleural movement. The reader is referred to a definitive text for a complete review of artifacts and their physical explanations [2]. The clinician-sonographer should consider the following issues related to artifact:

1. Obesity and edema degrade image quality. In this patient population, it is difficult to discern ultrasound interfaces and to judge the relative echogenicity tissue. Subcutaneous air causes intense reflection artifact and makes ultrasound examination difficult.

* Corresponding author. Division of Pulmonary and Critical Care Medicine, Beth Israel Medical Center, 7 Dazian MICU, 1st Avenue and 16th Street, New York, NY 10003.
E-mail address: pmayo@chpnet.org (P.H. Mayo).

2. Rib shadowing and lung aeration artifact are a constant challenge with pleural ultrasonography. Identification of the pleura–chest wall interface may be problematic because of near-field clutter.
3. Artifacts typically are visible in only one plane of scanning and often disappear or attenuate on changing probe angle. Artifacts often do not move with movement of adjacent body structures during the respiratory cycle; they are immobile or move with transducer movement.
4. Use of sufficient coupling medium between the skin and the transducer reduces some types of artifacts. Commercial ultrasound gel is effective. Water applied to the skin also is effective, although evaporative loss requires frequent re-application [3].

Discussion of the physics of ultrasonography must include a review of the controls of the ultrasound machine. With pleural ultrasonography, the operator needs to set the image marker on the screen in reference to the orientation of the transducer. Every ultrasound transducer has a groove or raised edge located on one side of the probe. Whichever direction the transducer indicator is pointed, it is projected to the side of the screen marker. The machine, by standard convention, should be set such that the image marker on the machine screen is to the left on the screen. This setup allows the operator to remain orientated to the anatomic axis of scanning, and it permits standardization of image projection for reporting purposes. In longitudinal scanning of the thorax, the probe always should be orientated such that the marker on the probe is pointed cephalad. This being the case, the cephalad direction always is projected to the left of the screen.

When the marker is set, the operator should set the appropriate gain. Machines allow for total gain setting, and most permit settings of individual gain levels within specific areas of the screen. Gain is adjusted so that the pleural and chest wall boundary is clearly visible and so that deeper structures of the image field are seen clearly, such as lung, liver, or spleen. The operator should set the machine for the proper depth penetration. Alteration of depth setting on the machine allows for more or less penetration of ultrasound waves for study purposes. Less penetration results in magnification of the image in the field. When the examiner wishes to visualize the actual pleural surface clearly, depth setting should be set for near-field magnification. This setting is important when examining the pleural surface for subtle findings, such as lung sliding. The depth setting should be increased to maximum when deeper structures that are crucial for defining the boundaries of a pleural effusion are relevant.

Transducer design is important to pleural ultrasonography. Higher frequency probes (7.5–10 MHz) generally are designed for vascular examination, but can be used for pleural ultrasonography. Their advantage is excellent resolution, but their disadvantage is poor penetration. The higher the frequency of the transducer, the better is its resolution, but the lower its penetration. In addition, most vascular probes are linear in design; in thin patients, this does not permit easy examination of the intercostal space in a longitudinal plane. High-frequency transducers have utility if the examiner wishes to do a detailed examination of the pleural surface, which is relatively close to the skin surface. The limited penetration of high-frequency probes prevents visualization of deeper structures, however, which are crucial in assessing pleural space pathology. Most general ultrasonography is performed with transducers with frequency of 3.5 to 5 MHz. Although there is a decline in fine resolution, penetration is superior so that deeper structures can be visualized. These probes are often of sector design so that they allow longitudinal scanning between interspaces in thin individuals. They may not allow detailed resolution of the individual parietal and visceral pleural surfaces. This has little relevance to the clinician, who is more interested in identifying the pleural lung interface and being able to observe structures deeper in the thorax and adjacent abdominal structures that are crucial to assessing pleural effusion and other pleural pathology and in guiding pleural interventions. The penetration and resolution of standard general ultrasound probes make them the ideal tool for pleural ultrasonography in clinical practice.

Ultrasound machine requirements for pleural ultrasonography

Pleural ultrasonography may be performed with a simple two-dimensional ultrasound machine. Doppler capability is not needed. Machines designed in the early 1990s are adequate for imaging pleural effusion or other pleural pathology. Just as a simple older machine suffices, a sophisticated high-end cardiac ultrasound machine also can image the pleura. An ultrasound machine that is capable of abdominal or cardiac imaging has utility in examining the pleural space. As discussed in the physics section, standard sector transducers with frequency of 3.5 to 5 MHz are preferred for clinical pleural ultrasonography. Higher frequency probes give excellent image resolution of the normal pleura, but lack the penetration required to examine deeper structures that are required for clinical applications.

Many different ultrasound machines are available on the market. Many of these machines are capable of performing pleural ultrasonography. Some of the small, handheld ultrasound units of modern design may lack adequate near-field resolution, however, which is needed for pleural ultrasonography. With some of these units, the inside of the chest wall is not clearly visualized when there is a pleural effusion present. As a result, the depth of needle penetration required to access the effusion cannot be determined accurately for performance of thoracentesis. In addition, recent generation ultrasound machines use extensive imaging processing for image smoothing. This processing may make subtle findings, such as lung sliding, more difficult to observe. Paradoxically, older ultrasound machines may be more suitable for pleural ultrasonography because they lack extensive image processing. This being said, pleural ultrasonography is so straightforward that any machine used for general ultrasound purposes would provide a useful image. In purchasing an ultrasound machine, the clinician should test the device carefully for its intended application.

Normal pleura

Ultrasound examination of the normal pleura is easy to perform. When the probe is applied to an interspace in longitudinal scanning plane between adjacent ribs, the normal pleura appears as a bright, highly echogenic line interposed between the chest wall and the air artifact of the lung. With small movement of the transducer, the examiner may orientate the rib shadows, such that the pleural line is centrally located on the screen. The marker on the probe should be pointed toward the head of the patient so that the cephalad direction is projected to the left of the machine screen. By sliding the transducer along the chest wall in a longitudinal direction, adjacent interspaces can be examined. When a longitudinal scan line is completed, the probe may be moved laterally or medially to an adjacent position, and another longitudinal scan line may be created. In this fashion, the costal pleura may be mapped almost completely. To view the diaphragmatic pleura, a transhepatic approach permits avoidance of lung air. On the left side, the full extent of diaphragmatic pleura may be blocked by lung air. The mediastinal pleura generally is not visible via a

transthoracic approach. A transesophageal probe allows visualization of some parts of the mediastinal pleura. This is a specialized technique and is not discussed further. Occasionally, consolidated lung or pleural effusion allows visualization of mediastinal pleural surfaces by virtue of acoustic wave transmission through the pleural effusion or the airless lung. The parietal pleura underlying rib may not be visible owing to rib shadowing. Breathing results in movement of the visceral pleura into the scanning field, however, allowing a complete examination of the visceral subcostal pleura. Approximately 70% of the pleural surface is accessible to ultrasound examination [4].

The normal pleura is 0.2 to 0.4 mm thick [5]. High-frequency probes may have sufficient resolution to allow visualization of the parietal and visceral pleura as separate linear structures that are closely opposed. The probes that are more commonly used for general ultrasonography application (3.5–5 MHz) may not offer sufficient resolution to separate the two pleural surfaces; rather, normal pleura appears as a single summation interface. The inability to visualize the separate pleural surfaces in the examination of normal pleura does not have any clinical relevance. Close apposition of the parietal and visceral pleura is normal. When a pleural effusion is present, the parietal pleura and the visceral pleura are separated. Only then are the two normal surfaces readily visualized by ultrasonography as two distinct echogenic structures when using a lower frequency probe.

A critical finding of the normal pleural examination is lung sliding. The examiner notes that the pleural line, interposed between the chest wall and the underlying aerated lung, has a mobile quality that cycles with respiration. This is called *lung sliding*. Careful observation also may reveal a subtle shimmering movement to the pleural line that coincides with cardiac pulsation; this is called *lung pulse*. The source of these movements of the pleural line is the visceral pleura moving or sliding along the parietal pleura. In spontaneously breathing patients, lung sliding is accentuated in the lower thorax because lung inflation is greatest in this area. Lung pulse may be accentuated most at pleural surfaces adjacent to the heart. Lung sliding and lung pulse are normal findings of the examination of the pleura. The identification of lung sliding indicates the absence of pneumothorax at the site of probe application [6]. Likewise, the presence of lung pulse excludes pneumothorax (Fig. 1) [7].

Most often, pleural ultrasonography is goal directed. A chest radiograph or chest CT scan identifies an abnormality that can be characterized further by

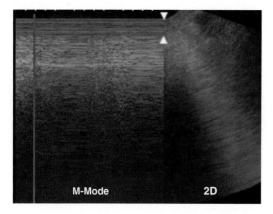

Fig. 1. Composite image of M-mode tracing and two-dimensional image of lung obtained through an intercostal space. Although a bright pleural reflection is not present in this image, the immobile chest wall between the arrows can be readily distinguished from the moving air artifact below. This "lung sliding" can be documented only on static images by using M-mode, but is readily visible during dynamic imaging. The presence of lung sliding excludes pneumothorax in the area of probe contact.

thoracic ultrasonography. In addition to examining the area of abnormality, a complete ultrasound examination of the costal pleura can be accomplished rapidly. For a complete examination of the costal pleura, the patient should be in an upright position with hands on head and arms abducted. This position enlarges the interspaces for better probe placement. The examiner can examine the pleura and underlying lung by moving the transducer along sequential longitudinal scan lines. If an area of abnormality is identified, the examiner can return to it for more detailed examination with the patient in a comfortable position. The anterior and lateral thorax of the supine patient may be examined using the same mapping technique.

The normal pleura should appear as a bright echogenic line interposed between the chest wall and the underlying lung. Lung sliding is a dynamic feature of normal pleural ultrasonography. Methodical examination of multiple adjacent interspaces results in a complete ultrasound evaluation of the costal pleura.

Pleural disease and pleural ultrasonography

Pleural effusions are seen easily with pleural ultrasonography. In addition, many types of less common pleural pathology may be identified.

Pleural effusion

Identification of pleural effusion is a straightforward application of pleural ultrasonography. Ultrasonography is ideally suited to the identification of fluid collections throughout the body because fluid is relatively echo-free compared with other body tissues. Taking advantage of this fact, the sonographer may readily identify pleural effusions of even small size. A minimum of 150 mL of pleural effusion is required for detection by standard upright chest radiography [8]. Effusions of 5 mL can be identified with careful pleural ultrasonography of the costophrenic angle in patients in the upright position [9]. Pleural ultrasonography is superior to standard upright chest radiography and supine chest radiography for detecting pleural effusion [9,10]. Identification of pleural effusion by pleural ultrasonography obviates the need for lateral decubitus chest radiographs, which commonly are ordered to verify pleural effusion after standard chest radiograph. Compared with chest CT scan, pleural ultrasonography has excellent performance characteristics in identifying pleural effusions in supine patients [11].

Identification of a pleural effusion with pleural ultrasonography in a patient who is in an upright position is straightforward. An important capability of pleural ultrasonography is identifying pleural effusions in a supine, critically ill patient on ventilatory support. Readers are well aware of the severe limitations of standard supine chest radiographs in the ICU. Penetration, rotation, and distance magnification artifacts are a consistent problem with these types of films. Also, pleural effusions accumulate in dependent fashion in the thorax, which results in a common problem, wherein thoracic opacities seen on standard supine chest radiographs in the ICU, particularly opacification in the lower chest region, derive from a summation of pleural effusion, compressed lung, and parenchymal lung disease. This nonspecific pattern of opacification is common in this type of chest radiograph. Pleural ultrasonography is able to characterize accurately the cause of the radiographic abnormality seen in the typical ICU chest radiograph. Ultrasonography can distinguish between pleural effusion and any contribution of abnormal lung aeration that contributes to the radiographic abnormality [11]. Pleural effusions are correlated closely with CT scan of the chest in this patient population.

A free-flowing effusion seeks a dependent position in the thorax by gravitational effect. Aerated lung assumes a nondependent position relative to the pleural effusion. Patient position determines where the pleural effusion is found by the sonographer. The predictable position of the effusion in a dependent position is a major advantage when the patient is scanned in an upright position; as a result, pleural ultrasonography is best accomplished with the patient in an upright position. Pleural ultrasonography is more difficult to perform in a supine patient, such as a critically ill patient whose hemodynamic status and multiplicity of support devices prohibit an upright position. In the supine position, the effusion is dependent and layers posteriorly with the lung assuming a nondependent or anterior position in the thorax. Unless the pleural effusion is very large and distributed laterally in the chest, the bed blocks easy viewing of smaller pleural effusions owing to the dependent position of the fluid. The examiner can place the transducer in the posterior axillary line and push down on the bed while angling the probe toward the center of the body; this permits visualization of smaller dependent effusions and defines ultrasound findings of coexisting lung disease. This probe position does not allow for a safe thoracentesis approach because the operator lacks adequate clearance from the bed to perform safe needle insertion.

If routine pleural ultrasonography identifies a pleural effusion that requires thoracentesis on clinical grounds, the examiner must be skilled in safely positioning a supine critically ill patient to find a safe path for thoracentesis. Several options are effective. In positioning a critically ill patient for thoracentesis, one team member must be assigned to monitor the airway if the patient is intubated. Unplanned extubation is always a risk when moving critically ill patients. One option is to bring the thorax to a near-vertical position using the bed controls. This position results in the pleural effusion collecting in the inferior thorax. Gentle adduction of the ipsilateral arm rotates and lifts the chest wall off of the bed, which may allow visualization of the pleural effusion by ultrasonography. This maneuver requires careful monitoring of the endotracheal tube position and an assistant to hold the patient's position during the thoracentesis. Patients who are hemodynamically unstable may not tolerate this position. An alternative to achieve pleural ultrasonography in a critically ill patient for the purpose of safe thoracentesis is to roll a supine patient to a full lateral decubitus position with the target hemithorax in the upper position. This position frequently allows good visualization of the pleural effusion and a suitable field for thoracentesis. Finally, for very unstable patients, carefully sliding a supine patient to the edge of the bed such that part of the hemithorax is exposed allows detection and sampling of small pleural effusions. To protect the patient, the authors use a sling made of bed sheets to hold the patient's body in place and prevent any possibility of the patient falling out of bed. The operator may choose to sit on the floor to perform the thoracentesis. These three techniques permit identification of a safe point for needle insertion that allows sufficient clearance with sterile technique for safe thoracentesis. Loculated pleural effusions or pleural masses that are anterior or lateral in position do not require any special positioning methods in a supine patient and are readily visualized with standard scanning technique.

Identification of a large free-flowing effusion in a thin echogenic patient is straightforward (Fig. 2). A patient who is less echogenic, such as a very muscular, obese, or edematous patient, and a patient who

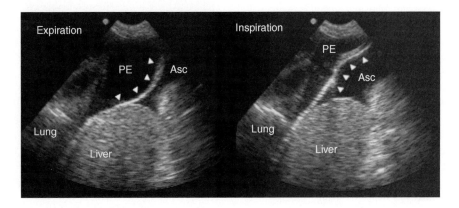

Fig. 2. Images of a hepatic hydrothorax and ascites (Asc) taken during expiration and inspiration. The diaphragm (*arrowheads*) moves cephalad during inspiration. This "paradoxical" diaphragmatic movement is commonly associated with severe dyspnea reversible with thoracentesis. The images also illustrate the importance of identification of the diaphragm before thoracentesis. Failure to do so may result in inadvertent puncture of the ascites. PE, pleural effusion.

is supine because of critical illness with only a small or moderate effusion is more challenging, particularly if thoracentesis is required. Across a continuum of difficulty, the principles of pleural ultrasonography for identification and sampling of a pleural effusion are the same. The three key findings that indicate the presence of a pleural effusion are as follows:

1. The operator should seek unequivocal identification of structures that define the boundaries of pleural anatomy and, in particular, the boundaries of any pleural effusion. This requires clear identification of the diaphragm and subdiaphragmatic organs, the liver on the right and the spleen on the left; identification of the chest wall and in particular its inner border; and identification of lung that is clearly distinguished from the pleural effusion.
2. The sonographer must identify whether a pleural effusion exists within the pleural space. A characteristic feature of pleural effusion is that it is relatively echo-free, and that it is demarcated by the usual anatomic boundaries—the lung, chest wall, and diaphragm.
3. The examiner must identify dynamic changes that are characteristic for pleural effusion.

With the probe held in the longitudinal plane and applied in the interspace, the operator notes two rib shadows, the upper rib on the left and the lower rib on the right of the screen with the inside of the chest wall visible about 5 mm below the origin of the rib shadows. With the patient in a seated position, the best starting position is to examine the posterior chest. In the supine patient, the posterior axillary line is most appropriate. The diaphragm is seen as a curvilinear structure that moves with the respiratory cycle. To confirm identification of the diaphragm, it is important to identify the liver or the spleen as structures that are clearly subdiaphragmatic (see Fig. 2). Rarely, a complex cellular pleural effusion has echogenicity that is similar to the liver or spleen; distinction between the two is crucial. When identified, a pleural effusion appears as a relatively echo-free space above the diaphragm with dynamic movement of the diaphragm occurring with the breathing cycle. The inside of the chest wall is not observed to undergo dynamic change because it is a relatively rigid structure. Underlying lung has a homogeneous gray aeration pattern or appears as a compressed tissue density structure owing to the compressive effect of the adjacent pleural effusion.

The airless lung frequently undulates spontaneously as it floats within the pleural effusion. The undulation of compressed lung is common in moderate-to-large pleural effusions and is termed *lung flapping* or the *jellyfish sign*. Smaller pleural effusions may not cause sufficient compression of the lung to yield these specific signs. Rather, the lung adjacent to the pleural effusion appears with tissue density. Dynamic changes in smaller effusions may include aerated lung that moves into the scanning field to obscure partially the pleural effusion and adjacent compressed lung during inspiration; this is called the *curtain sign*. Airless lung is common with pleural effusions secondary to compressive effect and has an ultrasound density similar to tissue. The term *sonographic hepatization of lung* has been applied to this finding of tissue-density airless lung (Fig. 3). Frequently, at the interface of the effusion and the visceral pleural line, there is a characteristic air artifact called *comet tail* that extends into the adjacent lung. By definition, comet tails start at the pleural interface, move with pleural movement, are sharp-bordered, and extend to the edge of the ultrasound screen. They indicate alveolar-interstitial lung abnormality [12] and often occur in conjunction with a curtain sign. M-mode ultrasound examination of the pleural surface often shows a "sinusoid" sign that is an indication of dynamic movement of the pleural surface within fluid-filled pleural space [13].

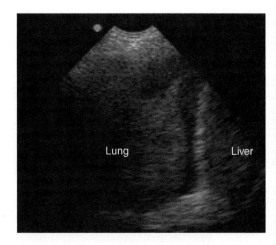

Fig. 3. Image of collapsed lung and normal liver with virtually identical echogenicity. This characteristic of collapsed lung has been named *hepatization* of lung. The bright band between lung and liver represents the diaphragm, and the dark area is a hypoechoic pleural effusion.

Box 1. Findings of importance to pleural sonography

Dynamic signs confirming the presence of pleural liquid

1. Lung flapping (jellyfish sign): Oscillating movement of collapsed lung in a pleural effusion
2. Swirling debris (plankton sign): Debris agitated by cardiac or respiratory motion in a pleural effusion
3. Undulating movements: Strands or fronds agitated by cardiac or respiratory motion in a pleural effusion

Pneumothorax

1. Lung sliding: Periodic movement of the pleural interface relative to chest wall as observed in two-dimensional mode. Indicates the absence of pneumothorax
2. Seashore sign: Equivalent of lung sliding in M-mode, used for documentation of lung sliding on static images
3. Stratosphere sign: Parallel lines representing chest wall and air reverberation artifact in M-mode, documents absence of lung sliding on static images

Miscellaneous

1. Comet tails: Air artifact consisting of a mobile ray-like effect emanating from the pleural surface and extending to the outer edge of the image. Role in pleural ultrasonography is mainly for the identification of air containing lung
2. Curtain sign: Refers to intermittent obscuration of underlying organs by intervening air-filled lung, also has been used to describe the moving air interface in a hydropneumothorax or lung abscesses
3. Hematocrit sign: Refers to the rare layering effect sometimes seen in hemothorax or other highly cellular effusions, the effusion is separated into two phases of different echogenicity

---

In searching for these three elements that are characteristic of a pleural effusion (Box 1), a relatively echo-free space with characteristic boundaries that undergoes characteristic dynamic changes, the examiner will need to move the probe widely over the thorax. A limited interspace examination is never sufficient to confirm the presence or absence of pleural effusion or to characterize fully the signs that are essential for its identification.

Beyond its simple identification, pleural ultrasonography allows characterization of a pleural effusion. The examiner should attempt to report features of the effusion as follows:

1. *Volume of the effusion*. The simplest approach for estimating the volume of a pleural effusion identified by pleural ultrasonography is a strictly qualitative approach. Based on the opinion and experience of the examiner, the pleural effusion is designated as small, moderate, or large. No particular rules apply to this definition. The

advantage of this approach is extreme simplicity. Its inherent inaccuracy is obvious. Another approach to estimating volume is to measure the thickness of the pleural effusion. This method has an inherent problem because the thickness of pleural effusion depends on transducer position. Eibenberger et al [14] reported a correlation between thickness and actual volume of the effusion. In this study, ultrasound methods were more accurate than estimates derived from standard chest radiography. Several authors have used more complex strategies to account for the complex geometry of the pleural space in developing methods of determining the volume of the pleural effusion by ultrasound. It is possible to estimate accurately the volume of a pleural effusion by using these methods [15].

2. *Echogenicity*. The examiner should characterize the echogenicity of the pleural effusion (Box 2). Transudates do not have constituents that serve as ultrasound reflectors and are echo-

free (anechoic). Swirling echoes, strands, fronds, or septations may be visible in exudates, and effusions with these findings are described as being heterogeneously echogenic. Highly cellular exudates, such as hemothorax or empyema, may show homogeneous echogenicity. Most effusions characterized by homogeneous or heterogeneous echogenicity are exudates. Exudative effusions also may be anechoic, however, whereas transudates are uniformly anechoic [16]. Swirling is suggestive of a cellular exudative effusion, such as associated with malignancy, but may occur with a transudate [17]. Increased density of the effusion reduces dynamic changes that are characteristic of pleural effusions, making ultrasound identification difficult. Effusions that are highly cellular may yield an obvious bilayer effect such that the more dependent part of the effusion is frankly echogenic as cells collect in dependent fashion by gravitational effect below an echogenic fluid component of the effusion. This is termed the *hematocrit sign*. If the patient has been immobile for a time, this interface can be quite distinct and suggests the presence of a hemothorax or a purulent pleural effusion.

3. *Stranding or septation.* Complex patterns of fibrinous stranding and frank septations are visualized easily by pleural ultrasonography (Fig. 4). These are found commonly in parapneumonic effusions and suggest the presence of complicated parapneumonic effusion or empyema [18]. Loculated effusions are readily detected by pleural ultrasonography as circular fluid collections that are separated one from the other by thick-walled echogenic structures. Isolated loculations may be located anywhere in the pleural space and are characterized by their atypical position and lack of movement with change of body position. They require careful ultrasound examination to confirm their location. When located, they may be drained under ultrasound guidance if clinically indicated. Pleural ultrasonography is superior to chest CT scan in visualizing septations with a pleural effusion [19]. Even with contrast enhancement, a chest CT scan is unable to clearly define stranding or septations in the pleural space.

Solid pleural abnormalities

Fluid within the pleural space is characteristically relatively nonechogenic. A variety of pleural diseases cause echogenic abnormalities within the pleural space, which are characterized as solid pleural abnormalities. Some of these may coexist with pleural effusions.

Benign and malignant tumors may involve the pleura. Pleural tumors, such as benign mesotheliomas, lipomas, chondromas, or thoracic splenosis, are rare diseases and not commonly found during pleural ultrasonography. They often are delineated by a distinct capsule and are echogenic. They are not seen to invade adjacent tissue planes, although this may be difficult to exclude with pleural ultrasonography. Pleural ultrasonography would not be a means to render a definitive diagnosis based on its nonspecific ultrasound morphology, although pleural ultrasonography can be used to guide biopsy of the lesion. Pleural malignancy may be primary, as in malignant mesothelioma, or metastatic. Pleural ultrasound findings of malignant mesothelioma include hypoechoic thickening of the pleural surface often with irregular or unclear borders (Fig. 5). It can cover large areas of the pleura and be nodular in character. Invasion of the chest wall and diaphragm can be discerned with ultrasonography. Pleural metastatic disease characteristically occurs with a coexisting pleural effusion. The presence of an ultrasound window through the pleural effusion makes the detection of pleural metastatic disease straightforward. Metastatic tumors are generally hypogenic to moderately echogenic and frequently multiple. They can assume a variety of shapes, such as circular, nodular, hemispheric, or broad-based. Frondlike protrusions may be present. Their size varies, and a characteristic feature is their

---

Box 2. Ultrasound characterization of pleural effusion

1. Anechoic (simple) effusion: Complete absence of internal echoes, black uniform appearance
2. Homogeneously echogenic (complex) effusion: Diffuse internal echoes, gray uniform appearance, occasionally may be seen in dependent parts of an effusion as a result of gravity acting on cellular constituents of an effusion (hematocrit sign)
3. Inhomogeneously echogenic (complex) effusion: Debris, strands, fronds, septations

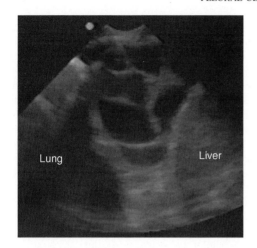

Fig. 4. Complex septate pleural effusion. Although typical for complicated parapneumonic effusion or empyema, this case actually represents spontaneous hemorrhage into a preexisting pleural effusion.

multiplicity. Chest wall or diaphragmatic invasion may be apparent as a disruption of normal tissue interfaces and by visualization of direct extension of the metastatic tumor into adjacent structures (Fig. 6).

Inflammatory diseases of the pleural space, particularly diseases involving infection, are well visualized by pleural ultrasonography. Pleuritis yields characteristic findings on pleural ultrasonography. The parietal pleura is thickened and hypoechoic. The

visceral pleura also may be thickened. Underlying lung may show consolidative changes in the subpleural area. As the pleuritis progresses, stranding within the pleural effusion may develop. Pleural ultrasonography identifies undulating, threadlike bands that float freely in the pleural effusion. In the later stage of pleuritis, these bands may thicken and divide the effusion into fluid-filled cavities. A complex network of septa then develop. Complicated parapneumonic effusions or true empyemas often have this septate pattern, with the pleural effusion that collects in each cavity being variably echogenic owing to accumulation of cellular debris (see Fig. 4). A densely echogenic but homogeneous empyema may have echogenicity similar to a subdiaphragmatic spleen or liver and not manifest with a septated pattern. This type of dense empyema does not exhibit dynamic changes that are important means of identifying pleural effusion. When this problem is a consideration, the sonographer should be especially attentive to clear identification of the position of the diaphragm before attempting a drainage procedure.

Pleural fibrosis may be the nonspecific end result of pleural injury. Its ultrasound pattern is characterized by obvious pleural thickening at the area of fibrosis. The echogenicity of pleural fibrosis varies. It may be hypoechoic, which makes distinction from small pleural effusion problematic. A finding that favors fibrosis is absent respiratory movement of the lung pleural interface. One of the few indications for color Doppler in pleural ultrasonography is to aid in distinguishing pleural fibrosis from a small pleural effusion [20]. Pleural fluid provides a color Dopp-

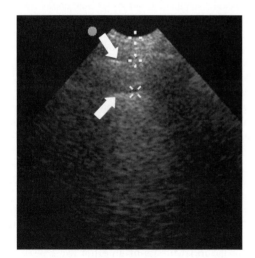

Fig. 5. Hypoechoic area interposed between chest wall and lung (between *arrows*). The distances have been marked for subsequent core biopsy. This echo pattern is not specific for mesothelioma, but can be seen in other malignancies and with pleural fibrosis or plaque.

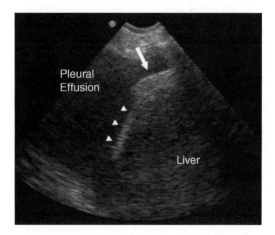

Fig. 6. Metastatic disease on the diaphragmatic pleura (*arrow*). The diaphragm (*arrowheads*) appears intact in this case. Metastasis may invade the diaphragm, and this may be visible with ultrasonography.

ler signal as small reflectors within the fluid move. Color signal from pleural fibrosis is generally absent. It is impossible to distinguish pleural fibrosis from neoplastic disease of the pleura with ultrasonography (see Fig. 5). Pleural calcification within areas of pleural fibrosis is difficult to distinguish because of underlying aerated lung artifact.

Pneumothorax

Pleural ultrasonography is an excellent means for excluding pneumothorax. The presence of sliding lung indicates that there is no possibility of pneumothorax at the site of the examination. The examiner can assess rapidly for sliding lung over a wide area of the thorax effectively excluding pneumothorax (see Fig. 1) [6]. The presence of lung pulse or comet tail artifact is another means of excluding pneumothorax [7,21]. Ultrasonography has special application to patients who are positioned in a supine position because standard chest radiographs may miss an anteriorly situated pneumothorax. For evaluation of pneumothorax, pleural ultrasonography is superior to standard chest radiography in critically ill patients and similar in performance to chest CT scan in this population [22]. The absence of lung sliding or lung pulse is strong, but not absolute, evidence for the presence of pneumothorax [6,7]. Inadequate visualization, pleural symphysis, or non-expanding lung may cause absent lung sliding without pneumothorax. The presence of lung sliding is a useful finding because it excludes pneumothorax absolutely. The value of sliding lung in pleural ultrasonography is in the emergency evaluation of critically ill patients. Another application is in routine use for invasive procedures that have risk of iatrogenic pneumothorax, such as transbronchial biopsy, subclavian vein cannulation, and thoracentesis. Patients may be examined before and immediately after the procedure to exclude pneumothorax promptly. This greatly reduces the need for post-procedure chest radiographs.

Ultrasound-guided thoracentesis and other pleural interventions

Ultrasound-guided thoracentesis is a valuable technique that can be mastered easily by the pulmonary critical care medicine clinician. It is associated with a very low risk of pneumothorax. A special application is in patients who are on mechanical ventilatory support. Supine chest radiographs do not permit deter-

mination of a safe thoracentesis site; iatrogenic pneumothorax in a patient on positive-pressure mechanical ventilatory support is particularly dangerous because there is a high risk of tension pneumothorax. Numerous reports of ultrasound guidance for thoracentesis using two-dimensional ultrasonography have been published since 1982 with a low rate of pneumothorax. A report by Jones et al [23] described 941 thoracenteses in nonintubated patients with a pneumothorax rate of 2.7%. Several studies have addressed the safety of ultrasound-guided thoracentesis in patients requiring mechanical ventilatory support [24–27]. Lichtenstein et al [28] reported 45 procedures in this patient population with a pneumothorax rate of 0%. Mayo et al [29] reported 232 procedures with a pneumothorax rate of 1.3% in a population of patients who were on mechanical ventilatory support. These two reports have interest to pulmonary critical care medicine clinicians because all procedures were performed by nonradiologists. This is strong support for the concept that pleural ultrasonography is a skill that is readily and appropriately acquired by nonradiologists. Findings of thoracentesis in critically ill patients had an impact on their clinical management [30,31]. There is no study that compares the rate of pneumothorax with and without ultrasound guidance of thoracentesis. Diacon et al [32] addressed this issue by comparing standard physical examination and chest radiographs with ultrasonography to identify the best site for thoracentesis. Their results indicate superiority of ultrasound over standard physical examination and chest radiographs for determination of the best site of thoracentesis.

To perform ultrasound-guided thoracentesis, the patient must be positioned properly. Proper positioning with a clear field of action is essential for success. Positioning is a challenge in critically ill patients. The operator likewise must be positioned for ease of operation; this includes orientating the ultrasound machine for easy viewing throughout the procedure and clearing monitoring and support devices from the area of interest in the cluttered environment of the ICU. When all of this is accomplished, the examiner determines the best site, angle, and depth of needle penetration to perform thoracentesis. The site is marked. The needle inserter memorizes the angle of needle penetration. After preparation of the site, needle insertion is performed at the marked point with the insertion assembly held at the same angle as was the probe. The thoracentesis is performed immediately after the ultrasound study without any patient movement because movement may cause shift of the effusion in relationship to the planned insertion site. The shortest possible time should be allowed between the scan and needle insertion so that the operator maintains a clear memory of probe angle. The authors have no formal lower limit for thickness of effusion below which thoracentesis cannot be attempted. Incursions of the lung or the diaphragm during the respiratory cycle into the ultrasound window are specific contraindications to thoracentesis. Unequivocal positive identification of the diaphragm and underlying spleen or liver is required to avoid puncture of these organs.

A dangerous error of the inexperienced sonographer is to mistake the liver or spleen for an echogenic effusion with potentially catastrophic consequence on thoracentesis attempt. This error may be perpetuated if the examiner falsely identifies the curvilinear aspect of Morison's pouch as the diaphragm, when in fact it lies between the liver and kidney. Meticulous attention to clear identification of the diaphragm avoids this error.

The authors routinely perform thoracentesis with freehand technique after marking of the site for needle insertion. It is not necessary to observe the needle in real time with the ultrasound transducer. Although this observation is possible, it complicates the procedure because it requires use of a sterile probe cover and an additional assistant. Real-time needle guidance is not required for safety purposes, as has been shown in a large study of ultrasound-guided pericardiocentesis [33]. Before and after ultrasound-guided thoracentesis, it is appropriate to check for sliding lung. This check permits prompt diagnosis of any procedure-related pneumothorax and avoids the need for postprocedure chest radiographs.

A common problem in performing ultrasound-guided thoracentesis is transducer compression artifact [34]. A probe pressed firmly to the skin indents the skin. The distance between skin surface and the pleural effusion is measured with the probe compressing the skin. On removal of the probe from the skin surface, however, the skin rebounds, assuming its normal configuration; and the actual distance between skin and pleura is greater than that measured during skin indentation. This artifact is especially problematic with patients in severe edema states, where a firmly applied probe may indent the skin several centimeters. The operator needs to be aware of this common problem and recognize that needle insertion may require a greater depth of penetration than was actually measured.

A variety of pleural interventions may be performed using ultrasound guidance. These include insertion of large-bore chest drainage devices, insertion of long-term indwelling drainage catheters for management of malignant effusions, mechanical

septal lysis, and guidance of pleural biopsy. Ultrasonography also can assist in access site selection for pleuroscopy. The principles of inserting large-bore drainage devices into a pleural effusion are similar to the performance of a thoracentesis. The best site for insertion is determined by standard criteria, but the operator may choose to use real-time ultrasound guidance to place the device into the appropriate position. Ultrasound guidance requires the use of a sterile probe cover and an assistant to hold the probe during the procedure. If a wire is being used to insert the catheter, its position can be ascertained by ultrasonography (Fig. 7). Likewise, the catheter can be directed into the appropriate position if a trocar-based system is used. If the pleural space is air-filled, the position of the drainage device is impossible to determine owing to air artifact. The main application of ultrasonography in the case of an air-filled pleural space is to locate a safe site for chest tube insertion in reference to diaphragmatic position and possible pleural symphysis.

Ultrasound guidance of pleural biopsy is possible [35]. The forceps is introduced into the pleural space and guided to the pleural-based lesion under real-time ultrasound guidance.

Mechanical septolysis is an application to which pleural ultrasonography is ideally suited. Complex septate effusions present a therapeutic challenge. Ideally, it is advantageous to disrupt them to achieve adequate drainage of the pleural space because

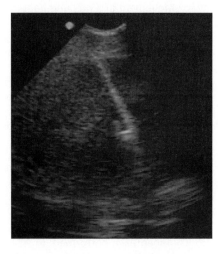

Fig. 7. Hardware may be imaged in real time with ultrasonography. Guidewires, as in this image, are particularly echogenic and can be visualized easily before introducing dilators or catheters. Needles and other hardware are at times more difficult to visualize, but even smooth needles generally have a bright echo at their tip.

thrombolytics may not be effective in this situation. If a trocar-based catheter is introduced into a pleural space that has a multiseptated effusion, pleural ultrasonography allows the operator to break down the walls of the septa with mechanical lysis. The procedure is performed under direct ultrasound guidance and consists of targeting individual walls of septa and breaking them apart with gentle movement of the trocar and catheter assembly. After lysis of multiple septa has been achieved, the catheter is left in the space after removal of the trocar. The authors have had success in mechanical septolysis using this technique under direct real-time ultrasound guidance.

Box 3. Basic skills and technique for ultrasound-guided thoracentesis

1. Identification of anatomic boundaries characteristic of a pleural effusion
   Inner border of the chest wall
   Diaphragm with identification of underlying liver or spleen
   Underlying lung
2. Dynamic changes of the anechoic space characteristic of a pleural effusion
   Movement of the diaphragm with respiratory cycle
   Movement of lung (lung flapping, jellyfish sign, curtain sign)
   Mobile echoic material within the anechoic space (plankton sign)
3. Identification of a site for needle insertion that permits sterile technique and adequate syringe-needle clearance for thoracentesis
4. Stable patient and operator position
5. Site, angle, and depth of needle insertion determined by ultrasonography that avoids any risk of needle injury to the lung, diaphragm, intercostal vessels, or other critical structure throughout the respiratory cycle
6. Thoracentesis performed in standard fashion immediately after ultrasound examination without any patient movement between the ultrasound examination and needle insertion

---

Training in pleural ultrasonography

Training in ultrasonography requires factual knowledge of the field, skill in image acquisition, and skill in image interpretation (Box 3):

1. *Factual knowledge*. This article provides an overview of the field of pleural ultrasonography. To introduce ultrasonography into clinical practice, the authors recommend reviewing a standard textbook and atlas of chest ultrasonography [2].
2. *Image acquisition*. Implicit to clinical application of pleural ultrasonography is that the physician personally performs the study, interprets the results, and applies them to the problem at hand. This being the case, the physician scanner must be skilled in image acquisition. Image acquisition in pleural ultrasonography is a relatively straightforward task, suitable for an autodidactic approach, provided that image interpretation skills have been acquired. An operator familiar with the concepts and interpretation of ultrasound images of the chest achieves proficiency in a short time.
3. *Image interpretation*. A large anechoic effusion is not a challenge to a trainee with even minimal experience. The challenges of poor image quality, complex echo patterns, and risks inherent to procedure guidance require that the trainee be prepared for difficult image interpretation. Articles and textbooks display only static images and are not adequate for full training in image interpretation. As always, the trainee learns the most from hands-on training with an experienced thoracic ultrasonographer. The shortcomings of static imagery in textbooks can be overcome, however, by using archived and commented video clips. The authors currently are using this approach in their respective fellowship training programs, in addition to hands-on training [36].

References

[1] Lichtenstein DA. Lung. In: General ultrasound in the critically ill. Berlin: Springer-Verlag; 2005. p. 116–28.
[2] Schuler A. Image artifacts and pitfalls. In: Mathis G, Lessnau KD, editors. Atlas of chest sonography. Berlin: Springer-Verlag; 2003. p. 137–45.
[3] Lichtenstein DA. The ultrasound equipment. In: General ultrasound in the critically ill. Berlin: Springer-Verlag; 2005. p. 9–12.

[4] Reuss J. Sonographic imaging of the pleura: nearly 30 years experience. Eur J Ultrasound 1996;3:125–39.

[5] Reuss J. The pleura. In: Mathis G, Lessnau KD, editors. Atlas of chest sonography. Berlin: Springer-Verlag; 2003. p. 17–35.

[6] Lichtenstein DA, Menu Y. A bedside ultrasound sign ruling out pneumothorax in the critically ill: lung sliding. Chest 1995;108:1345–8.

[7] Lichtenstein DA, Lascols N, Prin S, et al. The "lung pulse": an early ultrasound sign of complete atelectasis. Intensive Care Med 2003;29:2187–92.

[8] Collins JD, Burwell D, Furmanski S, et al. Minimal detectable pleural effusions. Radiology 1972;105:51–3.

[9] Gryminski J, Krakowka P, Lypacewicq G. The diagnosis of pleural effusion by ultrasonic and radiologic techniques. Chest 1976;70:33–7.

[10] Kelbel C, Borner N, Schadmand S, et al. Diagnosis of pleural effusions and atelectasis: sonography and radiology compared. Rofo 1991;154:159–63.

[11] Lichtenstein D, Goldstein I, Mourgeon E, et al. Comparative diagnostic performances of auscultation, chest radiography, and lung ultrasonography in acute respiratory distress syndrome. Anesthesiology 2004;100:9–15.

[12] Lichtenstein D, Meziere G, Biderman P, et al. The comet-tail artifact: an ultrasound sign of alveolar-interstitial syndrome. Am J Respir Crit Care Med 1997;15:1640–6.

[13] Lichtenstein DA. Pleural effusion and introduction to lung ultrasound. In: General ultrasound in the critically ill. Berlin: Springer-Verlag; 2005. p. 96–104.

[14] Eibenberger KL, Dock WI, Ammann ME, et al. Quantification of pleural effusions: sonography versus radiography. Radiology 1994;191:681–4.

[15] Roch AMD, Bojan M, Michelet P, et al. Usefulness of ultrasonography in predicting pleural effusions >500 ml in patients receiving mechanical ventilation. Chest 2005;127:224–32.

[16] Yang PC, Luh KT, Chang DB, et al. Value of sonography in determining the nature of pleural effusion: analysis of 320 cases. AJR Am J Roentgenol 1992;159:29–33.

[17] Chian CF, Su WL, Soh LH, et al. Echogenic swirling pattern as a predictor of malignant pleural effusions in patients with malignancies. Chest 2004;126:129–34.

[18] Tu CY, Hsu WH, Hsia TC, et al. Pleural effusions in febrile medical ICU patients chest ultrasound study. Chest 2004;126:1274–80.

[19] McLoud TC, Flower CD. Imaging the pleura: sonography, CT, and MR imaging. AJR Am J Roentgenol 1991;156:1145–53.

[20] Wu RG, Yuan A, Liaw YS, et al. Image comparison of real-time gray-scale ultrasound and color Doppler ultrasound for use in diagnosis of minimal pleural effusion. Am J Respir Crit Care Med 1994;150:510–4.

[21] Lichtenstein D, Meziere G, Biderman P, Gepner A. The comet-tail artifact: an ultrasound sign ruling out pneumothorax. Intensive Care Med 1999;25:383–8.

[22] Lichtenstein DA, Meziere G, Lascols N, et al. Ultrasound diagnosis of occult pneumothorax. Crit Care Med 2005;33:1231–8.

[23] Jones PW, Moyers P, Rogers JT, et al. Ultrasound-guided thoracentesis: is it a safer method? Chest 2003;123:418–23.

[24] Gervais DA, Petersein A, Lee MJ, et al. US-guided thoracentesis: requirement for postprocedure chest radiography in patients who receive mechanical ventilation versus patients who breathe spontaneously. Radiology 1997;204:503–6.

[25] Petersen S, Freitag M, Albert W, et al. Ultrasound-guided thoracentesis in surgical intensive care unit patients [letter]. Intensive Care Med 2000;25:1029.

[26] Godwin JE, Sahn SA. Thoracentesis: a safe procedure in mechanically ventilated patients. Ann Intern Med 1990;113:800–2.

[27] McCartney JP, Adams JW, Hazard PB. Safety of thoracentesis in mechanically ventilated patients. Chest 1993;103:1920–1.

[28] Lichtenstein D, Hulot JS, Rabiller A, et al. Feasibility and safety of ultrasound-aided thoracentesis in mechanically ventilated patients. Intensive Care Med 1999;25:955–8.

[29] Mayo PH, Golst HR, Tafreshi M, et al. Safety of ultrasound-guided thoracentesis in patients receiving mechanical ventilation. Chest 2004;125:1059–62.

[30] Fartoukh M, Azoulay E, Galliot R, et al. Clinically documented pleural effusions in medical ICU patients: how useful is routine thoracentesis? Chest 2002;121:178–84.

[31] Yu CJ, Yang PC, Chang DB, et al. Diagnostic and therapeutic use of chest sonography: value in critically ill patients. AJR Am J Roentgenol 1992;159:695–701.

[32] Diacon AH, Brutsche MH, Solèr M. Accuracy of pleural puncture sites: a prospective comparison of clinical examination with ultrasound. Chest 2003;123:436–41.

[33] Tsang TSM, Enriquez-Serrano M, Freeman WK, et al. Consecutive 1,127 therapeutic echocardiographically guided pericardiocenteses: clinical profile, practice patterns, and outcomes spanning 21 years. Mayo Clin Proc 2002;77:429–36.

[34] Lichtenstein DA. Interventional ultrasound. General ultrasound in the critically ill. Berlin: Springer-Verlag; 2005. p. 170–4.

[35] Reuss J. Interventional chest sonography. In: Mathis G, Lessnau KD, editors. Atlas of chest sonography. Berlin: Springer-Verlag; 2003. p. 147–62.

[36] Doelken P, Mayo P. Ultrasonography of pleural effusion. Charleston (SC): DM&C Electronic Publishing; 2003 [Customflix No: 205020].

ELSEVIER
SAUNDERS

Clin Chest Med 27 (2006) 229–240

CLINICS
IN CHEST
MEDICINE

Pleural Manometry

John T. Huggins, MD*, Peter Doelken, MD

Division of Pulmonary, Critical Care, Allergy, and Sleep Medicine, Medical University of South Carolina, PO Box 250625, Charleston, SC 29425, USA

Therapeutic thoracentesis is a commonly performed procedure. The goal of therapeutic thoracentesis is to remove the maximum amount of pleural fluid to improve dyspnea and facilitate the diagnostic evaluation of large pleural effusions. Clinicians do not routinely perform pleural manometry during large-volume thoracentesis today. Pleural manometry may be useful, however, for immediately detecting an unexpandable lung, which may coexist with any pleural fluid accumulation. In addition, pleural manometry may improve patient safety when removing large amounts of pleural fluid.

Pleural manometry was performed during the first half of the twentieth century in the management of pulmonary tuberculosis. Before the development of antituberculous chemotherapy, collapse therapy was performed routinely in the treatment of pulmonary tuberculosis [1–3]. One form of collapse therapy involved inducing an intentional pneumothorax. To determine if the needle was placed properly in the pleural space, pressures were monitored as the needle was inserted through the chest wall. When negative pressure was detected, the clinician was confident that the pleural space was entered. Air was introduced to induce the pneumothorax.

To maintain lobar collapse, therapeutic air refills had to be performed frequently. Clinicians performing these refills quickly recognized that trapped lung was a complication of pneumothorax therapy for tuberculosis. Approximately 5% of patients treated with therapeutic pneumothoraces developed an unexpandable lung characterized by a failure of the lung to expand between therapeutic refills. The failure to expand was due to parenchymal fibrosis or formation of scar tissue along the visceral pleura. Manometry performed during the refills revealed more negative pleural pressure than was usually encountered. Untreated, an effusion ex vacuo developed in response to the persistent pleural space [1–4]. This article discusses pleural space mechanics in relation to a normal pleural space and pleural effusion associated with expandable and unexpandable lung; discusses the concept of unexpandable lung and its varied underlying clinical condition; describes the instrumentation required to perform bedside manometry; discusses how manometry may improve patient safety when large amounts of fluid are removed; and discusses the diagnostic capabilities of manometry, including detecting an unexpandable lung and predicting pleurodesis success.

Pleural space mechanics

An understanding of the mechanics of a normal pleural space is essential for the understanding of the mechanics of the diseased pleural space. It is well known that the hydrostatic pressure within the normal pleural space is slightly negative when measured at functional residual capacity. This negative pressure serves to couple the chest wall and lung; it counterbalances the inward recoil of the lung and the outward recoil of the chest wall recoil [5–9]. Extensive research using animal models and techniques to mea-

* Corresponding author.

E-mail address: hugginjt@musc.edu (J.T. Huggins).

0272-5231/06/$ – see front matter © 2006 Elsevier Inc. All rights reserved.
doi:10.1016/j.ccm.2005.12.007

sure intrapleural pressure within a normal pleural space has been performed over the past 40 years. Based on the observations derived from these studies, pleural pressure is not uniform throughout the pleural space. Pleural pressure becomes more negative with increasing distance from the base to the apex of the lung. Also, pleural pressure does not behave as a simple hydrostatic column of fluid, decreasing by 1 cm H_2O pressure for each 1 cm of vertical distance above the lung base. The vertical gradient is approximately 0.5 cm H_2O pressure per 1 cm vertical distance. Two models—hydrostatic equilibrium versus viscous flow—have been proposed to explain why the vertical gradient is less than 1 [6].

In the hydrostatic model, proposed by Setnikar and colleagues [10] and Agostoni and colleagues [11–17], pleural liquid, similar to capillary blood, is in hydrostatic equilibrium with a vertical pressure gradient equal to 1 cm H_2O/1 cm height. The investigators postulated that hydrostatic equilibrium was achieved by absorption of pleural liquid into the blood until equilibrium was achieved between the oncotic and hydrostatic forces between the pleural liquid and capillary blood. Negative intrapleural pressure develops because fluid is reabsorbed until points of contact are established between the parietal and visceral pleurae. These points of contact resist further deformation of the pleural space [11–17].

Pleural liquid pressure varies as a hydrostatic column of fluid. Because there are more points of contact at the top of the lung, however, the vertical gradient of pleural pressure is less than 1. Pleural liquid pressure would be more negative than pleural surface pressure [11,12]. Animal models evaluating pleural space thickness suggest, however, that pleural fluid covers the entire lung as a continuous layer and is devoid of these points of contact [18,19].

Viscous flow is the alternative and is currently the most plausible model, which proposes that pleural liquid pressure and pleural surface pressure are identical [5,7,20–22]. The vertical pressure gradient is a consequence of the viscous flow generating a continuous column of fluid throughout the pleural space. Fluid filtered through the parietal pleura flows toward the dependent regions of the lung and is removed by lymphatics found on the parietal pleura. Maintaining flow through the pleural space and uniformity of pleural space thickness requires continuous recirculation of fluid. Recirculation of pleural fluid is driven by gravity, ventilatory, and cardiogenic forces [5].

The hydrostatic pressure gradient is dissipated with resistance to viscous flow. As the pleural space widens in the setting of a pleural effusion, however,

resistance to flow decreases. The gradient in pleural pressure becomes the hydrostatic pressure gradient.

The direct measurement of pleural pressures in the normal pleural space is technically challenging because of the close approximation of the two pleural surfaces. A device introduced into a normal pleural space would lead to geometric distortion and result in deformation forces that are not representative of the pressure before the introduction of the device. In the presence of a pleural effusion, an introduced catheter would not result in geometric distortion of the local pleural space, creating local deformation forces that influence measured pressure. An abnormally wide pleural space filled with fluid represents a hydrostatic gradient when viscous flow resistance becomes negligible. Pressure measured with a catheter residing in a pleural effusion is representative of the actual pressure at that particular level of the effusion. Changes of pressure during respiration represent pressure changes throughout the effusion. Pressure measured in this manner and referenced to an external vertical level reflects recoil forces of the lung and chest wall and vertical extent of the pleural effusion [23].

Under dynamic conditions, pressure changes result from two different mechanisms: (1) forces developed by respiratory muscles attenuated by the inflow of air into the lung and (2) vertical displacement of the fluid collection secondary to periodical changes in geometric configuration of the chest. Pressure changes as a result of fluid removal are due to (1) elastic forces of the lung and chest wall, which are altered by changes in the geometry of the pleural space; (2) vertical displacement of the fluid collection caused by the geometric changes; and (3) diminishing vertical extent of the fluid collection. At the end of drainage, local deformation forces around the catheter prevail and dominate other mechanisms.

The pressure inside a pleural effusion is determined by multiple factors. Obtaining information about the elastic properties of the pleural space is the primary objective of pleural manometry. When it is assumed that there is a relatively constant quantitative influence of the hydrostatic effects between patients, differences should be a result in differences of pleural space elastic recoil. With this assumption, the measured pressure changes reflect changes in recoil forces. Pleural liquid pressure changes, owing to fluid withdrawal, may be assessed in relation to the amount of fluid withdrawn, and true pleural space elastance may be calculated. When using pleural manometry, however, the pressure in the pleural space without sufficient fluid for a catheter to float is representative

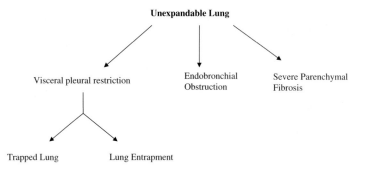

Fig. 1. Classification of unexpandable lung.

only of the pressure in the area immediately surrounding the catheter [23].

Unexpandable lung

An unexpandable lung is defined by the inability of the lung to expand to the chest wall allowing for a normal interaction between the visceral and parietal pleura. Several pathologic mechanisms can lead to an unexpandable lung, including (1) endobronchial obstruction leading to atelectasis, (2) severe parenchymal fibrosis, and (3) visceral pleural restriction (Fig. 1).

For practical purposes, unexpandable lung secondary to visceral pleural restriction is subdivided into two categories. The first category is *trapped lung,* which is considered a unique clinical diagnosis. The pathogenesis of trapped lung is related to a remote inflammatory process resulting in the formation of an irreducible pleural space owing to the formation of a fibrous visceral pleural peel. The inflammation must resolve to make the diagnosis of trapped lung. The clinical diagnosis of trapped lung is a chronic, undiagnosed pleural effusion that most often is asymptomatic, but may result in dyspnea. Pleural fluid formation in trapped lung results from an imbalance of hydrostatic forces. Pleural fluid analysis typically reveals a transudate. The chest radiograph shows no contralateral shift of the mediastinum. The initial

mean pleural liquid pressure is usually negative. The pressure/volume curve of trapped lung is linear with a steep slope over all intervals of fluid removal. Pleural space elastance, defined as the change in pressure to volume removed, is high (usually >25 cm H_2O/L) [4]. In the authors' unpublished pleural manometry database, pleural space elastance in the setting of a trapped lung may be only 16 cm H_2O/L (Table 1) (Huggins JT, Heidecker J, Sahn SA, et al, manuscript under review, 2005).

The second category includes any active inflammatory or malignant pleural disease leading to visceral pleural restriction preventing normal lung expansion. The term *lung entrapment* is used to describe this category. Lung entrapment, in the authors' definition, is a mechanical complication of active pleural disease. Lung entrapment occurs in the setting of malignancy, rheumatoid arthritis, uremia, and pleural space infection and after coronary artery bypass graft surgery. Lung entrapment is not considered a disease per se, but can be a complicating factor in these conditions. Lung entrapment secondary to active pleural disease, especially in malignancy, is more common than trapped lung. Lung entrapment may resolve with specific therapy directed at the underlying pleural disease. The active pleural process often dominates the clinical presentation of lung entrapment, and entrapment is evident only with pleural fluid removal. The chest radiograph may show contralateral medi-

Table 1
Characteristics of trapped lung versus lung entrapment

Criteria for comparison	Trapped lung	Lung entrapment
Pathogenesis	Remote inflammation; hydrostatic forces	Active inflammation; malignancy
Chest radiograph	Absence of contralateral shift	With or without contralateral shift
Pleural fluid analysis	Usually transudate	Exudate
Intial mean pleural liquid pressure	Always negative	Usually positive
Initial pleural elastance pressure	High elastance (>25 cm H_2O)	Normal or high elastance
Treatment	Observation; decortication	Specific treatment; decortication; palliation

astinal shift. Initial mean pleural liquid pressure is usually positive, and initial pleural space elastance may be normal or high. The initial slope of the pressure/volume curve may be normal (see Table 1). When a critical volume of pleural fluid is removed, the slope of the curve becomes steeper mimicking the slope of the pressure/volume curve of unexpandable lung, signifying a restricted pleural space at lower volumes. Fig. 2 illustrates the pressure/volume curves of a normally expanding lung, trapped lung, and lung entrapment secondary to malignancy.

The manometric findings of an atelectatic effusion in the setting of an endobronchial lesion or severe parenchymal fibrosis have not been described to the authors' knowledge. In a series of more than 200 patients at the authors' institution in which pleural manometry has been performed, these two clinical entities have not been seen.

An important modality to assist the clinician in distinguishing trapped lung from an atelectatic effusion secondary to endobronchial disease or underlying parenchymal fibrosis involves air-contrast chest CT. Visceral pleural thickness, underlying lung parenchyma, and the airways can be visualized directly by air-contrast CT.

Instrumentation

Pleural liquid pressure can be measured using either a simple water column manometer or more elaborate physiologic systems employing hemodynamic transducers. In the authors' institution, pleural manometry routinely is performed simultaneously with an overdamped vertical column water manometer and a hemodynamic transducer connected to a standard physiologic system [23]. An understanding of the technical aspects, advantages, and disadvantages of these systems in measuring pleural liquid pressure is presented.

Previous investigators performing pleural manometry used an underdamped, U-shaped water manometer and reported pressures as a mean of the oscillating water column [24–27]. The advantage of the water manometers is that they can be assembled easily and inexpensively. The disadvantages are related primarily to the difficulty in reading accurate values from an oscillating water column and the unfavorable physical characteristics of water manometers. It is impossible to construct a water manometer with the frequency response required to measure pleural pressure oscillations accurately. These difficulties are related to inertia and flow resistance when water is used as an indicator. Water manometry may be used, however, to measure accurate mean pleural liquid pressures when the manometer is overdamped by an interposed resistor. Pressure oscillations may not be measured.

Manometry systems useful for measuring pressure oscillations require a transducer element with minimal displacement if aqueous solutions are used as a coupling medium. Hemodynamic transducers used

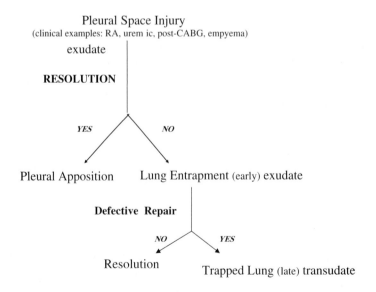

Fig. 2. Proposed pathogenic model for trapped lung versus lung entrapment. Post-CABG, post–coronary artery bypass graft; RA, rheumatoid arthritis.

in an intensive care unit setting are adequate for this purpose and are supplied with appropriate sterile connecting tubing. If measurement of mean pleural liquid is all that is needed, an overdamped water manometer is all that is required.

When measuring pressure oscillations, a hemodynamic transducer connected to a physiologic measuring system consisting of a signal conditioner and a data acquisition system can be used. This system needs proper calibration and is not readily available to most clinicians. Alternatively, standard hemodynamic monitors may be substituted. These monitors circumvent the unfamiliar calibration and zeroing procedures necessary in a reference system, but pose inherent problems. The software of hemodynamic monitors cannot process negative pressures, and numerical values may be erroneous owing to software optimized for positive hemodynamic signals. Transducing negative pressure can be achieved by creating an offset by moving the transducer by a known distance to a lower level after first zeroing the system. The fluid column in the tubing between the patient and the transducer creates a pressure offset proportional to the vertical distance that the transducer is moved. If the transducer is moved downward by a sufficient distance, negative pressures are not transmitted during any part of the respiratory cycle. The offset created must be subtracted from the recorded signal if absolute values are needed; however, changes in pressure are unaffected by the offset. A correction factor is needed if hemodynamic pressures are used because they record in mm Hg, whereas pleural pressure traditionally is reported in cm H_2O.

The authors described the technique of using an overdamped water manometer and electronic transducer system in acquiring pleural liquid pressure [23]. The water manometer is needed for calibration of the electronic system and is a convenient device for real-time display of mean pleural liquid pressure when a resistor is interposed. The water manometer may be used alone if an operator experienced with the electronic system is unavailable.

All patients undergoing manometric measurements are placed in the sitting position. A flexible thoracentesis catheter is inserted using standard technique. The thoracentesis catheter is placed in the most dependent portion of the pleural effusion as determined by thoracic ultrasonography.

The authors' water manometer consists of two lengths of intravenous tubing connected through a 22G needle inserted into an injection terminal. The tubing from the thoracentesis catheter to the measuring scale extends 40 to 50 cm below the level of the catheter insertion into the chest similar to a U-shaped

water manometer. The system is purged of air with normal saline and connected to the zeroing port of pressure transducer. The thoracentesis catheter and transducer assembly are purged of air before connection to the water manometer.

The transducer is connected to a signal conditioner for electronic signal generation. A personal computer data acquisition system is used to store and record the electronic signal (Fig. 3). The electronic signal is calibrated against the water signal. The vertical reference point for a pressure of zero is arbitrarily defined at the level at which the thoracentesis catheter is inserted into the chest.

Data acquisition is terminated after a satisfactory tracing is obtained and the water manometer is stabilized. The water manometer stabilizes in 30 seconds, and the mean pleural liquid pressure is recorded. The water column oscillates with amplitude of 2 to 4 mm H_2O around the mean. For the electronic method, a satisfactory tracing is defined by a group of at least four consecutive respiratory cycles in which the end-expiratory pressure returns to the same baseline. The last pressure measurement is valid when fluid can be seen on ultrasonography or at least 20 mL of pleural fluid can be withdrawn at the conclusion. Measurements are performed initially and for every 250 mL of fluid withdrawn thereafter. If unexpandable lung is suspected, smaller aliquots of 50 to 100 mL are removed.

The authors published the accuracy of the water manometer in obtaining mean pleural liquid pressure. In this study, 40 consecutive patients undergoing therapeutic thoracentesis had simultaneous recordings of mean pleural liquid pressure by the water manometer and the electronic system. For the 40 thoracenteses, a total of 325 pressure measurements were obtained by the electronic system, and 291 measurements were obtained by the water manometer. Mean pleural liquid pressure for 34 thoracenteses could not be recorded by the water manometer because of the development of cough. Linear regression analysis found a strong correlation for the mean pleural liquid pressure between the water manometer and the electronic system [23].

Re-expansion pulmonary edema

One of the complications of therapeutic thoracentesis is re-expansion pulmonary edema. Re-expansion pulmonary edema is a well-recognized clinical syndrome characterized by the development of unilateral pulmonary edema in a lung that has been reinflated rapidly after a variable period of collapse

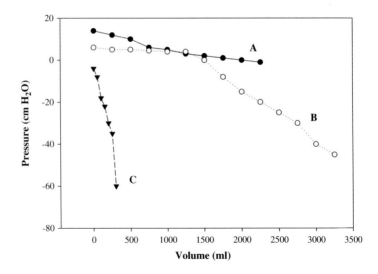

Fig. 3. Three pressure/volume (P/V) curves. P/V curve A (*closed circles*) illustrates a normally expandable lung in a patient with hepatic hydrothorax. The curve is monophasic with a calculated pleural space elastance of 6 cm H_2O/L. P/V curve B (*open circles*) is lung entrapment associated with pleural malignancy. The curve is biphasic. The pleural space elastance during the first 1500 mL of fluid removal was normal and calculated at 4 cm H_2O/L. After the first 1500 mL of fluid removal, the slope of the curve becomes steep with a calculated pleural space elastance of 26 cm H_2O/L. This signifies lung entrapment and predicts poor pleurodesis success. P/V curve C (*inverted closed triangles*) illustrates a trapped lung. The initial mean pleural liquid pressure is negative. The curve is monophasic with increased pleural space elastance. The calculated pleural space elastance was 180 cm H_2O/L.

from a pleural effusion or pneumothorax [28–35]. The clinical presentation of re-expansion pulmonary edema can be relatively benign or present as a life-threatening event [31]. Because of this dreaded complication, recommendations for fluid removal have been established arbitrarily not to exceed 1 to 1.5 L.

Clinical and experimental studies showed the pathogenesis of re-expansion pulmonary edema to be related to increase in microvascular permeability [36–38]. In a study published by Suzuki and colleagues [36], edema fluid in two cases of re-expansion pulmonary edema during thoracotomy was analyzed. A high value of fluid-to-serum protein concentration ratio indicated an increase in pulmonary microvascular permeability. There were marked increases in polymorphonuclear leukocyte counts and proinflammatory mediators, such as thromboxane B_2 and 6-keto-prostaglandin $F_1\alpha$, suggesting that inflammation plays a role in the increased vascular permeability [36]. Risk factors for the development of re-expansion pulmonary edema are related to the size of the effusion, duration of the effusion, and development of excessively negative pleural pressures.

Two well-controlled animal models published in the 1970s found that the duration of effusion and the development of excessively negative pleural pressures

were correlated with the development of re-expansion pulmonary edema. Based on their observations, mean pleural pressures not exceeding −20 cm H_2O pressure were relatively safe, whereas pleural pressures of −40 cm H_2O pressure placed the animals at high risk for the development of pulmonary edema [39,40].

It is reasonable to assume that pleural manometry can be used to monitor pleural pressures and improve patient safety when large volumes of pleural fluid are withdrawn. In a study published by Villena and colleagues [26], 57 unselected patients underwent therapeutic thoracentesis with an aim to remove as much fluid as possible. Reasons to terminate fluid removal included (1) no more fluid could be removed, (2) the patient developed symptoms related to fluid removal (ie, chest pain, cough, or chest tightness), or (3) mean pleural liquid pressure became −20 cm H_2O or lower. In 51% of cases, more than 1.5 L of pleural fluid was aspirated. Therapeutic thoracentesis had to be discontinued in approximately 50% of cases because clinical symptoms developed during the procedure. In 28% (16 of 57) of the cases, the cause of the interruption was the decrease in pleural liquid pressure without clinical symptoms. In 10 patients, the procedure was terminated because no more fluid could be removed. In two cases, the operator terminated the procedure for concerns that too much fluid had been evacuated. Clinical signs of hypo-volemia or re-expansion pulmonary edema were not seen [26]. In a similar study published by Light and colleagues [24], pleural pressures were measured initially and serially as pleural fluid was withdrawn in 52 patients undergoing therapeutic thoracentesis. Pleural fluid aspiration was continued until the pleural pressure decreased to less than -20 cmH$_2$O, the patient developed excessive symptoms, or no more fluid could be withdrawn. Mean pleural fluid removed was greater than 1 L, and in four patients, greater than 3 L of fluid was removed. None of the patients developed re-expansion pulmonary edema or signs of intravascular fluid depletion after thoracentesis.

In the authors' institution, pleural manometry is performed routinely during all therapeutic thora-centeses. To date, the authors have performed more than 200 therapeutic thoracenteses with pleural ma-nometry. Current guidelines in terminating fluid removal are (1) negative pleural pressure of -20 cm H$_2$O or less, (2) chest pain, or (3) intractable cough. Using these guidelines, one case of unilateral re-expansion pulmonary edema has been noted. Although pleural manometry did not prevent a single case of pulmonary edema, it may have prevented more cases of re-expansion pulmonary edema because the authors routinely exceed 1 L of fluid removal during these procedures.

Malignant pleural effusion

The estimated annual incidence of malignant pleural effusions in the United States is 200,000 cases. Malignant pleural effusions remain a therapeutic chal-lenge to pulmonologists and oncologists [41–43]. The primary goal in treating this condition is palliation with relief of dyspnea. In a meta-analysis of 417 patients with malignant pleural effusions, the median survival was 4 months [44]. Therapeutic op-tions for patients with recurrent, symptomatic pleural effusions should be tailored to their short survival. Current options for treating a recurrent, symptomatic malignant effusion include therapeutic thoracentesis, chemical pleurodesis through a thoracostomy tube, talc poudrage, pleuroperitoneal shunt, parietal pleur-ectomy, and long-term indwelling pleural catheters.

Chemical pleurodesis through a chest tube and talc poudrage are common modalities used to palliate these patients. Greater than 90% success has been reported when talc is used. Success with pleurodesis varies with agent employed, technique, and patient

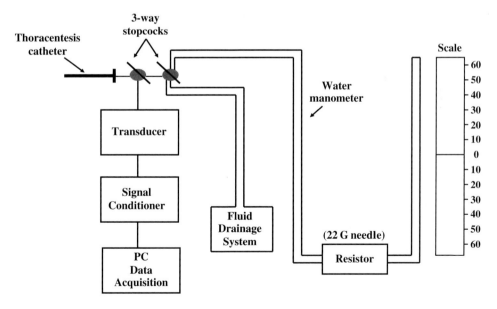

Fig. 4. Pleural manometry setup. Two three-way stopcocks are connected in series and attached to the side port of the thoracentesis catheter. The transducer is attached to the stopcock closest to the patient. The water manometer and pleural drainage system is attached to the other stopcock. When pressure measurements are acquired, the drainage system is closed, while the water manometer and transducer are opened to the patient. The interposed resistor (22G needle) connecting the intravenous tubing is part of the water manometer system. (*Adapted from* Doelken P, Huggins JT, Pastis N, et al. Pleural manometry: technique and clinical implications. Chest 2004;126:1764–9; with permission.)

selection [45–48]. More importantly, apposition of the visceral and parietal surfaces must occur for pleural symphysis. To exclude malignancy-associated lung entrapment, chest radiography is commonly used after fluid drainage to determine if appropriate apposition of the pleural surface is seen. Chest radiography is an insensitive modality for diagnosing lung entrapment, however.

In malignancy, lung entrapment develops when a large tumor burden or tumor-induced fibrosis encases the lung, preventing its expansion to the chest wall. Lung entrapment often is not appreciated until removal of pleural fluid has been performed. In the absence of an endobronchial lesion, a malignancy-associated lung entrapment should be suspected if any of the following is found: (1) failure of the lung

to expand completely on chest radiograph after most of the fluid has been removed by therapeutic thoracentesis; (2) initial negative mean pleural pressure; (3) decrease in pleural liquid pressure to -20 cm H_2O or less after 1 L of fluid is removed; or (4) a pleural space elastance of 19 cm H_2O or greater after removing 500 mL of fluid [25].

Performing pleural manometry in this setting can help the clinician predict the efficacy of pleurodesis. In a prospective cohort study of 65 patients with a malignant pleural effusion, 11 of 14 (79%) patients with a pleural space elastance of 19 cm H_2O/L or greater had lung entrapment. None of the 14 patients with a pleural space elastance of 19 cm H_2O/L or greater and none of patients with lung entrapment had a successful pleurodesis with bleomycin. In contrast,

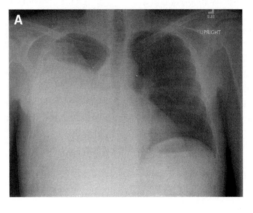

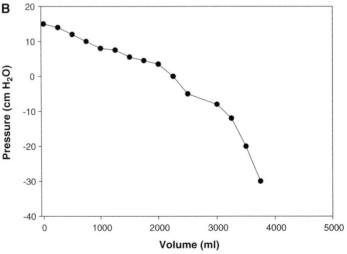

Fig. 5. (*A*) Posterior-anterior chest radiograph of a patient with stage IIIB non–small cell lung cancer. A massive right pleural effusion with absence of contralateral shift is seen. (*B*) The pressure/volume curve is biphasic with increased pleural space elastance during the terminal phase of the therapeutic thoracentesis. The patient was palliated successfully with the placement of a long-term indwelling pleural catheter.

42 or 43 (98%) patients with a pleural space elastance of 19 cm H_2O/L or less who did not have a lung entrapment had a successful bleomycin pleurodesis. Pleural space elastance was calculated from the first 500 mL of fluid removed [25].

Three pressure/volume curves can be seen in the setting of malignant pleural effusions. First, the pressure/volume curve can be monophasic with a normal pleural space elastance. This pressure/volume curve would signify a normal expandable lung. Terminal negative pressure deflections when minimal amounts of pleural fluid remain are seen and attributed to local deformation forces around the catheter. Second, the pressure/volume curve can be monophasic with an increased pleural space elastance. Finally, the pressure/volume curve can be biphasic revealing normal pleural space elastance during the initial fluid drainage; however, with increased fluid removal, the slope of the curve becomes steep signifying increased pleural space elastance. In the authors' experience and a review of their unpublished pleural manometry of malignant pleural effusions, a biphasic curve is seen more commonly than a monophasic curve with an increased pleural space elastance. The frequency of malignant pleural effusion associated with lung entrapment may have been underrepresented in the series published by Lan and colleagues [25].

Pleural fluid formation in this setting is driven primarily by parietal pleura capillary leak. Hydrostatic and oncotic pressure gradients established between the parietal pleural capillaries and pleural space also contribute to pleural fluid formation. Finding either a monophasic curve with increased pleural space elastance or a biphasic curve in which the terminal slope shows increased pleural space elastance suggests lung entrapment and poor pleurodesis success (Fig. 4).

Trapped lung

Trapped lung represents the sequela of fibrinous pleuritis in which a fibrous membrane develops on the visceral pleura while the lung is separated from the chest wall [3,4]. In a simplistic way, trapped lung can be thought of as a form of defective healing of the pleural space with the formation of scar tissue on the visceral pleura while the lung is collapsed. The diagnosis of trapped lung requires chronicity and stability over time. Pleural fluid formation in the presence of a trapped lung is the result of a pure mechanical mechanism.

Stead and colleagues [3] published a case series of 24 patients with tuberculous pleurisy who underwent thoracotomy for various reasons. Nine of the 24 patients did not have histologic evidence of tuberculosis. Two of the nine had large amounts of fibrous tissue completely obliterating the pleural space. The other seven cases shared the findings of a chronic pleural effusion and a thin fibrous peel preventing normal lung expansion. On histology, a nonspecific fibrous pleuritis was seen [3].

Moore and Thomas [49] reported four cases of persistent pleural effusions resulting from nonspecific pleuritis and trapped lung. A series of persistent pleural effusion after coronary artery bypass graft requiring surgical decortication was reported. In this series, the investigators described diminishing cellularity and increasing pleural peel with increased time from the coronary artery bypass graft [50].

The development of a trapped lung requires the presence of blood or inflammation of the pleura leading to a pleural effusion. The pleural effusion must persist long enough to allow fibrous tissue to develop along the visceral surface while the parietal and visceral pleural surfaces are separated. Several conditions have been associated with the development of a trapped lung. The predisposing conditions associated with the development of a trapped lung include coronary artery bypass graft, post–cardiac syndrome, empyema, uremic pleuritis, hemothorax, rheumatoid pleurisy, tuberculous pleurisy, and historically pneumothorax therapy for pulmonary tuberculosis. Because of the vast numbers of cardiac surgical procedures being performed today, cardiac surgery is considered one the most common causes of trapped lung today.

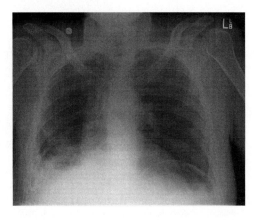

Fig. 6. Posterior-anterior chest radiograph of a man with long-standing uremia and chronic right-side pleural effusion. After placement of a small-bore chest tube, his right lower lobe failed to re-expand. This is the radiographic finding of a trapped lung.

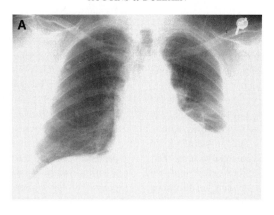

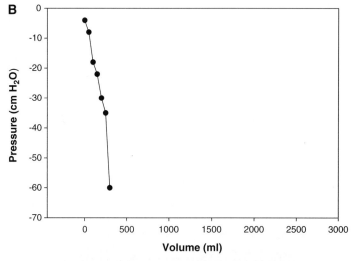

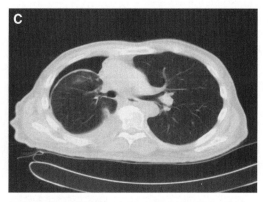

Fig. 7. (*A*) Posterior-anterior chest radiograph of a patient with end-stage renal disease with a moderate pleural effusion on the left. (*B*) The pressure/volume curve was consistent with the diagnosis of trapped lung and had a calculated pleural space elastance of 135 cm H_2O/L. (*C*) Air-contrast chest CT performed immediately after therapeutic thoracentesis shows the fibroelastic membrane along the visceral pleural surface, which is impeding normal lung expansion.

Pleural fluid formation and removal in trapped lung occurs under similar conditions found in a normal pleural space when oncotic and hydrostatic pressure gradients are intact. The pleural fluid in trapped lung persists when forces of pleural fluid formation and removal are in equilibrium.

With loss of lung volume, pleural pressure decreases leading to a decrease in thoracic volume on the affected side. Moderate decreases in thoracic volume after lobectomy and lobar atelectasis do not result in pleural effusions. Why a trapped lung with moderate volume loss results in pleural effusions requires explanation. In the case of a lobectomy, the remaining lung expands, the diaphragm is displaced upward, and the pleural space assumes its usual shape relative to the chest wall. In the case of a trapped lung, a fibroelastic membrane covers the visceral pleura, preventing a normal geometric alignment of the lung and chest wall. Although this fibroelastic membrane can cover the entire visceral surface, it most commonly involves the most dependent portion of the lung (Fig. 5). The presence of this visceral pleural membrane prevents the lung from conforming to the shape of the thoracic cavity. The unaffected part of the lung expands relatively normally during respiration and could fill the void left by the trapped lung. For an effusion to persist in the setting of a partially trapped lung, the shape of the trapped lung must be sufficiently different from the chest wall shape. The unaffected lung must be mechanically prevented from filling the space created by the unexpandable lung. Otherwise the space would be obliterated with re-establishment of negative pleural pressures when the inflammatory process has resolved (Fig. 6).

The conditions in trapped lung pleural effusions are similar to the mechanical conditions that exist along the lobar margins in the normal pleural space. Along the lobar margins, wider separation of the parietal and visceral pleural surface exists, creating more negative pleural pressures [4–6]. Mean pleural liquid pressures in patients with trapped lung typically are negative initially and decrease rapidly with fluid removal. Light and colleagues [24] reported the manometric findings in series of 52 patients undergoing therapeutic thoracentesis. Negative initial pleural pressures or rapid changes in the pressure as fluid was withdrawn suggested malignancy-associated entrapment or trapped lung. There is considerable overlap of initial pleural pressures in trapped lung and other pleural diseases. Initial negative mean pleural pressures may be seen in malignancy and transudative and exudative effusions without entrapment. This situation limits the diagnostic utility of initial pleural pressure measurements for diagnosing a trapped lung. In contrast, the finding of a positive mean initial pleural pressure would render the diagnosis of trapped lung highly unlikely.

The elastance of the pleural space in trapped lung was found to be consistently higher compared with other transudative or exudative effusions when pleural malignancy and endobronchial obstruction were excluded. The finding of negative initial mean pleural pressure and increased elastance is not surprising given the increased risk for concomitant lung entrapment in this condition. A negative initial mean pleural pressure and a pleural space elastance of greater than 16 cm H_2O/L in the absence of endobronchial obstruction and malignancy support the diagnosis of trapped lung (Fig. 7).

References

[1] Farber JE, Lincoln NS. The unexpandable lung. Am Rev Tuberc 1939;40:704–9.

[2] Douglas BE, Carr DT, Bernatz PE. Diagnostic thoracotomy in the study of "idiopathic" pleural effusion. Am Rev Tuberc Pulm Dis 1956;74:954–7.

[3] Stead WW, Eichenholz A, Stauss H-K. Operative and pathologic findings in twenty-four patients with syndrome of idiopathic pleurisy with effusion, presumably tuberculous. Am Rev Tuber Pulm Dis 1955; 71:473–502.

[4] Doelken P, Sahn SA. Trapped lung. Semin Respir Crit Care Med 2001;22:631–5.

[5] Lai-Fook SJ. Mechanics of the pleural space: fundamental concepts. Lung 1987;165:249–67.

[6] Lai-Fook SJ. Pleural mechanics and fluid exchange. Physiol Rev 2004;84:385–410.

[7] Boggs DS, Kinasewitz GT. Pathophysiology of the pleural space. Am J Med Sci 1995;309:53–9.

[8] Sahn SA. The pleura. Am Rev Respir Dis 1988;138: 184–234.

[9] Light RW, Lee YCG. Textbook of pleural diseases. London: Arnold; 2003.

[10] Setnikar I, Taglietti A, Agostoni E. La cinetica del liquido pleurico studiata per mezza di albumina marcata con. Boll Soc Ital Biol Sper 1990;70:1750–2.

[11] Agostoni E. Mechanics of the pleural space. Physiol Rev 1972;52:57–128.

[12] Agostoni E. Mechanics of the pleural space. In: Handbook of physiology: the respiratory system: mechanics of breathing, sect. 3, vol. III, pt. 2. Bethesda (MD): American Physiology Society; 1986. p. 531–60.

[13] Agostoni E, D'Angelo E. Thickness and pressure of pleural liquid at various heights and with various hydrothoraces. Respir Physiol 1969;6:330–42.

[14] Agostoni E, D'Angelo E. Pleural liquid pressure. J Appl Physiol 1991;71:393–403.

[15] Agostoni E, D'Angelo E, Bonanni MV. Measurements of pleural liquid without cannula. J Appl Physiol 1969; 26:258–60.

[16] Agostoni E, Miserocchi G, Bonnani MV. Thickness and pressure of the pleural liquid in some mammals. Respir Physiol 1969;6:245–56.

[17] Agostoni E, Zocchi L. Mechanical coupling and liquid exchanges in the pleural space. Clin Chest Med 1998;19:241–60.

[18] Albertine KH, Wiener-Kronish JP, Bastacky J, et al. No evidence for mesothelial cell contact across the costal pleural space of sheep. J Appl Physiol 1991;70: 123–34.

[19] Lai-Fook SJ, Kaplowitz MR. Pleural space thickness in situ by light microscopy in five mammalian species. J Appl Physiol 1985;59:603–10.

[20] Lai-Fook SJ. Mechanics of the pleural space: fundamental concepts. Lung 1987;165:249–67.

[21] Lai-Fook SJ, Rodarte JR. Pleural pressure distribution and its relationship to lung volume and interstitial pressure. J Appl Physiol 1991;70:967–78.

[22] Lai-Fook SJ, Beck KC, Southorn PA. Pleural liquid pressure measured by micropipettes in rabbits. J Appl Physiol 1984;56:1633–9.

[23] Doelken P, Huggins JT, Pastis N, et al. Pleural manometry: technique and clinical implications. Chest 2004;126:1764–9.

[24] Light RW, Jenkinson SG, Vu-Dinh M, et al. Observation of pleural fluid pressures as fluid is withdrawn during thoracentesis. Am Rev Respir Dis 1980;121: 799–804.

[25] Lan R-S, Lo SK, Chuang M-L, et al. Elastance of the pleural space: a predictor for the outcome of pleurodesis in patients with malignant pleural effusion. Ann Intern Med 1997;126:768–74.

[26] Villena V, Lopez-Encuentra A, Pozo F, et al. Measurement of pleural pressure during therapeutic thoracentesis. Am J Respir Crit Care Med 2000;162: 1534–8.

[27] Light RW, Standbury DW, Brown SE. The relationship between pleural pressures and changes in pulmonary function after therapeutic thoracentesis. Am Rev Respir Dis 1986;133:658–61.

[28] Carlson RJ, Classen F, Gollan WG, et al. Pulmonary edema following the rapid re-expansion of a totally collapsed lung due to a pneumothorax. Surg Forum 1959;9:367–71.

[29] Childress ME, Moy G, Mottram M. Unilateral pulmonary edema resulting from treatment of spontaneous pneumothorax. Am Rev Respir Dis 1971;104:119–21.

[30] Ratcliffe JL, Chavez CM, Jamechuk A, et al. Re-expansion pulmonary edema. Chest 1973;64:654–6.

[31] Sautter RD, Dreher WH, MacIndoe JH, et al. Fatal pulmonary edema and pneumonitis after re-expansion of chronic pneumothorax. Chest 1971;60:399–401.

[32] Shanahan MX, Monk I, Richards HJ. Unilateral pulmonary oedema following re-expansion of pneumothorax. Anaesth Intensive Care 1975;3:19–30.

[33] Steckel RJ. Unilateral pulmonary edema after pneumothorax. N Engl J Med 1973;289:621–2.

[34] Trapnell DH, Thurston JGB. Unilateral pulmonary oedema after pleural aspiration. Lancet 1970;1:1367–9.

[35] Waquaruddin M, Bernstein A. Re-expansion pulmonary oedema. Thorax 1975;30:54–60.

[36] Suzuki S, Tanita T, Koike K, et al. Evidence of acute inflammatory response in reexpansion pulmonary edema. Chest 1992;101:275–6.

[37] Sprung CL, Loewenherz JW, Baier H, et al. Evidence for increased permeability in reexpansion pulmonary edema. Am J Med 1981;71:497–500.

[38] Koike K, Ono S, Sakuma T, et al. Collapse and reexpasion of lungs increase microvascular permeability in sheep. Tohoku J Exp Med 1989;157:19–29.

[39] Miller WC. Experimental pulmonary edema following re-expansion of pneumothorax. Am Rev Respir Dis 1973;108:664–6.

[40] Pavlin J, Cheney FW. Unilateral pulmonary edema in rabbits after re-expansion of collapsed lung. J Appl Physiol Respirat Environ Exerc Physiol 1979; 46:31–5.

[41] Antony VB, Loddenkemper R, Astoul P, et al. Statement of the American Thoracic Society: management of malignant pleural effusions. Am J Respir Crit Care Med 2000;162:1987–2001.

[42] Sahn SA. Malignant pleural effusions. Semin Respir Crit Care Med 2001;22:607–15.

[43] Sahn SA. Malignant pleural effusions. In: Fishman AP, Elias JA, Fishman JA, et al, editors. Pulmonary disease and disorders. 3rd edition. New York: McGraw-Hill; 1998. p. 1429–38.

[44] Heffner JE, Nietert PJ, Barbieri MS. Pleural fluid pH as a predictor of survival for patients with malignant pleural effusions. Chest 2000;117:79–86.

[45] Walker-Renard PG, Vaughn LM, Sahn SA. Chemical pleurodesis for malignant pleural effusions. Ann Intern Med 1994;120:56–64.

[46] Sorensen PG, Svendsen TL, Enk B. Treatment of malignant pleural effusion with drainage, with and without instillation of talc. Eur J Respir Dis 1984; 65:131–5.

[47] Kennedy L, Sahn SA. Talc pleurodesis for the treatment of pneumothorax and pleural effusion. Chest 1994;106:1215–22.

[48] Kennedy L, Rusch VW, Strange C, et al. Pleurodesis using talc slurry. Chest 1994;106:342–6.

[49] Moore PJ, Thomas PA. The trapped lung with chronic pleural space: a cause of recurring pleural effusion. Milit Med 1967;132:998–1002.

[50] Lee YCG, Vaz MAC, Ely KA, et al. Symptomatic persistent post-coronary artery bypass graft pleural effusions requiring operative treatment: clinical and histologic features. Chest 2001;119:795–801.

ELSEVIER
SAUNDERS

Clin Chest Med 27 (2006) 241 – 252

CLINICS
IN CHEST
MEDICINE

Discriminating Between Transudates and Exudates

John E. Heffner, MD

Center of Clinical Effectiveness and Patient Safety, Medical University of South Carolina, 169 Ashley Avenue, PO Box 250332, Charleston, SC 29426, USA

Because numerous conditions may present with pleural effusions, clinicians traditionally have simplified their diagnostic approach by first dichotomizing pleural fluid as transudates or exudates [1]. This approach allows subsequent diagnostic testing to pursue the conditions that most commonly are associated with one or the other of these two types of effusions [2,3]. Transudates occur as an ultrafiltration of serum across pleural membranes and result from imbalances of hydrostatic or osmotic pressure. Most transudates occur in the setting of clinically apparent conditions, such as heart failure, cirrhosis with ascites, and nephrosis. The presence of a transudate usually allows clinicians to treat the underlying condition and observe the effusion for resolution. Exudative effusions develop as a consequence of inflammatory or malignant disorders, such as pneumonia, cancer, or tuberculosis, which increase capillary permeability and allow large-molecular-weight compounds to enter the pleural space. Detection of an exudate often requires additional testing that may be invasive in nature. Because the classification of pleural fluid as an exudate or transudate has important implications for patient care, clinicians require a clear understanding of the diagnostic performance of available tests and testing strategies used for pleural fluid classification.

Pleural fluid tests

The presence of high concentrations of various large-molecular-weight compounds in pleural fluid defines the presence of an exudative effusion. Pleural

fluid tests used in clinical practice detect the presence of these compounds or measure the effects of their presence on pleural fluid specific gravity.

Pleural fluid specific gravity, protein, and lactate dehydrogenase

Pleural fluid specific gravity was the first test used in clinical practice to define an exudative effusion. Values for pleural fluid specific gravity greater than 1.015 measured by a hydrometer (>1.020 by a refractometer) corresponded to a pleural fluid protein concentration greater than 3 g/dL and established an exudate [4]. As chemical assays became readily available in clinical practice, pleural fluid protein values greater than 3 g/dL replaced specific gravity as the primary test to classify pleural effusions [5]. Subsequent reports emphasized the improved performance of pleural fluid lactate dehydrogenase (LDH) testing compared with pleural fluid protein in establishing the presence of an exudate [6].

Light's criteria

To enhance diagnostic accuracy further, investigators examined the utility of using various test combinations to classify pleural fluid. Light and colleagues [7] studied the diagnostic performance of three pleural fluid tests combined in an "or rule," meaning that a positive finding from any one of the tests established the presence of an exudate:

- Pleural fluid-to-serum protein ratio >0.5, *or*
- Pleural fluid-to-serum LDH ratio >0.6, *or*
- Pleural fluid LDH concentration >200 U/L (later changed to two thirds the upper limit of normal for serum LDH)

E-mail address: heffnerj@musc.edu

Light's criteria were designed to approach 100% sensitivity and 100% specificity for detecting exudates to avoid misclassifying any pleural effusions. The original derivation study evaluated 150 patients with pleural effusions, of whom only 2 patients were misclassified, which resulted in a sensitivity of 99% and a specificity of 98% for identifying exudates [7]. Subsequent studies confirmed the high sensitivity of Light's criteria, but reported a lower specificity of 65% to 85% [2,8–10].

Several explanations exist for the lower specificity of Light's criteria reported in validation studies. First, the original retrospective study by Light and colleagues [7] excluded 33 of the 183 initially evaluated patients on the basis of rigorous study inclusion criteria. This strategy limited false-positive results and false-negative results and contributed to the lower specificity of the rule in unselected patient populations examined in subsequent studies [2]. Second, the original recommendation to use a value of 200 U/L as the cutoff for pleural fluid LDH concentration decreased reproducibility because of the variation in LDH assay techniques used in different laboratories. The LDH criterion cutoff point in Light's criteria was modified later to two thirds the upper limits of a laboratory's normal serum LDH value [11]. Third, validation studies of Light's criteria showed a lower specificity compared with the original report because of the nature of all strategies that use multiple tests combined in an "or rule." As the number of tests increase, the likelihood of correctly identifying a target condition (ie, sensitivity) increases, but the likelihood of incorrectly identifying another condition (false-positive test result) also increases and lowers specificity.

This reciprocal relationship between sensitivity and specificity is analogous to a trout fisherman who casts his fishing line into a lake filled with trout and bottom-dwelling catfish. He has an increasing likelihood of catching an increasing proportion of the trout in the lake (*sensitivity*) the more often he casts his line. The fisherman also has an increasing likelihood of bringing in an unintended catfish (*false positive*) the more often he casts his line, decreasing the *specificity* of his fishing technique. As a general rule, combining single, independent tests with an "or rule" always results in an increased sensitivity and a decreased specificity. Consequently, the use of Light's criteria—or any other combination of two or more pleural fluid tests—has the disadvantage of misclassifying some transudates as exudates. This problem is most notable for patients with transudative effusions secondary to heart failure who undergo diuretic therapy, which causes more rapid reabsorp-

tion of water from the pleural space compared with the large-molecular-weight constituents assayed in pleural fluid tests and increases the constituents' concentration [12,13]. Changing the cutoff point of a test also invokes the reciprocal relationship between sensitivity and specificity. Lowering the cutoff point for pleural fluid LDH increases the sensitivity of the test for identifying exudates, but simultaneously lowers the test's specificity by including more transudates with LDH values just below the initial cutoff point.

Serum-to-pleural fluid albumin gradient

To address the decreased specificity of Light's criteria shown in validation studies, investigators examined the discriminative properties of other pleural fluid tests to find a test or test combination with a higher specificity and equivalent sensitivity compared with Light's criteria. Roth and colleagues [9] applied observations made in peritoneal fluid to the pleural space and evaluated the performance of the serum-to-pleural fluid albumin gradient. In 59 patients with pleural effusions, an albumin gradient 12 g/dL or less correctly classified 57 of 59 patients (95% sensitivity, 100% specificity for exudates). A validation study by Burgess and colleagues [14] of 393 patients showed a sensitivity of 87% and specificity of 92% for the albumin gradient. The studies by Roth and colleagues [9] and Burgess and colleagues [14] decreased the misclassification rates of transudates as exudates among patients with heart failure who received diuretic therapy. This observation prompted recommendations to perform albumin gradient testing for patients who seem clinically likely to have a transudate secondary to heart failure, but have borderline evidence of exudates when tested by Light's criteria [11]. One more recent study did not show improved performance of the albumin gradient, however, compared with Light's criteria in this clinical setting [15]. Also, the improved specificity of the albumin gradient may result from the use of a single test compared with a combination test (Light's criteria), the latter of which has a lower specificity as a result of the reciprocal relationship between sensitivity and specificity discussed earlier.

Pleural fluid cholesterol

Hamm and colleagues [16] showed that exudates have a higher cholesterol concentration compared with transudates. The mechanisms for this difference has not been investigated, but likely explanations relate to breakdown of intrapleural cells with release of cellular content of cholesterol and to increased capillary permeability, which allows cholesterol in the bloodstream to enter the pleural space. In a group of 70 patients with pleural effusions using a cutoff for exudates of cholesterol greater than 60 mg/dL, Hamm and colleagues [16] showed a sensitivity of 100% and a specificity of 95% for exudates. Using a cutoff value of cholesterol greater than 55 mg/dL for exudates, Valdés and colleagues [17] showed a sensitivity of 91% and a specificity of 100%. These investigators also noted that the pleural fluid-to-serum ratio of cholesterol using a cutoff point of greater than 0.3 for exudates had a sensitivity of 93% and a specificity of 88% [17]. Other studies have reported varying performance of pleural fluid cholesterol and pleural fluid-to-serum cholesterol ratios in identifying exudative effusions [14,18,19].

Pleural fluid bilirubin

Meisel and colleagues [20] examined the discriminative properties of the pleural effusion-to-serum bilirubin ratio using a cutoff value greater than 0.6 for exudates. They showed in 51 patients a sensitivity of 96% and a specificity of 82%. Subsequent reports have not reproduced the high diagnostic accuracy of pleural fluid bilirubin [10,14], which is rarely used in clinical practice.

Other tests and approaches for identifying exudates

Investigators have evaluated other pleural fluid tests and imaging studies to identify exudates, but none has received widespread endorsement. Pleural fluid-to-serum cholinesterase ratios have been reported to have similar diagnostic accuracy compared with Light's criteria [21,22]. Cell-free DNA measured in pleural fluid has 91% sensitivity and 88% specificity for exudates [23]. Tests using aspartate transaminase, interleukin-1β, interleukin-6, uric acid, C-reactive protein, alanine transaminase, alkaline phosphatase, creatinine kinase, ferritin, interleukin-8, tumor necrosis factor-α, and γ-glutamyltransferase all have compared poorly with Light's criteria [14, 24–31].

Several studies evaluated the utility of imaging studies to obviate the need for thoracentesis. Gd-DTPA-enhanced MRI in a small study of 20 patients was reported to have a sensitivity of 83% and specificity of 100% [32]. Diffusion-weighted

MRI had a reported sensitivity of 91% and specificity of 85% [33]. Chest CT of 55 patients undergoing thoracentesis had a sensitivity of 50% and specificity of 100% [34]. Signs of an exudate included parietal pleural thickening, attenuation of extrapleural fat, and degree of loculation.

Analytic comparisons of tests and testing strategies

In an effort to improve on Light's criteria, multiple studies compared new pleural fluid tests or testing strategies with Light's criteria to determine if any of the new approaches had improved diagnostic performance. These studies almost always compared tests by reporting P values generated by χ^2 analysis, which does not describe relative diagnostic accuracies or test performance. Also, many of these studies had methodologic flaws, which have not been stated clearly in the literature [10]. Cutoff points for each test have been selected through informal techniques [10]. A series of reports of varying quality that resulted in marginal incremental improvement over Light's criteria resulted in a frustrated call from one editorialist that these continued efforts were of limited value [35].

Heffner and colleagues [10] performed a meta-analysis using the individual patient data provided by primary investigators who had published data on pleural fluid test results. In contrast to customary meta-analyses that use aggregated summary results of studies, analyses of full datasets of individual patient data received from primary investigators allow a more precise description and comparison of relative test performances [36]. The meta-analysis compared tests by calculating their diagnostic odds ratios for identifying exudates and their individual area under the curve (AUC) generated by receiver operating characteristics (ROC) analysis [37].

Diagnostic odds ratios describe the odds of positive test results in subjects with the target condition (exudate) compared with the odds of positive test results in subjects without the target condition (transudate) [38]. Higher diagnostic odds ratios identify better-performing tests. Comparing tests' diagnostic odds ratios with any accompanying overlap of their 95% confidence intervals (CI) allows a comparison of test performance and statistically significant differences. ROC analysis is used to depict the pattern of sensitivities and specificities observed when the performance of the test is evaluated at several different diagnostic thresholds (ie, cutoff points) [38]. The shape of the ROC curve describes the overall

Table 1
Commonly used pleural fluid tests to identify exudates with associated cutoff points from primary studies and a meta-analysis

Pleural fluid test	Meta-analysis ROC cutoff point [10]	Previously reported cutoff points [Ref.]
Pleural fluid protein	>2.9 g/dL	>3 g/dL [53]
Pleural fluid-to-serum protein ratio	>0.5	>0.5 [7]
Pleural fluid LDH	>0.45 of upper limits of normal when used in Light's criteria. >2/3 of normal when not combined with pleural fluid-to-serum LDH ratio	>200 IU/L [7,43] >2/3 of upper limit of normal [54]
Pleural fluid-to-serum LDH ratio	>0.6	>0.6 [7]
Pleural fluid cholesterol	>45 mg/dL	>45 mg/dL [43] >54 mg/dL [55,56] >55 mg dL [17] >60 mg/dL [16,18]
Pleural fluid-to-serum cholesterol ratio	>0.3	>0.3 [16–18,55]
Albumin gradient	≤1.2 g/dL	≤1.2 g/dL [9,14]
Pleural fluid-to-serum bilirubin ratio	>0.6	>0.6 [14,20]

Data from Heffner JE, Brown LK, Barbieri C. Diagnostic value of tests that discriminate between exudative and transudative pleural effusions. Chest 1997;111:970–9.

diagnostic performance of a test. Perfectly performing tests have an AUC of 1, and a test with no discriminative properties has an AUC of 0.5. ROC analysis also can provide a formal method for selecting cutoff points to maximize the performance of a diagnostic test [37].

The meta-analysis by Heffner and colleagues [10] examined cutoff points for individual pleural fluid tests reported in the literature (Table 1) and confirmed by formal ROC analysis the validity of most of the previously reported cutoff points. The meta-analysis found, however, that the cutoff point for pleural fluid LDH of greater than 0.45 of the upper limits of a laboratory's normal serum value had the best

discriminative properties when pleural fluid LDH is combined with the pleural-fluid-to-serum LDH ratio in Light's criteria [10]. This lower cutoff point for pleural fluid LDH results from the unique interaction between pleural fluid LDH and the pleural fluid-to-serum LDH ratio, both of which are highly correlated, as discussed subsequently.

The meta-analysis also compared the relative diagnostic accuracies of individual tests (Table 2), all pairwise combinations of tests (Fig. 1), and all triplet combinations of tests (including Light's criteria) (Fig. 2) [10]. In general, triplet test strategies had higher odds ratios than pair combinations, which had higher odds ratios than single tests. As shown in

Table 2
Diagnostic accuracy of individual pleural fluid tests for identifying exudative pleural effusions

Plerual fluid test	Sensitivity % (95% CI)	Specificity	OR	AUC
Pleural fluid protein: n=1187	91.5 (89.3–93.7)	83.0 (77.6–88.4)	52.6 (33.2–85.8)	94.2 (92.6–95.9)
Pleural fluid-to-serum protein ratio: n=1393	89.5 (87.4–91.6)	90.9 (87.4–94.5)	85.4 (53.6–141.8)	95.4 (94.3–96.7)
Pleural fluid LDH: n=1438	88.0 (85.8–90.3)	81.8 (77.1–86.6)	33.1 (22.7–49.0)	93.3 (91.8–94.8)
Pleural fluid-to-serum LDH ratio: n=1388	91.4 (89.4–93.3)	85.0 (80.6–89.4)	60.0 (39.7–92.9)	94.7 (93.4–96.0)
Pleural fluid cholesterol: n=1348	89.0 (86.8–91.2)	81.4 (76.6–86.2)	35.5 (24.3–52.8)	93.3 (91.7–94.8)
Pleural fluid-to-serum cholesterol ratio: n=1123	92.0 (90.1–93.9)	81.4 (76.6–86.2)	50.5 (33.9–76.6)	94.1 (92.5–95.7)
Albumin gradient: n=386	86.8 (82.2–91.4)	91.8 (86.4–97.3)	73.9 (34.2–180.9)	94.0 (91.3–96.6)
Pleural fluid-to-serum bilirubin ratio: n=303	84.3 (79.3–89.3)	61.1 (51.2–70.9)	8.4 (4.9–14.9)	81.3 (76.3–86.4)

Data from Heffner JE, Brown LK, Barbieri C. Diagnostic value of tests that discriminate between exudative and transudative pleural effusions. Chest 1997;111:970–9.

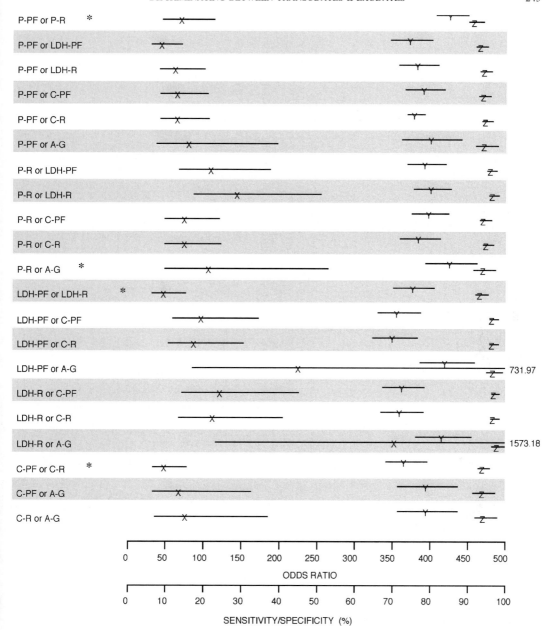

Fig. 1. Point estimates and 95% CI for odds ratios (*X*), sensitivity (*Y*), and specificity (*Z*) for paired test combinations. Asterisk denotes combinations that contain correlated test pairs ($R>|0.75|$). Numbers in the right-hand margin denote the upper 95% CI limits for odds ratios that fall off the figure. (*From* Heffner JE, Brown LK, Barbieri C. Diagnostic value of tests that discriminate between exudative and transudative pleural effusions. Chest 1997;111:970–9; with permission.)

Table 2, the overlapping 95% CI values show that all of the single tests have similar performance except for pleural fluid bilirubin, which had the poorest discriminative properties. As shown in Fig. 2 and Box 1, considerable overlap of the 95% CI values for the odds ratios did not allow identification of a superior combination of tests that had the highest significantly different discriminative properties. Several paired and triplet combinations that included pleural fluid albumin gradient had the highest point estimates for

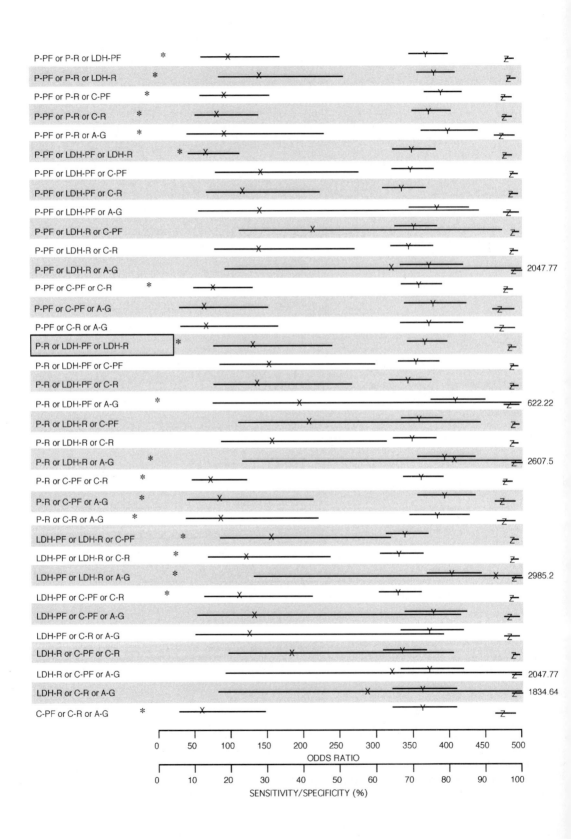

the odds ratio, however, suggesting that these combinations would be better performers if adequately powered studies were conducted.

The meta-analysis also examined pairwise correlations of each of the individual pleural fluid tests to determine the independence of each of these tests [10]. Tests used in combination test strategies should be independent with a low intertest correlation. Use of a correlated pair in a combined test strategy would be expected to identify the same subset of patients with each test and weaken test performance. The pleural fluid LDH test and the pleural fluid-to-serum LDH ratio had a Pearson coefficient of correlation of 0.84, indicating that the two tests were too closely correlated to function well in a diagnostic "or rule" strategy. This finding is expected considering the mathematical coupling evident by the presence of the value for pleural fluid LDH in both tests. The meta-analysis noted that the "abbreviated Light's criteria," which uses only two tests (pleural fluid-to-serum LDH ratio and the pleural fluid-to-serum protein ratio) performed as well as the classic three-test Light's criteria [10].

This high correlation between pleural fluid LDH and the LDH ratio explains why the meta-analysis identified a cutoff point of 0.45 for the LDH ratio as mentioned earlier. When used as a single test, a cutoff point of greater than two thirds normal had the highest diagnostic accuracy. When used in combination with pleural fluid LDH in Light's criteria, the high correlation between two mathematically coupled tests altered performance, resulting in a change in the optimal pleural fluid LDH cutoff point. The meta-analysis recommended the use of this lower pleural fluid cutoff point if the three-test Light's criteria were to be used (modified Light's criteria) [10].

The meta-analysis by Heffner and colleagues [10] showed that individual pleural fluid tests commonly used in clinical practice (except for pleural fluid bilirubin) had similar test performance, and that several test combinations had similar performance compared with Light's criteria. This finding is expected considering that all commonly used tests assess the same pathophysiologic event: the increased concentration of large-molecular-weight compounds in exudative effusions. The higher odds ratio and sensitivities of strategies that use test combinations encourage their use in clinical practice because of the greater importance of maximizing sensitivity to avoid missing some exudates (false-negative results) because of their diagnostic and prognostic importance. The similarity of performance of the various combinations allows selection of a testing strategy, however, that has the most clinical advantages. Light's criteria require pleural fluid and serum tests, which increases the cost and inconvenience of the test combination. The meta-analysis by Heffner and colleagues [10] showed good performance of several combinations that use only pleural fluid test results. Reasonable testing strategies include the two-test combination of pleural fluid LDH and pleural fluid cholesterol (sensitivity 97.5%, 95% CI 96.4–98.6%; specificity 71.9%, 95% CI 66.4–77.5%) and the three-test combination of pleural fluid protein, pleural fluid LDH, and pleural fluid cholesterol (sensitivity 98.4%, 95% CI 97.5–99.3%; specificity 70.4%, 95% CI 64.7–76%), which are statistically comparable to the three-test modified Light's criteria (sensitivity 97.9%, 95% CI 96.9–98.9%; specificity 74.3%, 95% CI 68.9–79.7%).

The strategy that combines pleural fluid LDH and pleural fluid cholesterol has been validated in several studies [39–41] and recommended as a cost-effective approach [42]. If Light's criteria are used, the two-test strategy with pleural fluid-to-serum LDH ratio and pleural fluid-to-serum protein ratio is preferred because of the high correlation between pleural fluid LDH and pleural fluid-to-serum LDH ratio. These "abbreviated" Light's criteria have been shown in an independent cohort to have good discriminative properties [43].

Bayesian approach to pleural fluid analysis

The traditional dichotomous approach to pleural fluid analysis that uses a single cutoff point loses much of the information contained within the available laboratory tests, which generate continuous integer results [44–46]. Dichotomization treats borderline abnormal and extremely abnormal test results the same, which underlies the observation that some patients with malignant effusions have transudates, and some patients with heart failure have

---

Fig. 2. Point estimates and 95% CI for odds ratios (X), sensitivity (Y), and specificity (Z) for triplet test combinations. Asterisk denotes combinations that contain correlated test pairs ($R > |0.75|$). Light's criteria combination is enclosed in a box. Numbers in the right-hand margin denote the upper 95% CI limits for odds ratios that fall off the figure. (*From* Heffner JE, Brown LK, Barbieri C. Diagnostic value of tests that discriminate between exudative and transudative pleural effusions. Chest 1997;111:970–9; with permission.)

Box 1. Use of likelihood ratios derived from pleural fluid tests to convert pretest to post-test probabilities of an exudate

The probability of an exudate can be computed with Bayes' theorem using likelihood ratios (LR):

- Based on the clinical presentation, a clinician might estimate the pretest probability (Preprob) of an exudate to be 10%
- Pretest odds = Preprob/ (1 − Preprob) = 0.11
- Thoracentesis returns the following pleural fluid test results:
  - LDH = 0.50 upper limits of laboratory normal
  - LDH ratio = 0.50
  - Protein ratio = 0.51

By Light's criteria, these results would establish the presence of an exudate:

- LR are calculated from pleural fluid values using equations in Table 3:
  - $LR_{LDH} = 0.42$
  - $LR_{LDH\ ratio} = 0.29$
  - $LR_{protein\ ratio} = 1.07$
- Post-test odds
  - = pretest odds × LR_{LDH} × $LR_{LDH\ ratio}$ × $LR_{protein\ ratio}$
  - = 0.11 × 0.42 × 0.29 × 1.07
  - = 0.014
- Post-test probability
  - = post-test odds/(1 + post-test odds)
  - = 1.4%

With the use of LR, the laboratory results have decreased the clinicians' 10% pretest probability of an exudate to an even lower value of 1%. The test results support the presence of a transudate. The clinician could have used the multilevel likelihoods in Table 4 that correspond to the pleural fluid test results to perform the above calculations.

Table 3
Exponential equations for calculating continuous likelihood ratios for discrete pleural fluid test criteria results

Pleural fluid test criteria	Continuous likelihood ratio equations
Pleural fluid protein	exp[1.68(ProPF test result − 3.263)]
Pleural fluid-to-serum protein ratio	exp[13.45(ProR test result − 0.505)]
Pleural fluid LDH	exp[4.97(LDHPF test result − 0.676)]
Pleural fluid-to-serum LDH Ratio	exp[4.24(LDHR test result − 0.792)]
Pleural fluid cholesterol	exp[0.08(CholPF test result − 52.208)]
Pleural fluid-to-serum cholesterol ratio	exp[13.98(CholR test result − 0.350)]
Pleural fluid-to-serum albumin gradient	exp[−2.43(AlbG test result − 1.307)]

Abbreviations: AlbG, pleural fluid-to-serum albumin gradient; CholPF, pleural fluid cholesterol; CholR, pleural fluid-to-serum cholesterol ratio; LDHPF, pleural fluid LDH as a fraction of the upper limits of the normal laboratory value; LDHR, pleural fluid-to-serum LDH ratio; ProPF, pleural fluid protein; ProR, pleural fluid-to-serum protein ratio.
Data from Heffner JE, Highland K, Brown LK. A meta-analysis derivation of continuous likelihood ratios for diagnosing pleural fluid exudates. Am J Respir Crit Care Med 2003;167:1591−9.

exudates [12,47,48]. These observations have resulted in reports suggesting a unique nature of these types of effusions that have prompted some authors to adopt the term *pseudoexudates* for false-positive exudates in patients with heart failure [12]. These findings represent borderline test results and the "false-positive" and "false-negative" misclassifications of some patients that nearly always occur with diagnostic tests. An examination of Light's criteria shows the diminished performance of dichotomous tests when they return results near cutoff points. Light's criteria have an overall diagnostic accuracy of greater than 95%. Diagnostic accuracy of the three-test combination decreases to 65% to 75%, however, when any one of the three tests returns results near their cutoff points (Table 5). As with most tests that return continuous integer results, diagnostic certainty decreases when patients have borderline test results.

A bayesian approach manages this uncertainty by encouraging clinicians to estimate a pretest probability that a patient has an exudate and calculate a post-test probability from the test result using likelihood ratios. A likelihood ratio describes how many

Table 4

Multilevel likelihood ratios for pleural fluid protein, pleural fluid-to-serum protein ratios, pleural fluid lactate dehydrogenase, and pleural fluid-to-serum fluid lactate dehydrogenase ratios

P-PF	LR	P-R	LR	LDH-PF	LR	LDH-R	LR
>5.0	47.30	>0.70	168.70	>1.00	44.30	>1.10	38.90
4.6–5.0	32.80	0.66–0.70	53.30	0.91–1.00	10.00	1.01–1.10	16.70
4.1–4.5	16.40	0.61–0.65	6.90	0.81–0.90	2.20	0.91–1.00	5.90
3.6–4.0	2.40	0.56–0.60	3.00	0.71–0.80	3.60	0.81–0.90	2.00
3.1–3.5	1.00	0.51–0.55	1.80	0.61–0.70	2.10	0.71–0.80	1.30
2.6–3.0	0.50	0.46–0.50	0.50	0.51–0.60	0.60	0.61–0.70	1.00
2.1–2.5	0.20	0.41–0.45	0.30	0.41–0.50	0.40	0.51–0.60	0.50
1.6–2.0	0.10	0.36–0.40	0.10	0.31–0.40	0.30	0.41–0.50	0.20
≤1.5	0.04	0.31–0.35	0.10	0.21–0.30	0.10	0.31–0.40	0.10
—	—	≤0.30	0.04	≤0.20	0.04	≤0.30	0.05

Abbreviations: LDH-PF, pleural fluid lactate dehydrogenase as a fraction of the upper limit of the serum value for the primary laboratory; LR, likelihood ratio, P-PF, pleural fluid protein in g/dL; P-R, pleural fluid to serum protein ratio.
Data from Heffner JE, Heffner JN, Brown LK. Multilevel and continuous pleural fluid pH likelihood ratios for evaluating malignant pleural effusions. Chest 2003;123:1887–94.

times more likely a specific test result would be found in a patient with an exudate as opposed to a transudate [49]. Converting a clinician's pretest probability to pretest odds, multiplying the pretest odds by the test result's likelihood ratio, and converting the resulting post-test odds to a post-test probability determines to what degree the test result increases or decreases the clinician's initial diagnostic suspicion that the patient has an exudative effusion. Pretest odds can be multiplied by two or more likelihood ratios before conversion to a post-test probability, which is done when combining several pleural fluid

Table 5

Diagnostic accuracies of Light's criteria when the value of each component test changes across its test result range

LDH-R test results	Diagnostic accuracy (%)	LDH-PF test results	Diagnostic accuracy (%)	P-R test results	Diagnostic accuracy (%)
≤0.30	94	≤0.20	94	≤0.3	91
0.31–0.35	95	0.21–0.25	94	0.31–0.35	94
0.36–0.40	92	0.26–0.30	84	0.36–0.40	65
0.41–0.45	83	0.31–0.35	81	0.41–0.45	84
0.46–0.50	65	0.36–0.40	82	0.46–0.50	70
0.51–0.55	73	0.41–0.45	88	0.51–0.55	84
0.56–0.60	76	0.46–0.50	79	0.56–0.60	91
0.61–0.65	76	0.51–0.55	74	0.61–0.65	94
0.66–0.70	71	0.56–0.60	76	0.66–0.70	99
0.71–0.75	79	0.61–0.67	86	>0.70	100
0.76–0.80	76	0.68–0.70	82	—	—
0.81–0.85	85	0.71–0.75	87	—	—
0.86–0.90	89	0.76–0.80	89	—	—
0.91–0.95	92	0.81–0.85	86	—	—
0.96–1.00	97	0.86–0.90	93	—	—
>1.00	98	>0.90	98	—	—
Overall accuracy	**92**		**92**		**92**

Binary cut off values as follows: LDH-R >0.6, LDH-PF >0.67 (2/3 upper limits of laboratory normal value), and P-R >0.5.
Abbreviations: LDH-PF, pleural fluid LDH as fraction of normal value; LDH-R, pleural fluid-to-serum LDH ratio; P-R, pleural fluid-to-serum protein ratio.
Data from Heffner JE, Highland K, Brown LK. A meta-analysis derivation of continuous likelihood ratios for diagnosing pleural fluid exudates. Am J Respir Crit Care Med 2003;167:1591–9.

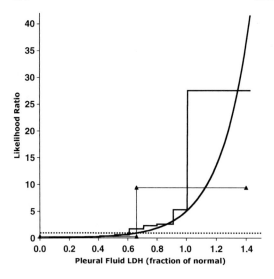

Fig. 3. Binary (*lines with triangle at intersects*), multilevel (*multiple stepped lines*), and continuous (*curved line*) likelihood ratios for the range of values for pleural fluid LDH (as depicted by the multiple of the upper limits of laboratory normal). As shown by the considerable separation of the three lines at a value for pleural fluid LDH of 1 of the upper limits of laboratory normal, binary and multilevel likelihood levels can overestimate or underestimate the true likelihood ratio, which is represented by the continuous likelihood ratio. (*Data from* Heffner JE, Highland K, Brown LK. A meta-analysis derivation of continuous likelihood ratios for diagnosing pleural fluid exudates. Am J Respir Crit Care Med 2003;167:1591–9.)

tests in a diagnostic strategy, such as Light's criteria (Fig. 3).

Likelihood ratios can be calculated for dichotomous pleural fluid tests using the cutoff points in Table 1. This approach does not remedy the problem of dichotomous testing, however, which misclassifies many patients with borderline test results. Multilevel likelihood ratios represent an advance that quantifies the degree of uncertainty that exists with borderline results. These ratios are generated by stratifying test results along their entire range at multiple, equal intervals and generating likelihood ratios for each interval. Use of multilevel likelihood ratios captures more of the information contained within continuous integer test results because extremely abnormal results have a greater effect on the post-test probability than borderline results. Heffner and colleagues [50] reported multilevel likelihood ratios for commonly performed pleural fluid tests that identify exudates (Tables 4 and 6). Continuous likelihood ratios derived by logistic regression represent a further advance over multilevel likelihood ratios because they provide a discrete likelihood ratio for every possible test result [51]. This increased precision allows all of the information available in a test result to be used in clinical decision making. As shown in Fig. 3, binary and multilevel likelihood ratios at some test result values considerably overestimate or underestimate the true likelihood ratio as derived by the calculation of continuous likelihood ratios. Continuous likelihood ratios have the additional benefit of being easily calculated by laboratory software or bedside personal digital assistants using simple exponential equations (Table 3) [52].

Table 6
Likelihood ratios for pleural fluid cholesterol, pleural fluid-to-serum cholesterol ratios, and pleural fluid albumin gradients

Chol-PF (mg/dL)	LR	Chol-R	LR	Albumin-gradient (g/L)	LR
>90	106.50	>0.55	44.40	≤0.8	74.90
81–90	12.40	0.51–0.55	15.70	0.9–1.0	11.80
71–80	6.60	0.46–0.50	7.20	1.1–1.2	6.20
61–70	3.70	0.41–0.45	3.70	1.3–1.4	0.40
51–60	1.30	0.36–0.40	1.40	1.5–1.6	0.30
41–50	0.40	0.31–0.35	0.80	1.7–1.8	0.10
31–40	0.20	0.26–0.30	0.30	1.9–2.0	0.10
21–30	0.10	0.21–0.25	0.10	>2.0	0.04
11–20	0.00	0.16–0.20	0.10	—	—
≤10	0.09	0.11–0.15	0.04	—	—
—	—	0.05–0.10	0.04	—	—
—	—	≤0.05	0.14	—	—

Abbreviations: Chol-PF, pleural fluid cholesterol; Chol-R, pleural fluid-to-serum cholesterol ratio; LR, likelihood ratio.
Data from Heffner JE, Heffner JN, Brown LK. Multilevel and continuous pleural fluid pH likelihood ratios for evaluating malignant pleural effusions. Chest 2003;123:1887–94.

Summary

Despite advances in chest imaging and other diagnostic modalities, the discrimination between exudates and transudates remains an important first step in evaluating patients with pleural effusions. Multiple tests and test combinations provide acceptable and similar discriminative properties. The three-test Light's criteria represent the traditional approach. Because pleural fluid LDH and the pleural fluid-to-serum LDH ratio have a high degree of correlation, performance of Light's criteria is not significantly diminished by using a paired test approach with the inclusion of the pleural fluid-to-serum protein ratio with one or the other test that incorporates LDH ("abbreviated" Light's criteria). Other test combinations may be preferred clinically, however, because they obviate the need to measure a serum value. The two-test combination of pleural fluid LDH and pleural fluid cholesterol and the three-test combination of pleural fluid protein, pleural fluid LDH, and pleural fluid cholesterol compare favorably with Light's criteria. Clinicians should recognize that considerable diagnostic uncertainty exists with borderline laboratory results and adopt a bayesian approach to classifying pleural effusions. In the future, refined approaches to pleural fluid testing will identify specific diseases and diminish the importance of categorizing effusions as transudates and exudates.

References

[1] Paddock FK. The diagnostic significance of serous fluid in disease. N Engl J Med 1940;223:1010–5.

[2] Peterman TA, Speicher CE. Evaluating pleural effusions: a two-stage laboratory approach. JAMA 1984; 252:1051–3.

[3] Sahn SA. State of the art: the pleura. Am Rev Respir Dis 1988;138:184–234.

[4] Paddock FK. The relationship between the specific gravity and the protein content in human serous effusions. Am J Med Sci 1941;201:569–74.

[5] Carr DT, Power MH. Clinical value of measurement of concentration of protein in pleural fluid. N Engl J Med 1958;259:926–7.

[6] Chandrasekhar AJ, Palatao A, Dubin A, et al. Pleural fluid lactice acid dehydrogenase activity and protein content. Arch Intern Med 1969;123:48–50.

[7] Light RW, MacGregor I, Luchsinger PC, et al. Pleural effusion: the diagnostic separation of transudates and exudates. Ann Intern Med 1972;77:507–13.

[8] Hirsch A, Ruffie P, Nebut M. Pleural effusion: laboratory tests in 300 cases. Thorax 1979;34:106–12.

[9] Roth BJ, O'Meara TF, Cragun WH. The serum-effusion albumin gradient in the evaluation of pleural effusions. Chest 1990;98:546–9.

[10] Heffner JE, Brown LK, Barbieri C. Diagnostic value of tests that discriminate between exudative and transudative pleural effusions. Chest 1997;111:970–9.

[11] Light RW. Pleural diseases. 3rd edition. Baltimore: Williams & Wilkins; 1995.

[12] Chakko SC, Caldwell SH, Sforza PP. Treatment of congestive heart failure: its effect on pleural fluid chemistry. Chest 1989;95:798–802.

[13] Romero-Candeira S, Fernandez C, Martin C, et al. Influence of diuretics on the concentration of proteins and other components of pleural transudates in patients with heart failure. Am J Med 2001;110:681–6.

[14] Burgess L, Maritz FJ, Taljaard JJF. Comparative analysis of the biochemical parameters used to distinguish between pleural transudates and exudates. Chest 1995;107:1604–9.

[15] Romero-Candeira S, Hernandez L, Romero-Brufao S, et al. Is it meaningful to use biochemical parameters to discriminate between transudative and exudative pleural effusions? Chest 2002;122:1524–9.

[16] Hamm H, Brohan U, Bohmer R, et al. Cholesterol in pleural effusions: a diagnostic aid. Chest 1987;92: 296–302.

[17] Valdés L, Pose A, Suàrez J, et al. Cholesterol: a useful parameter for distinguishing between pleural exudates and transudates. Chest 1991;99:1097–102.

[18] Romero S, Candela A, Martín C, et al. Evaluation of different criteria for the separation of pleural transudates from exudates. Chest 1993;104:399–404.

[19] Guleria R, Agarwal SR, Sinha S, et al. Role of pleural fluid cholesterol in differentiating transudative from exudative pleural effusion. Natl Med J India 2003;16: 64–9.

[20] Meisel S, Shamiss A, Thaler M, et al. Pleural fluid to serum bilirubin concentration ratio for the separation of transudates and exudates. Chest 1990;98:141–4.

[21] Garcia-Pachon E, Padilla-Navas I, Sanchez JF, et al. Pleural fluid to serum cholinesterase ratio for the separation of transudates and exudates. Chest 1996;110: 97–101.

[22] Sharma M, Gupta KB, Goyal KM, et al. Evaluation of cholinesterase to differentiate pleural exudates and transudates. J Assoc Physicians India 2004;52: 387–90.

[23] Chan MH, Chow KM, Chan AT, et al. Quantitative analysis of pleural fluid cell-free DNA as a tool for the classification of pleural effusions. Clin Chem 2003;49:740–5.

[24] Kjeldsberg CR, Knight JA. Body fluids. Chicago: American Society of Clinical Pathologists Press; 1993.

[25] Uzun K, Vural H, Ozer F, et al. Diagnostic value of uric acid to differentiate transudates and exudates. Clin Chem Lab Med 2000;38:661–5.

[26] Yilmaz Turay U, Yildirim Z, Turkoz Y, et al. Use of pleural fluid C-reactive protein in diagnosis of pleural effusions. Respir Med 2000;94:432–5.

[27] Gazquez I, Porcel JM, Vives M, et al. Pleural alkaline phosphatase in separation of transudative and exudative pleural effusions. Chest 1997;112:569–70.

[28] Metintas M, Alatas O, Alatas F, et al. Comparative analysis of biochemical parameters for differentiation of pleural exudates from transudates Light's criteria, cholesterol, bilirubin, albumin gradient, alkaline phosphatase, creatine kinase, and uric acid. Clin Chim Acta 1997;264:149–62.

[29] Alexandrakis MG, Kyriakou D, Alexandraki R, et al. Pleural interleukin-1beta in differentiating transudates and exudates: comparative analysis with other biochemical parameters. Respiration (Herrlisheim) 2002; 69:201–6.

[30] Alexandrakis MG, Coulocheri SA, Bouros D, et al. Evaluation of ferritin, interleukin-6, interleukin-8 and tumor necrosis factor alpha in the differentiation of exudates and transudates in pleural effusions. Anticancer Res 1999;19:3607–12.

[31] Alexandrakis MG, Kyriakou DS, Bouros D, et al. Interleukin-6 and its relationships to acute phase proteins in serous effusion differentiation. Oncol Rep 2001;8:415–20.

[32] Frola C, Cantoni S, Turtulici I, et al. Transudative vs exudative pleural effusions: differentiation using Gd-DTPA-enhanced MRI. Eur Radiol 1997;7:860–4.

[33] Baysal T, Bulut T, Gokirmak M, et al. Diffusion-weighted MR imaging of pleural fluid: differentiation of transudative vs exudative pleural effusions. Eur Radiol 2004;14:890–6.

[34] Wolek R, Mason BJ, Reeser P, et al. Pleural fluid: accuracy of computed tomography in differentiating exudates from transudates. Conn Med 1998;62: 259–65.

[35] Bartter T, Santarelli RJ, Pratter MR. Transudate vs exudate: genug! Chest 1996;109:1419–21.

[36] Sutton AJ, Abrams KR, Jones DR, et al. Methods for meta-analysis in medical research. New York: John Wiley & Sons; 2000.

[37] Hanley JA. Receiver operating characteristic (ROC) methodolgy: the state of the art. Crit Rev Diagn Imaging 1989;29:307–35.

[38] Deeks JJ. Systematic reviews in health care: systematic reviews of evaluations of diagnostic and screening tests. BMJ 2001;323:157–62.

[39] Jimenez Castro D, Diaz Nuevo G, Perez-Rodriguez E. [Comparative analysis of Light's criteria and other biochemical parameters to distinguish exudates from transudates]. Rev Clin Esp 2002;202:3–6 [in Spanish].

[40] Yilmaz A, Tunaboyu IK, Akkaya E, et al. A comparative analysis of the biochemical parameters used to distinguish between pleural exudates and transudates. Respirology 2000;5:363–7.

[41] Gazquez I, Porcel JM, Vives M, et al. Comparative analysis of Light's criteria and other biochemical parameters for distinguishing transudates from exudates. Respir Med 1998;92:762–5.

[42] Porcel JM, Vives M, Vicente de Vera MC, et al. Useful tests on pleural fluid that distinguish transudates from exudates. Ann Clin Biochem 2001;38(Pt 6):671–5.

[43] Costa M, Quiroga T, Cruz E. Measurement of pleural fluid cholesterol and lactate dehydrogenase: a simple and accurate set of indicators for separating exudates from transudates. Chest 1995;108:1260–3.

[44] Heffner JE. Evaluating diagnostic tests in the pleural space: differentiating transudates from exudates as a model. Clin Chest Med 1998;19:277–93.

[45] Jaeschke R, Guyatt G, Sackett D. Users' guides to the medical literature: III. how to use an article about a diagnostic test. JAMA 1994;271:703–7.

[46] Sackett DL, Straus SE, Richardson WS, et al. Evidence-based medicine: how to practice and teach EBM. 2nd edition. Edinburgh: Churchill Livingstone; 2000.

[47] Moltyaner Y, Miletin MS, Grossman RF. Transudative pleural effusions: false reassurance against malignancy. Chest 2000;118:885.

[48] Ryu JS, Ryu ST, Kim YS, et al. What is the clinical significance of transudative malignant pleural effusion? Korean J Intern Med 2003;18:230–3.

[49] Deeks JJ, Altman DG. Diagnostic tests 4: likelihood ratios. BMJ 2004;329:168–9.

[50] Heffner JE, Sahn SA, Brown LK. Multilevel likelihood ratios for identifying exudative pleural effusions(*). Chest 2002;121:1916–20.

[51] Simel DL, Samsa GP, Matchar DB. Likelihood ratios for continuous test results—making the clinicians' job easier or harder? J Clin Epidemiol 1993;46:85–93.

[52] Heffner JE, Highland K, Brown LK. A meta-analysis derivation of continuous likelihood ratios for diagnosing pleural fluid exudates. Am J Respir Crit Care Med 2003;167:1591–9.

[53] Leuallen EC, Carr DT. Pleural effusion, a statistical study of 436 patients. N Engl J Med 1955;252(3): 79–83.

[54] Light RW. Pleural disease. 3rd edition. Baltimore: Williams & Wilkins; 1995.

[55] Suay VG, Moragón EM, Viedma EC, et al. Pleural cholesterol in differentiating transudates and exudates: a prospective study of 232 cases. Respiration (Herrlisheim) 1995;62:57–63.

[56] Heffner JE, Heffner JN, Brown LK. Multilevel and continuous pleural fluid pH likelihood ratios for evaluating malignant pleural effusions. Chest 2003; 123:1887–94.

ELSEVIER
SAUNDERS

Clin Chest Med 27 (2006) 253 – 266

CLINICS
IN CHEST
MEDICINE

The Approach to the Patient with a Parapneumonic Effusion

Najib M. Rahman, BM, BCh, MA, MRCP*,
Stephen J. Chapman, BM, BCh, MA, MRCP, Robert J.O. Davies, DM, FRCP

Oxford Pleural Diseases Unit, Oxford Centre for Respiratory Medicine, Churchill Hospital Site, Oxford Radcliffe Hospital, Headington, Oxford OX3 7LJ, UK

Pleural effusion in the context of a pneumonic illness is a frequent clinical problem. Pneumonia is a common illness, with an estimated annual incidence of between 5 and 11 cases per 1000 population [1], translating to around 50,000 hospital admissions in the United Kingdom per year. Between 40% and 57% of cases of pneumonia [2] are associated with pleural effusion. Up to one third of exudative pleural effusions occur in association with a pneumonic illness. Each year, there are approximately 60,000 cases of pleural infection in the United Kingdom and United States [3], and 20,000 of these patients need surgery or die.

Although most patients with a parapneumonic effusion respond to antibiotic therapy, a significant number develop complex intrapleural collections that progress to become frankly purulent, known as empyema at this stage. The mortality and morbidity of this condition are high, with 15% of UK cases resulting in surgery and a mortality rate of greater than 20% [4]. The current treatment strategy involves antibiotics and drainage of the pleural space, with intrapleural thrombolytic agents and surgery used in certain cases. The timing of interventional treatment and which options to choose are unclear, however. Several recent trials have addressed some of the key issues in this area, but much is still unknown.

This review seeks to discuss the diagnosis and management of patients with parapneumonic effusion and empyema on basis of current available evidence.

---

* Corresponding author.
E-mail address: naj_rahman@yahoo.co.uk
(N.M. Rahman).

Background

The first description of pleural infection has been ascribed to the Egyptian physician Imhotep around 3000 BC, but it was more famously described by Hippocrates in 500 BC. Until the early twentieth century, the only treatment available was open surgical drainage, with associated high mortality; at that time, closed-tube drainage became widely practiced. The principles of treatment established during the flu pandemic of 1917 through 1919 have remained in place up to the present time.

Pathogenesis and definitions

Empyema is defined as pus within the pleural space. In its development, pleural fluid passes through stages of increasing host defense activity and bacterial invasion. Not all infected pleural effusions progress to empyema.

Infection within the pulmonary parenchyma is usually contained as pneumonia. If the inflammatory process extends to the visceral and parietal pleura, pleuritic chest pain may be felt and a pleural rub may be heard. Many patients with pneumonia complain of pleuritic chest pain but do not go on to develop an effusion. This fact implies that pleural inflammation alone is insufficient to cause parapneumonic effusion. The presence of pleural fluid is probably required for the development of empyema. Data from animal models suggest that direct inoculation of infected material into a dry pleural space results in over-

chestmed.theclinics.com

whelming sepsis or recovery rather than persisting infection in the form of empyema [5].

The formation of an infected pleural space is a complicated interaction of host defense mechanisms and organisms. There are three distinct pathophysiologic stages in empyema, reflecting changing physiology within the pleural space.

Exudative stage

In response to bacterial infection and continued inflammation within the lung parenchyma and pleural membranes, proinflammatory cytokines, such as interleukin (IL)-8 and tumor necrosis factor (TNF)-α are released locally [6,7]. These act on mesothelial cells and capillaries within the visceral and parietal pleura, leading to increased tissue and capillary permeability. Fluid accumulates within the pleural space (a combination of interstitial tissue fluid and a microvascular exudate) and is not infected, having normal biochemical characteristics (vide infra). The effusion is free flowing, and the pleural membranes are not thickened.

Fibrinopurulent stage

The fibrinopurulent stage occurs in response to bacterial invasion. Early on, the normal profibrinolytic state of the pleural cavity is altered, allowing the formation of fibrin clots and fibrinous septae. Clotting factors from the serum enter the pleural space in abundance, promoting the fibrotic process. This results in a heavily loculated pleural space that may be resistant to drainage with a single intercostal tube. As infection progresses, bacterial invasion promotes neutrophil migration and high levels of metabolic activity. As bacteria and inflammatory cells are lysed, pus is formed.

Organizational stage

The final organizational stage is characterized by fibroblast proliferation and subsequent deposition of thick rinds of fibrous tissue on the inner surface of the pleural membranes, the inelastic "pleural peel." The lung is unable to expand fully, leading to impaired gas exchange, lung function abnormalities, and the potential for chronic infection. The further course after organization is variable; some individuals undergo spontaneous healing with resolution of the pleural thickening [8], whereas others progress to chronic lung function defects and chronic infection of the pleural space [9]. This may result in a lung abscess, bronchopleural fistula, and infected material penetrating the chest wall (empyema necessitans) [9]. The process of organization is known to be driven by mediators, such as transforming growth factor (TGF)-β and platelet-derived growth factor (PDGF) from animal model data [10]. Recent experiments in a well-established animal model of empyema have shown a decrease in the amount of pleural thickening after intrapleural administration of anti-TGFβ antibodies [11].

Pleural fluid changes

The characteristics of pleural fluid pass through distinct changes in the evolution of empyema (Table 1). Initially, pleural fluid accumulates but is not infected (corresponding to the exudative phase). The fluid is sterile and clear with a normal pH. Lactate dehydrogenase (LDH) and glucose levels are normal, and the cell count is not altered. This stage is referred to as "simple parapneumonic effusion," because most of these cases resolve with antibiotics alone [2].

Table 1
Table of pleural fluid characteristics

	Simple parapneumonic effusion	Complicated parapneumonic effusion	Empyema
Appearance	May be slightly turbid	Cloudy	Pus
Biochemical markers	pH >7.30	pH <7.20	n/a
	LDH maybe slightly elevated	LDH >1000 IU/L	
	Glucose >60 mg/dL or pleural/serum ratio >0.5	Glucose <35 mg/dL	
Nucleated cell count	Neutrophils usually <10,000 cells/μL	Neutrophils + + (usually >10,000 cells/μL)	n/a
Microbiology: Gram stain	Negative	May be positive	May be positive
Microbiology: culture	Negative	May be positive	May be positive

Abbreviations: LDH, lactate dehydrogenase; n/a, not applicable.
Data from Davies CW, Gleeson FV, Davies RJ. BTS guidelines for the management of pleural infection. Thorax 2003;58 Suppl 2:ii20.

As inflammation of the pleural space continues, bacterial invasion occurs via leaky capillaries and damaged lung tissue. This encourages further neutrophil migration and cell lysis, leading to release of bacterial proteins and a highly metabolically active pleural space. The characteristic biochemical features of infection develop; low pH (secondary to lactate and carbon dioxide [CO_2] production), low glucose (secondary to white cell and bacterial glycolysis), and high LDH (secondary to cell turnover) [2,12–15]. The effusion is referred to as "complicated parapneumonic effusion," correlating to the early fibrinopurulent stage in which features of infection are present but the fluid is not frankly purulent. The fluid may be turbid, contains high numbers of neutrophils, and may reveal organisms on Gram stain or culture. Most of these effusions do not resolve with antibiotics alone, requiring tube drainage (vide infra).

The appearance of pus in the pleural space correlates to the late fibrinopurulent stage and is diagnostic of empyema, regardless of biochemical markers (ie, macroscopically visible evidence of bacterial and leukocyte cell death). It is generally accepted that tube drainage is required for resolution. Once again, Gram stain and culture may be positive or negative.

The presence of bacteria promotes the coagulation cascade in favor of fibrin deposition and inhibition of fibrinolysis, eventually resulting in fibroblast proliferation (the organizing stage) [16,17]. Factors like tissue plasminogen inhibitor (PAI)-1 and PAI-2 and TNFα are increased in empyema and complicated parapneumonic effusions compared with effusions from malignancy and other causes [18], with direct evidence of mesothelial cell release [19]. Effusions of other causes may become loculated, but the depression of the fibrinolytic system (as demonstrated by elevated PAI and depressed tissue-type plasminogen activator [tPA]) has not been shown in effusions secondary to malignancy or transudative causes [18,20].

Epidemiology

Empyema occurs more commonly during childhood and in the elderly [21,22]. Pleural infection is most commonly a complication of bacterial pneumonia; hence, patients at risk for pneumonia are also at risk of pleural infection. Independent risk factors for empyema include diabetes mellitus, alcohol abuse, gastroesophageal reflux disease, and intravenous drug abuse [4]. Poor dental hygiene and aspiration predispose to infection with anaerobic organisms [23].

Up to one third of cases occur without as yet identified risk factors [4].

The remaining cases of pleural infection unrelated to pneumonia are largely iatrogenic, including thoracic (20%) and esophageal surgery, esophageal perforation, and trauma (5%) [24–26]. Infection may be introduced into a pleural effusion of any cause by thoracocentesis (2% of cases of empyema) or during intervention for primary spontaneous pneumothorax (2%), underlining the importance of appropriate use of invasive pleural procedures for these conditions. Abdominal sepsis or spontaneous bacterial peritonitis may cause empyema (1%), which is sometimes seen after complications in laparoscopic cholecystectomy or splenectomy. Rarely, a primary infection of the pleural space may occur.

Although most pleural infections occur in the context of adjacent consolidated lung, it is increasingly recognized that a minimal amount of consolidation may be seen. This theory is supported by the frequent finding of oropharyngeal organisms in infected pleural fluid.

Bacteriology

The microbiology of pleural infection shows substantial variation according to clinical context and the reported series [20]. There are clear differences in the pathogen pattern between hospital- and community-acquired infections in a manner analogous to pneumonia but with markedly different organisms.

Gram-positive aerobic bacteria are by far the most common cause of pleural infection regardless of setting, with streptococcal species most commonly found, followed by staphylococci [20]. The incidence of *Streptococcus pneumoniae* as a cause of pleural infection has markedly decreased, presumably with widespread use of β-lactam antibiotics, to represent approximately 10% of cases at the present time [27], although use of the polymerase chain reaction (PCR) suggests a figure closer to 25% (R.J.O. Davies, DM, unpublished data, 2005). Gram-negative aerobes are also a common cause of pleural infection, although occurring more frequently in the hospital-acquired setting; organisms in this group include *Haemophilus influenzae*, *Escherichia coli*, *Pseudomonas*, and *Klebsiella*, to which diabetic patients seem to be particularly susceptible [28]. Resistant organisms (particularly methicillin-resistant *Staphylococcus aureus* [MRSA]) are a common cause of hospital-acquired pleural infection [27]. The incidence of anaerobic bacteria causing pleural infection is variably reported to range from 14% to 32% [20].

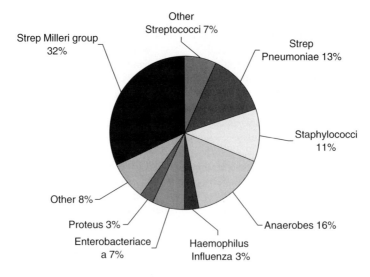

Fig. 1. MIST 1 cohort microbiology in those with positive cultures, community-acquired infections.

In the recently published report on the Multicenter Intrapleural Sepsis Trial (MIST 1) [29], 454 patients with pleural infection were recruited, of whom 300 (66%) achieved a microbiologic diagnosis using conventional methods [27]. In this cohort (Figs. 1–3), community-acquired infections were caused by streptococcal species (most commonly *Streptococcus milleri* and *S pneumoniae*), followed by staphylococci and a number of gramnegative organisms, with anaerobes in only 16% of cases. Of hospital-acquired cases, almost 50% were caused by staphylococci (of which almost two thirds were MRSA), with most of the remain-

der caused by gram-negative organisms. This translates to frequent infection with organisms resistant to standard antibiotics in the hospital-acquired setting (eg, MRSA, Enterobacteriaceae, enterococci, and *Pseudomonas* responsible for 60% of such cases) [27].

One third of the MIST 1 cohort did not achieve a microbiologic diagnosis with conventional methods, a figure typical for pleural infection [27]. This implies that empiric therapy is required in many cases; it seems likely that the culture-negative cases are caused by streptococcal species partially treated with antibiotics, although this is not proven. Blood cul-

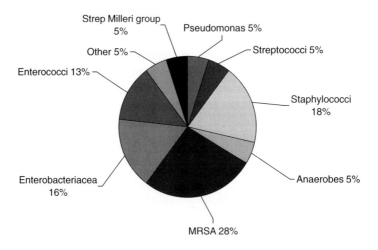

Fig. 2. MIST 1 cohort microbiology in those with positive cultures, hospital-acquired infections.

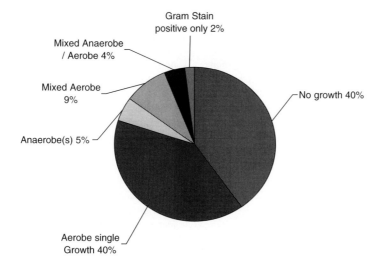

Fig. 3. MIST 1 cohort: summary of microbiology.

tures are positive in a few cases of pleural infection (12%); when positive, such a blood culture is often the only microbiologic test with a positive result [27].

These results have implications for empiric therapy, underline the important differences between hospital- and community-acquired infections, and demonstrate the poor yield of standard microbiologic tests.

Clinical features and differential diagnosis

Patients with pleural infection most commonly present with the clinical picture of pneumonia: acute onset of cough, fever, purulent sputum, and dyspnea. Pleuritic chest pain (implying parietal pleural involvement) is by no means universal, and its absence does not exclude the diagnosis of pleural infection [2]. Anaerobic infections often present in an indolent manner with weight loss, anorexia, and malaise [30]. The average time from symptom onset to assessment in secondary care is 14 days [4], however, suggesting substantial delay in presentation.

Pleural infection should be suspected in any case of nonresolving pneumonia on antibiotics, a situation requiring prompt clinical and radiologic evaluation. An assessment of risk factors for empyema is of importance, because coexistent alcohol abuse has been found to be associated with empyema in a substantial number of cases [29,31,32]. Anaerobic infection is associated with poor oral hygiene and presumed aspiration of oral contents; hence, a predisposition to aspiration (eg, after an episode of im-

paired consciousness) is likely to increase the chance of infection.

The diagnosis is normally made on the basis of specific tests, but there are important differential diagnoses to consider. Pulmonary embolus with associated pulmonary infarction may present in a similar manner, as may tuberculous pleuritis, rheumatoid pleuritis, lupus pleuritis, or effusion secondary to pancreatitis. In the case of indolent infection, empyema may initially present as possible lung malignancy.

Several studies have shown that there are no clinical criteria able to distinguish between those with pneumonia and those with parapneumonic effusion or to identify those with parapneumonic effusion that requires drainage [21,33]. No differences have been demonstrated in age, temperature, the presence of pain, the presence of infiltrate on a chest radiograph, or white cell count between patients responding to medical treatment and those requiring further interventions [2]. Although large effusion size [4] and pleural fluid purulence [34] were previously observed to be associated with a worse outcome, the MIST 1 cohort did not support these findings [29].

Diagnosis of parapneumonic effusion or empyema

There are no clinical features (including blood tests and radiology) reliably able to predict which patients with parapneumonic effusion require drainage. Hence, it is recommended that all patients in whom pleural infection is suspected should have a pleural aspirate for diagnostic purposes [20]. The exception to this is a small pleural effusion (defined as <10 mm on a lateral decubitus chest radiograph), because clinical experience suggests that such effusions resolve with antibiotics alone [2,35]. For small effusions, ultrasound-guided aspiration is recommended as a safer and more accurate method, reducing patient discomfort [36]. The presence of frank pus on thoracocentesis is diagnostic of empyema, and no further tests are needed to confirm the diagnosis. A gram-positive stain or positive culture of nonpurulent pleural fluid is diagnostic of a complicated parapneumonic effusion, which should be managed similar to empyema.

Pleural fluid analysis

Pleural fluid from parapneumonic effusions and empyemas is an exudate; the presence of a transudate on the basis of the criteria of Light and colleagues [37] suggests an alternative diagnosis. The absolute value of the protein level is of no value in determining the outcome [33]. The presence of a predominance of lymphocytes (as opposed to neutrophils) should raise the possibility of malignancy or tuberculosis.

In the absence of purulent fluid and positive microbiology results, biochemical markers are used as surrogates for evidence of active pleural infection, with the characteristic changes in pH, LDH, and glucose (vide supra).

Parapneumonic effusions with an acidic pH (<7.20) are at increased risk of developing multiseptated collections and frank empyema if intercostal drainage is not instituted, in contrast to effusions with a nonacidic pH, which tend to resolve without drainage [2,13]. Many trials have assessed the value of various biochemical markers in predicting which patients require tube drainage [20]. Inherent in this strategy is the assumption that those patients who run a "complicated" course with antibiotics alone (ie, develop septations and frank empyema) benefit from early institution of tube drainage; although this seems likely and biologically sensible, there is no direct supportive evidence.

A meta-analysis [15] critically assessed the markers best able to separate effusions that are likely to run a simple course from those that are likely to run a complicated course (ie, become frankly purulent, nonpurulent fluid requiring drainage, and nonpurulent fluid progressing to frank pus later in the clinical course or at autopsy) using area under the curve receiver operating characteristic (ROC) statis-

tical techniques. Pleural fluid pH emerged as the best predictor of a complicated course, with the exact value determined by pretest probability, prevalence, and cost issues (7.29 for low clinical suspicion and 7.21 for high-risk patients). In this analysis, pleural fluid glucose and LDH did not improve diagnostic accuracy in addition to pH, and reliance on these values (glucose <35 mg/dL and LDH >1000 IU/L) is only recommended when accurate pH values are not available.

Current guidelines [20,35] therefore recommend institution of tube drainage in the appropriate clinical context with a pH less than 7.20. Those patients with a pH greater than 7.20 usually respond to antibiotics alone, although in patients not responding to treatment, repeat sampling is recommended. Support for this strategy comes from data indicating that some patients with pleural fluid with an initial pH greater than 7.20 eventually progress to requiring surgical intervention for empyema [21]; hence, a single pH level greater than 7.20 should be used to predict patients who are likely to respond to antibiotics alone in 100% of cases. The presence of gram- or culture-positive pleural fluid should be taken as diagnostic of pleural infection, and appropriate treatment should be instituted regardless of pleural pH. It should be noted that a lower threshold for intervention is probably required in older patients with more comorbidities, given their increased mortality [15].

Pleural fluid pH should be collected in a heparinized syringe, separately from syringes containing lignocaine (which is acidic [38]), and analyzed immediately using a blood gas analyser. Measuring pH via litmus paper has been shown to be unreliable [39], and substantial clinical experience suggests that measuring pH on nonpurulent pleural fluid using blood gas analyzers does not cause damage to the equipment. The pH should not be measured in frankly purulent pleural fluid, because tube drainage should be instituted regardless of the pH value.

Caution is needed in overinterpreting a single pleural fluid pH measurement in the diagnosis of pleural infection, especially if the clinical context is not consistent. Several other conditions result in an acidic pleural space, including malignant effusion, rheumatoid, lupus pleuritis, and tuberculosis. One study has shown variable pH measurements in different loculations of the same parapneumonic effusion greater than and less than the generally agreed action threshold of 7.20 [40]. Conversely, some patients with a parapneumonic pleural pH greater than 7.20 proceed to surgery despite drainage [21]; hence, the test is not 100% sensitive and cannot be used to predict those requiring surgery. Occasionally, a urea-splitting organism (eg, *Proteus* species) may result in an alkalotic pleural fluid pH [41].

Recent data suggest the use of pleural fluid TNFα levels as a reliable differentiator of simple parapneumonic effusion from complex parapneumonic effusion or empyema [42,43]. In an analysis of 80 patients, a TNFα level greater than 80 pg/mL was shown to be as useful in diagnosing pleural infection as pH, glucose, and LDH as well as being useful in guiding management decisions [42]. In a study of 81 patients, a pleural fluid-serum TNFα gradient of 9.0 pg/mL accurately discriminated between complicated and simple parapneumonic effusion, with sensitivity and specificity greater than 95% [43].

Pleural fluid microbiology

Standard pleural fluid culture is positive in approximately 60% of cases of pleural infection but is less efficient in the diagnosis of anaerobic infection [27]. Pleural fluid is normally sent for microbiologic analysis in a sterile container. Inoculation of pleural fluid into growth medium (ie, "blood culture bottles") may increase diagnostic yield, perhaps specifically when anaerobic infection is concerned, in an analogous way to spontaneous bacterial peritonitis [44]. One study exists in support of this theory in aerobic infection, but larger trials are needed to establish its role and address the minimum volume of inoculate required [45].

Radiology

The radiologic changes of pleural infection are covered in detail in the article on imaging of pleural disease in this issue.

The chest radiograph usually confirms the clinical suspicion of pleural fluid with or without parenchymal consolidation. The effusion is often loculated and may show evidence of air-fluid levels. The presence of an encapsulated effusion in a nondependent position makes empyema likely [46]. Empyema may present as a pleural mass or loculated area of fluid within the fissure, being mistaken for a pleural or pulmonary malignancy.

Small effusions may be identified using lateral decubitus views [35]. If less than 1-cm thick on decubitus films, effusions may resolve without drainage [2], and therefore do not require sampling, although the need for a lateral decubitus view rather than a standard lateral view has recently been called

into question [47]. With the advent of widely available ultrasound (US), decubitus views are largely being superseded, because US permits assessment of effusion location and character (eg, septations) and allows accurate diagnostic sampling and therapeutic drainage with a low complication rate [36,48,49]. US is able to identify exudative effusions, is more sensitive in estimating the amount of pleural fluid, and is successful in 97% of attempted pleural fluid aspirations [50]. The presence of dense echogenicity in a series of 320 cases predicted empyema and hemorrhage [51]. Loculations on thoracic US have been shown to predict a poor outcome, but whether this should promote prompt chest tube drainage is unknown [52,53].

Contrast-enhanced thoracic CT is a useful tool in differentiating pulmonary abscess from empyema, with empyema displaying the "split pleura sign" with enhancement of visceral and parietal pleura around an infected collection [54,55]. The absence of pleural thickening in suspected empyema is important, because 86% to 100% of empyemas are associated with pleural thickening [56]. CT is not reliably able to differentiate pleural thickening from a malignant or infective etiology [57], however, for which fluorodeoxyglucose (FDG) positron emission tomography is likely to be effective [58].

MRI in pleural infection may be of value in identifying loculations [59] and is able to identify infiltration of the chest wall [59], although it is unable to differentiate malignant from infective disease.

Treatment

Treatment of patients with pleural infection relies on rapid recognition of the condition, appropriate antibiotic use, chest drainage when appropriate, and attention to good basic care, including nutrition.

Nutrition

Patients with empyema enter a catabolic state; hence, good nutrition is vital. It has been observed that patients with low serum albumin have a worse outcome from empyema [4], although no trials have addressed this issue with aggressive nutritional support.

Antibiotics

All patients suspected of having pleural infection should be given antibiotics [20]. When possible, this should be based on the results of pleural and blood microbiology, but treatment should not be delayed until these results are available. "Empiric" antibiotic regimens are therefore recommended until the culture results are available or patients remain culture-negative (as seen in 40% of cases) [27].

In community-acquired infection, likely organisms include *S milleri*, *S pneumoniae*, staphylococci, and *H influenzae*. Although the *S milleri* group is highly sensitive to B-lactams, a substantial proportion of the others are resistant to B-lactams [60], and anaerobic infection occurs in approximated 10%. Antibiotic choice is dictated by local policy, but a suggested regimen for community-acquired infection is a second-generation cephalosporin (eg, cefuroxime) or aminopenicillin with a β-lactamase inhibitor plus anaerobic coverage (eg, metronidazole).

For patients sensitive to penicillins or cephalosporins, a combination of ciprofloxacin plus clindamycin covers all likely pathogens. So-called "atypical" bacteria are an exceedingly rare cause of pleural infection, although they may cause a simple parapneumonic effusion [61].

To cover resistant gram-positive and gram-negative bacteria, broad-spectrum antibiotics are required in hospital-acquired infection or in those patients who have had a prior transthoracic procedure. Staphylococcal infection is an important cause of hospital-acquired empyema, with MRSA in 25% of the MIST cohort [27]. A combination of carbapenems (eg, meropenem) and a drug with anti-MRSA activity (eg, vancomycin) is likely to be needed. The incidence of MRSA infections suggests that recent hospital admission is a major risk factor [62]; hence, any patient with a recent admission to the hospital or with a prior transthoracic procedure should be given an appropriate antibiotic.

Pleural penetration of most antibiotics is excellent [63], and intrapleural antibiotics are not necessary. Although gentamicin has good antistaphylococcal and anti-MRSA activity, its use is not recommended in empyema; its pleural space penetration is poor and drug activity is poor in acidic environments [64].

Any antibiotic regimen should be rationalized once culture results become available, although given the difficulty in culturing anaerobic organisms, continuation of antianaerobic therapy may be necessary in the absence of a positive anaerobic culture.

There exist no direct data on how long to treat empyema. Most authorities consider treatment for at least 3 weeks, with at least 1 week of intravenous antibiotics. Support for this comes from treatment of intraparenchymal lung abscesses [60]; however, if the adopted drainage strategy is successful, it may be that a shorter course of antibiotics is adequate.

Closed intercostal drainage

The first reported account of treatment for pleural infection was by Hippocrates in 400 BC [65]. Drainage of an infected pleural space has long been a guiding principle in successful treatment, especially after mortality was much reduced in the influenza epidemic of 1917 with the introduction of closed-tube drainage as opposed to open surgical drainage [66].

There is consensus of opinion that frank pus within the pleural space requires prompt tube drainage [20,35]. The pleural space should be drained in cases of complicated parapneumonic effusion, as defined by a low pH or positive microbiologic findings [15]. Parapneumonic effusions with a pH greater than 7.30, even if large, usually resolve with antibiotic treatment. The evidence supports using pleural fluid pH as the best predictor of effusions requiring drainage, regardless of size [15,20]. Large uncomplicated parapneumonic effusions may be drained or undergo large-volume thoracocentesis for symptomatic relief of dyspnea.

Repeated thoracocentesis may be an alternative strategy to intercostal drain insertion, with advantages of increased mobility and lower complication and infection rates. This management strategy has been shown to be effective in a rabbit model of empyema [67] and has been reported in two nonrandomized series in adults [68,69] and one in children [70]. No randomized evidence to date has compared this strategy directly with tube drainage, and this strategy is not as yet widely practiced. It may become a valuable tool in the outpatient management of highly selected cases in the future.

Many authorities believe that a large-bore chest drain (>20 French) is necessary to drain the pleural space in empyema adequately. There is no randomized definitive evidence to guide which size of chest drain is optimal in management [71,72]; many series have reported success with smaller bore catheters (eg, 14 French) [36,72–75], which are associated with less discomfort and a low rate of complications. Furthermore, the role of suction and flushes (sterile saline, 30 mL, administered every day) has not been adequately studied, although clinical experience suggests that small-bore chest tubes should be used in conjunction with a suction and flush regimen applied by trained nurses. Flushing and suction of large-bore chest tubes is unlikely to confer any advantage in terms of maintaining drain patency, and because these tubes are usually not connected to a three-way tap system, this has potential complications.

The optimal timing of drain removal is unknown, although clinical response in the patient is clearly the most important parameter. Some authorities suggest removing the drain once pleural fluid is being produced at a rate less than 150 mL/d.

Radiologic insertion of chest drains is likely to offer significant advantages if available [36,76], because the complication rate is lower, accidental insertion of drains into the liver or spleen is avoided in the case of an unsuspected raised hemidiaphragm, and the presence of a multiloculated pleural space is established, allowing insertion of the drain into the largest locule.

In those effusions failing to resolve with a single chest drain, further radiologic assessment allows confirmation of correct placement, repositioning, and further chest drain insertion into nonaccessed loculations [77]. Contrast-enhanced CT is a valuable tool to assess visceral pleural thickening preventing adequate lung expansion. Intriguingly, there are no CT criteria reliably able to predict outcome from tube drainage [54]. Failure of chest tube drainage heralds increased morbidity and mortality [78], and should therefore prompt swift further evaluation and consideration of further therapies.

Intrapleural fibrinolytics

The progress of infected pleural collections into the fibrinopurulent stage heralds the establishment of a heavily septated pleural space with multiple loculations. This is well seen at thoracic US and directly demonstrated at thoracoscopy. The loculations prevent easy drainage of the pleural fluid via a single chest tube and are thought to be the reason for failure of "medical treatment."

More than 50 years ago, Tillett and Sherry [79] instilled broth from streptococcal cultures containing bacterial enzymes into the pleural space of patients with resistant empyema, with some benefits in drainage. Although the enzymes contained fibrinolytic and DNAse activity, most subsequent practice has focused on the use of fibrinolytic agents to break up fibrin adhesions.

There are many observational studies showing the apparent benefit of fibrinolytics (the reader is referred to the article by Davies and colleagues [20] for a comprehensive set of references). These observations are supported by five randomized studies in adults [80–84] showing high success rates of between 60% and 95%. These studies have different inclusion criteria and outcome measures (one study compares streptokinase with urokinase [85]), and the total number of patients recruited is small (N = 207). None of these studies were individually powered to assess the need for surgery or mortality, and their

designs were different. Similar small controlled trials exist in the pediatric literature [86,87]. A Cochrane review conducted in 2004 [88] concluded that although fibrinolytics conferred some benefits (eg, decreased hospital stay, improved radiographic appearance, decreased rate of surgery), these were not consistent across the studies. On the basis of the available randomized data, benefit from use of fibrinolytics in empyema was unproven, and therefore not recommended [88].

The MIST 1 [29] study recruited 454 patients with empyema (on the basis of pH, microbiology, or fluid purulence) across 52 UK hospitals and, in addition to normal treatment of antibiotics and chest drainage, randomized to blind treatment with intrapleural streptokinase or intrapleural saline. No difference was found in the rates of death or surgery at 3 or 12 months (primary outcome measure), together occurring in approximately 30% of patients. Subgroup analysis demonstrated that regardless of the characteristic studied (purulence, radiographic appearance, or parapneumonic effusion) no difference was demonstrated between streptokinase and placebo. There were also no differences in the secondary outcome measures of radiographic changes, length of hospital stay, or lung function. Overall, there was no associated increase is systemic activation of the thrombolytic cascade, and a small increase in adverse events was mainly associated with immunologic reactions [29].

Hence, the only randomized study powered to address the question of mortality and need for surgery [29] found no benefit from using streptokinase or any benefit in terms of radiology, lung function, or length of hospital stay. There was no appreciable increase in serious adverse events; therefore, although the data suggest that the use of intrapleural fibrinolytics is safe, their routine use is not supported by the evidence. Nevertheless, intrapleural fibrinolytics probably aid in thoracic decompression in the case of large infected pleural collections and are a useful treatment for respiratory embarrassment in this case [29].

It is well documented that fibrinous septae are dissolved by intrapleural streptokinase; hence, an explanation for the lack of benefit in the MIST 1 trial is needed. It is possible that the fibrin adhesions were divided by the streptokinase, but the fluid remaining was so viscid that it was unable to drain out via the chest tube. The original isolate used by Tillett and Sherry [79] contained bacterial deoxyribonuclease (DNAse), an enzyme able to lyse strands of DNA. It is thought that these strands give pus its viscosity, and DNAse has been used with success in the context of viscid secretions in cystic fibrosis [89,90]. In vitro data suggest that although DNAse is highly effective in reducing pus viscosity, thrombolytics have no such effect [91,92]. There is one case report [93] and a series of 15 cases [94] (using streptokinase plus strepdornase) of DNAse being used to treat empyema, and further studies are needed to clarify its role.

Surgical treatment

Medical therapy fails in up to 30% of patients with empyema [29,32], and these patients are generally referred for surgical options. The optimum timing of surgery and indications for referral are unknown [20], and no good-quality data exist to guide the clinician. Although observational studies [33,34,53,95] suggest that those with purulent pleural fluid and those with loculations are more likely to need surgery, there are data suggesting that these parameters are not predictive [29,54], and many such patients make a complete recovery without recourse to surgery. It is generally accepted that patients who are not improving clinically and radiologically after 7 days of standard treatment should be discussed with a surgical center experienced in the management of empyema [20,96].

Video-assisted thoracoscopic surgery (VATS) is a possible next step in the treatment of empyema when tube drainage has failed. The adhesions and septae can be divided to aid drainage, although this may need to be done early [97]. This approach is not always adequate, requiring conversion to formal decortication in up to 40% of cases [98,99], implying that the facility to convert to thoracotomy must be in place. More recent series report a higher success rate using VATS [100,101], and a similar retrospective evidence base supports the use of VATS or early thoracotomy in children [102]. There are no randomized trials comparing VATS with thoracotomy, and its role in the treatment of early disease and in chronic empyema is yet to be defined [103].

The outcome from thoracotomy and decortication is generally good, with a success rate of up to 95% [32] in this highly selected group, with associated complications in a significant number [104]. Most deaths from pleural infection occur in old and frail patients. In patients unfit for general anesthesia, local anesthetic rib resection and open surgical drainage are possible. This is a lengthy process, with chest drains being slowly withdrawn over a period of months, with a significant risk of chronic pneumothorax and respiratory failure.

A retrospective review of 93 patients treated for empyema found no difference in mortality between patients treated surgically and medically, although surgical treatment was associated with a longer delay in definitive treatment but a shorter hospital stay [105]. Several retrospective studies suggest that early surgical treatment may hasten recovery and decrease complications in pediatric empyema [106–108].

Only one randomized trial has been conducted comparing VATS with intrapleural streptokinase in 20 patients [109]. Surgery was associated with a shorter hospital stay and shorter drainage times, but in light of the MIST 1 negative results and because of methodologic problems, replication of the study is needed. A Cochrane review evaluating surgical versus nonsurgical treatment of empyema in 2002 [110] included only one study (as cited previously [109]), questioned the validity and size of the study, and concluded that further randomized trials were needed to address this question.

In cases of chronic empyema with persistent sepsis and pleural fibrosis, decortication is likely to be the only treatment option [111], although 40% of these patients may require additional surgery [111]. Given that spontaneous recovery of lung function and resolution of pleural peel [8] are reported weeks after empyema in some cases, the compelling reason to operate on such patients is chronic sepsis rather than lung function derangement. As discussed previously, there are no established predictors of which patients are likely to recover. Decortication for poor lung function alone is probably only justified in those with persistent and severe impairment.

Long-term survival from empyema is good [21] if the patient survives the first year. Longer term sequelae include residual pleural thickening [112], which is seen in up to 13% of patients (more commonly in those with purulent pleural fluid and delayed drainage of more than 15 days) but is not usually associated with significant functional impairment.

Summary

Pleural infection is a common disease with high morbidity and mortality. Although advances have been made in understanding the process, development, and microbiology of this disease, treatment still relies on principles established 100 years ago. Chest drainage is vital in established pleural infection but often fails once loculations develop. The current evidence suggests that intrapleural fibrinolytics do not change the outcome in pleural infection. Surgery remains an important treatment option in many patients, but timing of referral and surgery as well as which surgical modality to choose is not well defined.

References

[1] MacFarlene J, Boswell T, Douglas G, et al. BTS guidelines for the management of community acquired pneumonia in adults. Thorax 2001;56(Suppl 4): IV1–64.

[2] Light RW, Girard WM, Jenkinson SG, et al. Parapneumonic effusions. Am J Med 1980;69(4):507–12.

[3] Sahn SA. Management of complicated parapneumonic effusions. Am Rev Respir Dis 1993;148(3): 813–7.

[4] Ferguson AD, Prescott RJ, Selkon JB, et al. The clinical course and management of thoracic empyema. QJM 1996;89(4):285–9.

[5] Sahn SA, Taryle DA, Good Jr JT. Experimental empyema. Time course and pathogenesis of pleural fluid acidosis and low pleural fluid glucose. Am Rev Respir Dis 1979;120(2):355–61.

[6] Broaddus VC, Hebert CA, Vitangcol RV, et al. Interleukin-8 is a major neutrophil chemotactic factor in pleural liquid of patients with empyema. Am Rev Respir Dis 1992;146(4):825–30.

[7] Kroegel C, Antony VB. Immunobiology of pleural inflammation: potential implications for pathogenesis, diagnosis and therapy. Eur Respir J 1997;10(10): 2411–8.

[8] Neff CC, van Sonnenberg E, Lawson DW, et al. CT follow-up of empyemas: pleural peels resolve after percutaneous catheter drainage. Radiology 1990; 176(1):195–7.

[9] Hamm H, Light RW. Parapneumonic effusion and empyema. Eur Respir J 1997;10(5):1150–6.

[10] Sasse SA, Jadus MR, Kukes GD. Pleural fluid transforming growth factor-beta1 correlates with pleural fibrosis in experimental empyema. Am J Respir Crit Care Med 2003;168(6):700–5.

[11] Kunz CR, Jadus MR, Kukes GD, et al. Intrapleural injection of transforming growth factor-beta antibody inhibits pleural fibrosis in empyema. Chest 2004; 126(5):1636–44.

[12] Sahn SA, Reller LB, Taryle DA, et al. The contribution of leukocytes and bacteria to the low pH of empyema fluid. Am Rev Respir Dis 1983;128(5): 811–5.

[13] Light RW, MacGregor MI, Ball Jr WC, et al. Diagnostic significance of pleural fluid pH and PCO2. Chest 1973;64(5):591–6.

[14] Potts DE, Taryle DA, Sahn SA. The glucose-pH relationship in parapneumonic effusions. Arch Intern Med 1978;138(9):1378–80.

[15] Heffner JE, Brown LK, Barbieri C, et al. Pleural fluid chemical analysis in parapneumonic effusions. A meta-analysis. Am J Respir Crit Care Med 1995; 151(6):1700–8.

[16] Idell S, Girard W, Koenig KB, et al. Abnormalities of pathways of fibrin turnover in the human pleural space. Am Rev Respir Dis 1991;144(1):187–94.

[17] Kroegel C, Antony VB. Immunobiology of pleural inflammation: potential implications for pathogenesis, diagnosis and therapy. Eur Respir J 1997;10(10): 2411–8.

[18] Aleman C, Alegre J, Monasterio J, et al. Association between inflammatory mediators and the fibrinolysis system in infectious pleural effusions. Clin Sci (Lond) 2003;105(5):601–7.

[19] Idell S, Zwieb C, Kumar A, et al. Pathways of fibrin turnover of human pleural mesothelial cells in vitro. Am J Respir Cell Mol Biol 1992;7(4):414–26.

[20] Davies CW, Gleeson FV, Davies RJ. BTS guidelines for the management of pleural infection. Thorax 2003;58(Suppl 2):ii18–28.

[21] Davies CW, Kearney SE, Gleeson FV, et al. Predictors of outcome and long-term survival in patients with pleural infection. Am J Respir Crit Care Med 1999;160(5 Part 1):1682–7.

[22] Givan DC, Eigen H. Common pleural effusions in children. Clin Chest Med 1998;19(2):363–71.

[23] Brook I, Frazier EH. Aerobic and anaerobic microbiology of empyema. A retrospective review in two military hospitals. Chest 1993;103(5):1502–7.

[24] Smith JA, Mullerworth MH, Westlake GW, et al. Empyema thoracis: 14-year experience in a teaching center. Ann Thorac Surg 1991;51(1):39–42.

[25] Snider GL, Saleh SS. Empyema of the thorax in adults: review of 105 cases. Dis Chest 1968;54(5): 410–5.

[26] Yeh TJ, Hall DP, Ellison RG. Empyema thoracis: a review of 110 cases. Am Rev Respir Dis 1963;88: 785–90.

[27] Maskell NA, Davies CW, Jones E, et al. The characteristics of 300 patients participating in the MRC/BTS multicentre intra-pleural streptokinase vs. placebo trial (ISRCTN-39138989). Presented at the American Thoracic Society Meeting. Atlanta (GA), 2002.

[28] Chen KY, Hsueh PR, Liaw YS, et al. A 10-year experience with bacteriology of acute thoracic empyema: emphasis on Klebsiella pneumoniae in patients with diabetes mellitus. Chest 2000;117(6):1685–9.

[29] Maskell NA, Davies CW, Nunn AJ, et al. UK controlled trial of intrapleural streptokinase for pleural infection. N Engl J Med 2005;352(9):865–74.

[30] Bartlett JG, Finegold SM. Anaerobic infections of the lung and pleural space. Am Rev Respir Dis 1974;110(1):56–77.

[31] Alfageme I, Munoz F, Pena N, et al. Empyema of the thorax in adults. Etiology, microbiologic findings, and management. Chest 1993;103(3):839–43.

[32] LeMense GP, Strange C, Sahn SA. Empyema thoracis. Therapeutic management and outcome. Chest 1995;107(6):1532–7.

[33] Poe RH, Marin MG, Israel RH, et al. Utility of pleural fluid analysis in predicting tube thoracostomy/decortication in parapneumonic effusions. Chest 1991;100(4):963–7.

[34] Davies CW, Kearney SE, Gleeson FV, et al. Predictors of outcome and long-term survival in patients with pleural infection. Am J Respir Crit Care Med 1999;160(5 Part 1):1682–7.

[35] Colice GL, Curtis A, Deslauriers J, et al. Medical and surgical treatment of parapneumonic effusions: an evidence-based guideline. Chest 2000;118(4): 1158–71.

[36] Stavas J, van Sonnenberg E, Casola G, et al. Percutaneous drainage of infected and noninfected thoracic fluid collections. J Thorac Imaging 1987; 2(3):80–7.

[37] Light RW, MacGregor MI, Luchsinger PC, et al. Pleural effusions: the diagnostic separation of transudates and exudates. Ann Intern Med 1972;77(4): 507–13.

[38] Jimenez CD, Diaz G, Perez-Rodriguez E, et al. Modification of pleural fluid pH by local anesthesia. Chest 1999;116(2):399–402.

[39] Lesho EP, Roth BJ. Is pH paper an acceptable, low-cost alternative to the blood gas analyzer for determining pleural fluid pH? Chest 1997;112(5): 1291–2.

[40] Maskell NA, Gleeson FV, Darby M, et al. Diagnostically significant variations in pleural fluid pH in loculated parapneumonic effusions. Chest 2004; 126(6):2022–4.

[41] Pine JR, Hollman JL. Elevated pleural fluid pH in Proteus mirabilis empyema. Chest 1983;84(1):109–11.

[42] Porcel JM, Vives M, Esquerda A. Tumor necrosis factor-alpha in pleural fluid: a marker of complicated parapneumonic effusions. Chest 2004;125(1):160–4.

[43] Odeh M, Makhoul B, Sabo E, et al. The role of pleural fluid-serum gradient of tumor necrosis factor-alpha concentration in discrimination between complicated and uncomplicated parapneumonic effusion. Lung 2005;183(1):13–27.

[44] Runyon BA, Antillon MR, Akriviadis EA, et al. Bedside inoculation of blood culture bottles with ascitic fluid is superior to delayed inoculation in the detection of spontaneous bacterial peritonitis. J Clin Microbiol 1990;28(12):2811–2.

[45] Ferrer A, Osset J, Alegre J, et al. Prospective clinical and microbiological study of pleural effusions. Eur J Clin Microbiol Infect Dis 1999;18(4):237–41.

[46] Kirsch E, Guckel C, Kaim A, et al. [The findings and value of computed tomography in pleural empyema]. Rofo 1994;161(5):404–11 [in German].

[47] Metersky ML. Is the lateral decubitus radiograph necessary for the management of a parapneumonic pleural effusion? Chest 2003;124(3):1129–32.

[48] Eibenberger KL, Dock WI, Ammann ME, et al. Quantification of pleural effusions: sonography versus radiography. Radiology 1994;191(3):681–4.

[49] Jones PW, Moyers JP, Rogers JT, et al. Ultrasound-guided thoracentesis: is it a safer method? Chest 2003;123(2):418–23.

[50] O'Moore PV, Mueller PR, Simeone JF, et al. Sonographic guidance in diagnostic and therapeutic interventions in the pleural space. AJR Am J Roentgenol 1987;149(1):1–5.

[51] Yang PC, Luh KT, Chang DB, et al. Value of sonography in determining the nature of pleural effusion: analysis of 320 cases. AJR Am J Roentgenol 1992; 159(1):29–33.

[52] Himelman RB, Callen PW. The prognostic value of loculations in parapneumonic pleural effusions. Chest 1986;90(6):852–6.

[53] Huang HC, Chang HY, Chen CW, et al. Predicting factors for outcome of tube thoracostomy in complicated parapneumonic effusion for empyema. Chest 1999;115(3):751–6.

[54] Kearney SE, Davies CW, Davies RJ, et al. Computed tomography and ultrasound in parapneumonic effusions and empyema. Clin Radiol 2000;55(7):542–7.

[55] Stark DD, Federle MP, Goodman PC, et al. Differentiating lung abscess and empyema: radiography and computed tomography. AJR Am J Roentgenol 1983;141(1):163–7.

[56] Aquino SL, Webb WR, Gushiken BJ. Pleural exudates and transudates: diagnosis with contrast-enhanced CT. Radiology 1994;192(3):803–8.

[57] Waite RJ, Carbonneau RJ, Balikian JP, et al. Parietal pleural changes in empyema: appearances at CT. Radiology 1990;175(1):145–50.

[58] Duysinx B, Nguyen D, Louis R, et al. Evaluation of pleural disease with 18-fluorodeoxyglucose positron emission tomography imaging. Chest 2004;125(2): 489–93.

[59] Evans AL, Gleeson FV. Radiology in pleural disease: state of the art. Respirology 2004;9(3):300–12.

[60] Neild JE, Eykyn SJ, Phillips I. Lung abscess and empyema. Q J Med 1985;57(224):875–82.

[61] Sahn SA. Pleural effusions in the atypical pneumonias. Semin Respir Infect 1988;3(4):322–34.

[62] Lu PL, Chin LC, Peng CF, et al. Risk factors and molecular analysis of community methicillin-resistant Staphylococcus aureus carriage. J Clin Microbiol 2005;43(1):132–9.

[63] Taryle DA, Good Jr JT, Morgan III EJ, et al. Antibiotic concentrations in human parapneumonic effusions. J Antimicrob Chemother 1981;7(2):171–7.

[64] Shohet I, Yellin A, Meyerovitch J, et al. Pharmacokinetics and therapeutic efficacy of gentamicin in an experimental pleural empyema rabbit model. Antimicrob Agents Chemother 1987;31(7):982–5.

[65] Miller Jr JI. The history of surgery of empyema, thoracoplasty, Eloesser flap, and muscle flap transposition. Chest Surg Clin N Am 2000;10(1):45–53 [viii].

[66] Peters RM. Empyema thoracis: historical perspective. Ann Thorac Surg 1989;48(2):306–8.

[67] Sasse S, Nguyen T, Teixeira LR, et al. The utility of daily therapeutic thoracentesis for the treatment of early empyema. Chest 1999;116(6):1703–8.

[68] Simmers TA, Jie C, Sie B. Minimally invasive treatment of thoracic empyema. Thorac Cardiovasc Surg 1999;47(2):77–81.

[69] Storm HK, Krasnik M, Bang K, et al. Treatment of pleural empyema secondary to pneumonia: thoracocentesis regimen versus tube drainage. Thorax 1992; 47(10):821–4.

[70] Shoseyov D, Bibi H, Shatzberg G, et al. Short-term course and outcome of treatments of pleural empyema in pediatric patients: repeated ultrasound-guided needle thoracocentesis vs chest tube drainage. Chest 2002;121(3):836–40.

[71] Patz Jr EF, Goodman PC, Erasmus JJ. Percutaneous drainage of pleural collections. J Thorac Imaging 1998;13(2):83–92.

[72] Ulmer JL, Choplin RH, Reed JC. Image-guided catheter drainage of the infected pleural space. J Thorac Imaging 1991;6(4):65–73.

[73] Merriam MA, Cronan JJ, Dorfman GS, et al. Radiographically guided percutaneous catheter drainage of pleural fluid collections. AJR Am J Roentgenol 1988; 151(6):1113–6.

[74] Silverman SG, Mueller PR, Saini S, et al. Thoracic empyema: management with image-guided catheter drainage. Radiology 1988;169(1):5–9.

[75] Westcott JL. Percutaneous catheter drainage of pleural effusion and empyema. AJR Am J Roentgenol 1985;144(6):1189–93.

[76] Cantin L, Chartrand-Lefebvre C, Lepanto L, et al. Chest tube drainage under radiological guidance for pleural effusion and pneumothorax in a tertiary care university teaching hospital: review of 51 cases. Can Respir J 2005;12(1):29–33.

[77] van Sonnenberg E, Nakamoto SK, Mueller PR, et al. CT- and ultrasound-guided catheter drainage of empyemas after chest-tube failure. Radiology 1984; 151(2):349–53.

[78] Pothula V, Krellenstein DJ. Early aggressive surgical management of parapneumonic empyemas. Chest 1994;105(3):832–6.

[79] Tillett WS, Sherry S. The effects in patients of streptococcal fibrinolysin (streptokinase) and deoxyribonuclease on fibrous, purulent and sanguinous pleural exudates. J Clin Invest 2005;28:173–90.

[80] Davies RJ, Traill ZC, Gleeson FV. Randomised controlled trial of intrapleural streptokinase in community acquired pleural infection. Thorax 1997; 52(5):416–21.

[81] Bouros D, Schiza S, Patsourakis G, et al. Intrapleural streptokinase versus urokinase in the treatment of complicated parapneumonic effusions: a prospective, double-blind study. Am J Respir Crit Care Med 1997; 155(1):291–5.

[82] Bouros D, Schiza S, Tzanakis N, et al. Intrapleural urokinase versus normal saline in the treatment of complicated parapneumonic effusions and empyema. A randomized, double-blind study. Am J Respir Crit Care Med 1999;159(1):37–42.

[83] Diacon AH, Theron J, Schuurmans MM, et al. Intrapleural streptokinase for empyema and complicated parapneumonic effusions. Am J Respir Crit Care Med 2004;170(1):49–53.

[84] Tuncozgur B, Ustunsoy H, Sivrikoz MC, et al. Intrapleural urokinase in the management of parapneumonic empyema: a randomised controlled trial. Int J Clin Pract 2001;55(10):658–60.

[85] Bouros D, Schiza S, Patsourakis G, et al. Intrapleural streptokinase versus urokinase in the treatment of complicated parapneumonic effusions: a prospective, double-blind study. Am J Respir Crit Care Med 1997; 155(1):291–5.

[86] Singh M, Mathew JL, Chandra S, et al. Randomized controlled trial of intrapleural streptokinase in empyema thoracis in children. Acta Paediatr 2004; 93(11):1443–5.

[87] Thomson AH, Hull J, Kumar MR, et al. I. Randomised trial of intrapleural urokinase in the treatment of childhood empyema. Thorax 2002;57(4): 343–7.

[88] Cameron R, Davies HR. Intra-pleural fibrinolytic therapy versus conservative management in the treatment of parapneumonic effusions and empyema. Cochrane Database Syst Rev 2004;2:CD002312.

[89] Fuchs HJ, Borowitz DS, Christiansen DH, et al. Effect of aerosolized recombinant human DNase on exacerbations of respiratory symptoms and on pulmonary function in patients with cystic fibrosis. The Pulmozyme Study Group. N Engl J Med 1994; 331(10):637–42.

[90] McCoy K, Hamilton S, Johnson C. Effects of 12-week administration of dornase alfa in patients with advanced cystic fibrosis lung disease. Pulmozyme Study Group. Chest 1996;110(4):889–95.

[91] Light RW, Nguyen T, Mulligan ME, et al. The in vitro efficacy of varidase versus streptokinase or urokinase for liquefying thick purulent exudative material from loculated empyema. Lung 2000;178(1):13–8.

[92] Simpson G, Roomes D, Heron M. Effects of streptokinase and deoxyribonuclease on viscosity of human surgical and empyema pus. Chest 2000;117(6): 1728–33.

[93] Simpson G, Roomes D, Reeves B. Successful treatment of empyema thoracis with human recombinant deoxyribonuclease. Thorax 2003;58(4):365–6.

[94] Fujiwara K, Yasumitsu T, Nakagawa K, et al. [Intrapleural streptokinase-streptodornase in the treatment of empyema and hemothorax]. Kyobu Geka 2002;55(13):1115–9 [in Japanese].

[95] Lindstrom ST, Kolbe J. Community acquired parapneumonic thoracic empyema: predictors of outcome. Respirology 1999;4(2):173–9.

[96] Pothula V, Krellenstein DJ. Early aggressive surgical management of parapneumonic empyemas. Chest 1994;105(3):832–6.

[97] Sendt W, Forster E, Hau T. Early thoracoscopic debridement and drainage as definite treatment for pleural empyema. Eur J Surg 1995;161(2):73–6.

[98] Ridley PD, Braimbridge MV. Thoracoscopic debride-

ment and pleural irrigation in the management of empyema thoracis. Ann Thorac Surg 1991;51(3):461–4.

[99] Striffeler H, Gugger M, Im H, et al. Video-assisted thoracoscopic surgery for fibrinopurulent pleural empyema in 67 patients. Ann Thorac Surg 1998;65(2):319–23.

[100] Kim BY, Oh BS, Jang WC, et al. Video-assisted thoracoscopic decortication for management of postpneumonic pleural empyema. Am J Surg 2004;188(3):321–4.

[101] Luh SP, Chou MC, Wang LS, et al. Video-assisted thoracoscopic surgery in the treatment of complicated parapneumonic effusions or empyemas: outcome of 234 patients. Chest 2005;127(4):1427–32.

[102] Gates RL, Caniano DA, Hayes JR, et al. Does VATS provide optimal treatment of empyema in children? A systematic review. J Pediatr Surg 2004;39(3):381–6.

[103] Waller DA. Thoracoscopy in management of postpneumonic pleural infections. Curr Opin Pulm Med 2002;8(4):323–6.

[104] Melloni G, Carretta A, Ciriaco P, et al. Decortication for chronic parapneumonic empyema: results of a prospective study. World J Surg 2004;28(5):488–93.

[105] Anstadt MP, Guill CK, Ferguson ER, et al. Surgical versus nonsurgical treatment of empyema thoracis: an outcomes analysis. Am J Med Sci 2003;326(1):9–14.

[106] Chen CF, Soong WJ, Lee YS, et al. Thoracic empyema in children: early surgical intervention hastens recovery. Acta Paediatr Taiwan 2003;44(2):93–7.

[107] Hilliard TN, Henderson AJ, Langton Hewer SC. Management of parapneumonic effusion and empyema. Arch Dis Child 2003;88(10):915–7.

[108] Kalfa N, Allal H, Montes-Tapia F, et al. Ideal timing of thoracoscopic decortication and drainage for empyema in children. Surg Endosc 2004;18(3):472–7.

[109] Wait MA, Sharma S, Hohn J, et al. A randomized trial of empyema therapy. Chest 1997;111(6):1548–51.

[110] Coote N. Surgical versus non-surgical management of pleural empyema. Cochrane Database Syst Rev 2002;2:CD001956.

[111] Martella AT, Santos GH. Decortication for chronic postpneumonic empyema. J Am Coll Surg 1995;180(5):573–6.

[112] Jimenez CD, Diaz G, Perez-Rodriguez E, et al. Prognostic features of residual pleural thickening in parapneumonic pleural effusions. Eur Respir J 2003;21(6):952–5.

ELSEVIER
SAUNDERS

Clin Chest Med 27 (2006) 267 – 283

CLINICS
IN CHEST
MEDICINE

The Spectrum of Pleural Effusions After Coronary Artery Bypass Grafting Surgery

Jay Heidecker, MD*, Steven A. Sahn, MD

Division of Pulmonary, Critical Care, Allergy, and Sleep Medicine, Medical University of South Carolina, 171 Ashley Avenue, Charleston, SC 29425, USA

Coronary artery bypass grafting (CABG) is performed on more than 600,000 patients per year in the United States [1]. Patients commonly develop pleural effusions directly related to this operation, making this procedure one of the most common causes of a pleural effusion. The cause and management differ because of the varied pathogenesis and time course of these pleural effusions. These effusions can be best categorized by time intervals: (1) perioperative (within the first week), (2) early (within 1 month), (3) late (2–12 months), or (4) persistent (after 6 months). The pathophysiology of pleural effusion formation in the perioperative period after CABG can differ; however, these effusions usually resolve without intervention. The effusions that occur later than 1 week and within 1 month typically present with acute chest pain and fever and often require anti-inflammatory medication. The persistent effusions are the consequence of dysfunctional pleural healing, which results in a visceral pleural peel or fibrosis leading to a trapped lung, often requiring decortication.

Perioperative coronary artery bypass grafting pleural effusions

Pleural effusions have been reported to occur in the immediate postoperative period in 41% to 87% of patients [2–6]. These effusions are typically small and left-sided, but they can be bilateral. There are two distinct pleural effusions directly related to

* Corresponding author.
E-mail address: heidecj@musc.edu (J. Heidecker).

CABG in the perioperative period: effusions resulting from atelectasis from diaphragm dysfunction and hemorrhagic effusions resulting from internal mammary artery (IMA) harvesting. In addition, pleural effusions from congestive heart failure may occur after CABG. These pleural effusions are associated with different clinical characteristics, pathophysiology, pleural fluid (PF) analyses, management, and sequelae.

Pleural effusions from diaphragm dysfunction

Clinical characteristics

In the immediate postoperative period, patients often experience substantial chest pain and diaphragm dysfunction that results in a significant decrease in their forced vital capacity (FVC). With conventional chest tube placement, FVC falls by 66% during the first postoperative day and causes an average pain score of 5 of 10 during forced inspiration [7]. The decreased FVC is also likely related to decreased chest wall compliance, interstitial pulmonary edema, and poor bellows function from the median sternotomy. The drop in FVC, per se, may not produce symptoms; however, patients with decreased FVC often manifest a rapid and shallow breathing pattern with resultant atelectasis and small pleural effusions. The chest radiograph often reveals bibasilar-dependent atelectasis with blunting of the left costophrenic or bilateral costophrenic angles.

Pathophysiology

Atelectasis is extremely common after CABG and may be related to diaphragm paresis and/or paralysis. Fedullo and colleagues [8] observed left diaphragm dysfunction in 8 (16%) of 48 post-CABG patients as

chestmed.theclinics.com

detected by comparing right and left diaphragm excursion by ultrasonography. Using the right diaphragm as a control for the bilateral effects of splinting and global reduction in FVC, the presence of left-sided phrenic nerve dysfunction was found in 16% of these patients. Direct cold cardioplegia, associated with an increased incidence of left lower lobe atelectasis [9] and effusion [10], induced phrenic nerve paresis [10]. The phrenic nerve paresis lasted from 6 to 28 days [9]. Lower lobe atelectasis from phrenic nerve paralysis has been replicated in animal models by direct application of cold to the ipsilateral phrenic nerve [11]. Intraoperative electrophysiologic phrenic nerve monitoring during cardiac surgery has confirmed left phrenic nerve paralysis [12]. All cases occurred when moderate hypothermic cardiopulmonary bypass was used as opposed to off-pump CABG [12]. The role of direct cold cardioplegia has been further clarified. Patients with aortic root cooling and cardioplegia with intracoronary cooling without direct cooling of the myocardium did not develop phrenic nerve paresis and/or paralysis in one study [13]. Two of 6 patients with topical ice cooling of the myocardium developed intraoperative left phrenic nerve paresis and/or paralysis, however, as documented by phrenic nerve monitoring [13]. In a study of 30 patients, Vargas and colleagues [6] found an 87% incidence of atelectasis by CT scan 2 days after CABG. These effusions were small and often bilateral. They also found a significant correlation between the degree of atelectasis and presence of pleural effusion between postoperative days 2 and 7 ($r = 0.53$, $P = .0025$) [6]. Left-sided atelectasis with effusion persisted more often than right-sided atelectasis with effusion at hospital day 7. Therefore, the literature supports the concept that the most immediate post-CABG effusions are caused by atelectasis related to splinting from pain, poor chest wall compliance, and diaphragm dysfunction.

Diagnosis, management, and sequelae

The pleural effusions that result from diaphragm dysfunction are often diagnosed by their radiographic appearance. The effusions are small, with associated ipsilateral atelectasis on the left; thoracentesis is rarely performed on these effusions. Management of these effusions is conservative. Avoidance of direct topical cold cardioplegia may lessen the risk of phrenic nerve paresis and/or paralysis and atelectasis. Early mobilization, incentive spirometry, and effective pain control also minimize atelectasis. An improvement in postoperative pain and FVC has been documented with the use of subxiphoid chest tubes

[7]. These pleural effusions usually resolve spontaneously within 2 weeks without clinical sequelae.

Pleural effusions from internal mammary artery harvesting

Clinical characteristics

The surgical technique used can affect the development of pleural effusions after CABG in the immediate postoperative period. The use of an IMA graft [2,4,14,15] tends to result in an ipsilateral pleural effusion more often than a saphenous vein graft (87% versus 47% at postoperative day 6; $P < .05$; $n = 200$) [4]. These effusions usually present similar to the effusion from diaphragm dysfunction; the fluid appears in the immediate perioperative period, is usually small, is ipsilateral to the IMA harvesting, and may be associated with atelectasis. Large pleural effusions in the immediate postoperative period occur with an incidence of 0.5% to 8.5% [4,16,17]. Neither the operative time, number of grafts, nor type of cardioplegia (anterograde or retrograde) was found to be significantly different between patients with large effusions and those without effusions [18]. Most patients with large effusions had IMA harvesting (10.9% of 282 of patients with IMA ± saphenous venous graft (SVG) versus 4.5% of 67 patients with SVG alone, $P = .2$) [18].

Pathophysiology

The presumed cause of pleural effusions attributable to IMA harvesting is parietal pleural injury. The method of IMA harvesting affects the incidence of early post-CABG pleural effusions. When the IMA is harvested with the pleural and thoracic fascia intact, the reported incidence of postoperative pleural effusion is 5% to 11% [19–21]. When the IMA is harvested by incising the pleura and thoracic fascia, the incidence of postoperative pleural effusion increases from 20% [19] to 50% [21]. Furthermore, the chest tube drainage of patients with IMA harvesting with an open incision is significantly increased compared with the drainage of patients without an open incision [4,22] (1413 versus 1028 mL; $P < .01$) [4].

Diagnosis, management, and sequelae

These larger pleural effusions are typically hemorrhagic and inflammatory with elevated protein and lactate dehydrogenase (LDH) levels [18]. In a study of therapeutic thoracentesis for symptomatic patients after CABG, the early large effusions had a mean red blood cell (RBC) count of 706,000 cells/μL, mean white blood cell (WBC) count of 7000 cells/μL with an eosinophil predominance, and mean LDH level of

1368 U/dL [23]. In a prospective study of 602 consecutive patients with CABG, 63% had pleural effusions at 30 days. Most of these effusions were small and did not require any intervention at 3- and 6-month follow-ups, however [18]. Nevertheless, some patients developed larger pleural effusions in the immediate postoperative period that required drainage. Usually, only one or two thoracenteses were required for resolution [18]. In addition, two studies suggest that the use of small-bore intrapleural drains placed during surgery can decrease the incidence of symptomatic pleural effusions [24,25]. These drains remained in place for 3 to 5 days after the large-bore chest tubes were removed. Although the use of small-bore drains did not decrease the length of hospital stay or mortality, they did decrease the number of symptomatic pleural effusions (4 [3.5%] of 115 versus 41 [11.9%] of 345; P=.005) [24]. Diclofenac may decrease pleural effusions after CABG and could be considered to treat large effusions [26]. In the absence of definitive trials, however, the widespread use of anti-inflammatory drugs for symptomatic early pleural effusions cannot be advocated. Because some patients with a persistent pleural effusion after CABG can develop a trapped lung [27] (vide infra), patients with a symptomatic effusion should be followed after therapeutic thoracentesis to ensure resolution.

Other perioperative pleural effusions not directly related to the coronary artery bypass grafting

These pleural effusions may be related to perioperative factors, such as the systemic inflammatory response syndrome (SIRS), decreased ambulation, and secretion management. These pleural effusions are caused by congestive heart failure, pulmonary embolism, and pneumonia, respectively. Chylothorax is a rare complication of thoracic surgery that results from inadvertent thoracic duct injury. These pleural effusions can usually be distinguished by their clinical characteristics and PF analysis.

Congestive heart failure

After CABG, patients often have bilateral effusions; therefore, other mechanisms could be involved. After cardiac surgery, some patients develop a "stunned myocardium." During surgery, patients often require substantial volume loading because of redistribution of fluids secondary to increased vascular permeability. During cardiopulmonary bypass with or without cardioplegia, myocardial edema may

develop. The use of cardiopulmonary bypass causes increased filtration of fluid across myocytes from increased coronary perfusion as well as increased microvascular permeability. An increase in myocardial water by 3.5% has been shown to decrease cardiac output by 40% [28]. Thus, as fluid redistributes into the vascular space, patients with a transient stunned myocardium can develop pulmonary edema with bilateral pleural effusions. Another proposed cause is noncardiogenic pulmonary edema from a systemic inflammatory response. Massoudy and colleagues [29] found markedly increased levels of interleukin (IL)-6, IL-8, and IL-10 after reperfusion following cardiopulmonary bypass. Complement, neutrophils, and platelets may also play a role in acute lung injury [30]. These patients can develop reperfusion pulmonary edema with pleural effusions resulting from increased endothelial permeability and fluid movement into the pleural space. These pleural effusions are usually small and need no specific management. If signs and symptoms of heart failure are present, however, diuretics can be used for symptomatic relief.

Pleural infection

Infectious causes of pleural effusion in the postoperative period after CABG should be considered in the appropriate clinical context. Prolonged chest tube drainage can result in empyema [31,32], most commonly from *Staphylococcus aureus*. These patients usually have fever and purulent chest tube drainage. Empyema from direct infection of a chest tube is uncommon and occurs only when chest tubes remain in place for more than a week. Pleural infection from extension of postoperative pneumonia is a more common presentation. Of 380 cases of empyema, Weissberg and Refaely [33] found that 308 (81%) occurred because of progression of a parapneumonic effusion. Patients with postoperative atelectasis and difficulty in clearing secretions are at risk for pneumonia [29] and present with fever, productive cough, and a new alveolar infiltrate on chest radiography [34,35]. With inadequate treatment of pneumonia, parapneumonic effusions can occur from altered microvascular permeability [36]. Inflammatory mediators cause liquid and protein to leak across capillary barriers into the pleural space at a rate that exceeds the resorptive capacity of the parietal pleural lymphatics. A neutrophilic exudative pleural effusion develops, which, if untreated, can progress to frank empyema. With prompt recognition and appropriate treatment of the pneumonia, less than 2% of such cases progress to empyema [37].

Pulmonary emboli

A pulmonary embolism can also complicate the management of post-CABG patients. Small ipsilateral bloody effusions characterize pleural effusions from a pulmonary embolism. Thus, they can be difficult to distinguish from the bloody pleural effusions related to pleural injury from CABG.

Chylothorax

The thoracic duct, which originates at the cisterna chyle, enters the thorax through the right diaphragm and eventually drains into the left subclavian vein. Its position is usually protected from disruption during surgery; however, lymphatic collaterals, which are common, can be injured. Pego-Fernandes and colleagues [38] reported 12 patients with iatrogenic chylothorax from CABG. Thoracentesis typically reveals a milky exudate with high triglycerides and the presence of chymicrons on lipoprotein electrophoresis. Conservative management with a low-fat diet or parenteral nutrition is usually effective after 10 to 14 days. Serial thoracentesis in these patients can lead to malnutrition and immunologic compromise and should be avoided if possible. The causes of immediate post-CABG pleural effusions and their characteristics on PF analysis are listed in Table 1.

Early postcoronary artery bypass grafting pleural effusions

Postcardiac injury syndrome

History

The postcardiac injury syndrome (PCIS) has been described after myocardial infarction [39], myocardial incision [40], pacemaker implantation [41], penetrating chest trauma [42], and CABG. In 1953, Soloff and coworkers [43] described a constellation of symptoms suggestive of rheumatic fever after a mitral commissurotomy. Dressler [39], in 1958, described a syndrome characterized by fever, chest pain, electrocardiac evidence of pericarditis, pleurisy, and pneumonitis in 44 patients after myocardial infarction. The syndrome occurred within days of the myocardial infarction and was associated with frequent relapses. The term *postcardiac injury syndrome* was introduced by Sahn and his colleagues [44] in 1983 to include chest pain, fever, pericarditis or pleuritis, left-sided pleural effusions and infiltrates, and leukocytosis and increased erythrocyte sedimentation rate (ESR) after myocardial infarction, cardiac surgery, penetrating chest trauma, or pacemaker placement. PCIS after cardiac surgery is relatively

common. In a prospective study of 86 patients, the incidence was 30%, with the presence of antimyocardial antibodies in the serum being a sensitive and specific confirmatory test [45]. Patients who develop pleural effusions as a result of PCIS have a similar pathogenesis, clinical presentation, PF analysis, natural history, and treatment.

Clinical presentation

The true incidence of PCIS is unknown. Estimates range from 1% to 30%. In a series of 400 pediatric patients surviving intrapericardial surgery, the incidence of PCIS, clinically and with increased antimyocardial antibodies, was 27% [46]. After CABG, the incidence of complete PCIS with symptoms and antimyocardial antibodies has been reported at 13%, with 26% described as having the clinical syndrome only [47]. In a prospective study by Light and colleagues [18], chest pain and fever were uncommon and it was concluded that post-CABG pleural effusions from PCIS are likely uncommon. The disparity between these reports likely reflects different study designs. The studies by Engle and colleagues [41,48,49] and DeSchreeder and coworkers [47,50] were prospective and focused specifically on the presence of PCIS after cardiac surgery. In contrast, the study by Light and colleagues [18] followed a hospital database; however, specific symptoms of PCIS were not recorded. The presence of symptoms was ascertained by telephone follow-up 3 months after surgery. Because antimyocardial antibodies were discovered in all patients with the full PCIS syndrome, it is likely that PCIS after CABG is more common than reported by Light and colleagues [18]. If the syndrome is mild, however, the symptoms can be mistaken for postoperative surgical pain and fever that can readily be treated with anti-inflammatory medications. It is likely that PCIS is underreported in studies that did not specifically target PCIS.

PCIS effusions can occur within a few days to up to 1 year after CABG, with the most common appearance being at 3 weeks. Thus, PCIS can overlap with perioperative post-CABG effusions. Unlike patients with perioperative post-CABG effusions, however, patients with PCIS manifest characteristic clinical features. The typical syndrome includes pleuritic chest pain, fever, and dyspnea with associated pleural effusions as well as parenchymal infiltrates occurring within 3 weeks of CABG [44]. Of the 35 patients reported by Stelzner and coworkers [44], pleuritic chest pain occurred in 91%, fever in 66%, pericardial rub in 63%, dyspnea in 57%, crackles in 51%, and pleural rub in 41%. Chest radiography revealed a pleural effusion in 83% (most often uni-

Table 1
Perioperative pleural effusions after coronary artery bypass grafting (within 1 week of surgery)

	Clincal characteristics	Radiograph findings	Pleural fluid analysis	Proposed mechanism	Management	Sequelae
Atelectasis	Immediate postoperative period; often associated with splinting	Ipsilateral volume loss, small, left-sided effusion	Transudate	Phrenic nerve dysfunction; splinting	Spontaneous resolution	Resolution of diaphragm dysfunction can be slow (over weeks)
Bloody effusion	small to large effusion; within days of CABG	Left sided, small to large effusion	Bloody, neutrophilic, exudative	Pleural injury from IMA harvesting	Thoracentesis if symptomatic large effusion; usually resolves spontaneously;	Can progress to chronic lymphocytic effusion of unknown cause
Congestive heart failure	Dyspnea, lower extremity edema, PND, orthopnea	Bilateral effusions; right > left; pulmonary edema	Mononuclear predominant transudate	Myocardial edema from SIRS; underlying ischemia	CHF management	None
Rare effusions						
Pulmonary embolus	Ipsilateral chest pain; acute dyspnea	Small effusion; may have peripheral consolidation	Bloody, PMN predominant exudate; transudate (20%);	Ischemia/infarct; transudate from atelectasis	Anticoagulation	Usually, no sequelae
Empyema	Fever, chest pain, purulent drainage from chest tube	Moderate to large effusion; loculation; may have ipsilateral infiltrate	pus, neutrophil predominant exudates, pH <7.20; Gram stain may reveal organism	Contamination from chest tube; sequela of hospital acquired pneumonia	Antibiotics; drainage	Can progress to pleural sepsis and later trapped lung if untreated
Chylothorax	Dyspnea; immediate post-operative period	Usually left-sided; can be right-sided and massive	Exudative; milky, high triglycerides; chylomicrons present	Thoracic duct or collateral injury during surgery	Low-fat diet; parenteral nutrition; thoracic duct ligation or pleurodesis for severe cases	Malnutrition and infection with prolonged chest tube drainage

Abbreviations: CABG, coronary artery bypass grafting; CHF, congestive heart failure; IMA, internal mammary artery; PMN, polymorphonuclear cell; PND, paroxysmal nocturnal dyspnea; SIRS, systematic inflammatory response syndrome.

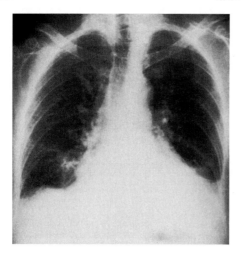

Fig. 1. Radiographic appearance of a patient with PCIS. Note the presence of pleural effusion with alveolar infiltrates. (*From* Stelzner TJ, King Jr TE, Antony VB, et al. The pleuropulmonary manifestations of the postcardiac injury syndrome. Chest 1983;84(4):385; with permission.)

lateral on the left), left lower lobe parenchymal infiltrates in 74%, and an enlarged cardiac silhouette in 49%. Fig. 1 illustrates a characteristic radiograph of PCIS. Leukocytosis was present in 49% of patients, and an elevated ESR (~62 mm/h) was present in 96% [44]. An electrocardiogram may reveal diffuse ST segment elevation consistent with pericarditis. Engle and colleagues [49] found elevated antimyocardial antibody levels in the serum of all patients with PCIS.

Pathogenesis

PCIS is likely caused by an exaggerated immune response. After myocardial injury, myocardial antigens seem to be released into the circulation. In some patients, an autoimmune response is evoked that follows a characteristic course. Why some patients are affected and others are not is unknown. In addition, viral infections may play a role, because PCIS seems to occur more often when the incidence of viral infection is highest [51]. Postoperative antiactin and antimyosin antibodies are also present in PCIS [47] in addition to antimyocardial antibodies. Antibodies against heart sarcolemma, skeletal muscle sarcolemma, and endothelium have been found in 16 (84%), 17 (90%), and 18 (95%) of 19 patients, respectively, after cardiac surgery with PCIS [52]. In contrast, 28 patients with cardiac surgery and without PCIS symptoms manifested these antibodies less commonly: 5(18%), 7 (25%), and 8 (29%), respectively

[52]. Antimyocardial antibodies seem to be generated locally within PF of patients with PCIS; a serum titer of 1:40 and a PF titer of 1:80 were reported in a patient with PCIS [53]. In addition, complement levels are decreased in the PF of patients with effusions from PCIS compared with serum. In a patient with the PCIS syndrome, the PF/serum C4/PF/serum protein ratio is less than 0.38, with an absolute C4/PF level of less than 8 [53]. Also, C1q binding was demonstrated in PF but not in serum, which is indicative of immune complexes within PF [53,54]. The natural history of serum antimyocardial antibody titers is elevation by postoperative day 14, with a gradual decline over 30 days. The rise and fall in antibody titers seem to mimic the clinical course of the patient [45]. The autoantibodies generated in the PCIS may play a role in graft failure. The presence of anticardiolipin antibody after CABG was associated with a doubling of the rate of graft occlusion in one series [55] and suggested in another [56]. In our opinion, the uncommon reporting of PCIS in the current literature may be attributable to masking by anti-inflammatory and antiplatelet medications.

Diagnosis, treatment, and sequelae

PF analysis can be useful in confirming the diagnosis of post-CABG PCIS effusion [44]. Other conditions in the differential diagnosis include congestive heart failure, immediate postoperative pleural effusion secondary to atelectasis, parapneumonic effusion, and pulmonary embolism. The presence of chest pain, fever, and leukocytosis makes congestive heart failure and immediate postoperative pleural effusion from atelectasis unlikely. Pulmonary embolism, parapneumonic effusion, and PCIS effusion can have similar clinical presentations. The PF from PCIS is characteristically a hemorrhagic exudate. The protein level is greater than 3.0 g/dL, the pH is usually greater than 7.40, and the LDH level is in the exudative range [44]. If PF analysis is performed within 10 days of clinical symptoms, the predominant cell should be the neutrophil; after 10 days, macrophages and lymphocytes predominate [44]. PF characteristics of the effusions that occur in the early post-CABG period are listed in Table 2.

Patients with PCIS usually require anti-inflammatory therapy for relief of symptoms, [40,44,57], including prednisone in some cases. Approximately 50% of patients relapse and need additional anti-inflammatory therapy. The current choice of anti-inflammatory medication has become problematic. With the recent data on an increased risk of myocardial infarction from rofexicob [58], cyclooxygenase (COX)-II inhibitors should be avoided in these

Table 2
Early pleural effusion after coronary artery bypass grafting (within 1 month after surgery)

	Clincal characteristics	Radiograph findings	Pleural fluid analysis	Proposed mechanism	Management	Sequelae
PCIS	Occurs weeks after CABG; chest pain, fever, rub, leukocytosis, elevated ESR	Moderate to large left pleural effusion; often left pulmonary infiltrates	Exudate; neutrophilic initially, then lymphocytic; bloody; anti-myocardial antibodies present	Immune response to myocardium antigens	Spontaneous resolution; NSAIDs and prednisone; often recurs	Can lead to constrictive pericarditis or trapped lung

Abbreviations: CABG, coronary artery bypass grafting; ESR, erythrocyte sedimentation rate; NSAID, nonsteroidal anti-inflammatory drug; PCIS, post-cardiac injury syndrome.

patients. In addition, indomethacin has been shown to impair ventricular healing after myocardial infarction [59,60]. Therefore, in the setting of recent myocardial ischemia, we would recommend ibuprofen or aspirin for anti-inflammatory treatment. Corticosteroids typically result in rapid resolution of symptoms [40,44,61]; however, the natural history of PCIS does not seem to be influenced by corticosteroids, because their withdrawal often results in recurrence [61]. Given the deleterious effect of corticosteroids on wound healing and the propensity of PCIS effusions to recur after their withdrawal, we reserve corticosteroids for patients with moderate to severe persistent symptoms. Narcotics should be considered for patients with severe chest pain. Therapeutic thoracentesis should be performed if clinically significant dyspnea is present; however, it does not alter the natural course of the disease.

Most patients have resolution of PCIS without clinically important sequelae. Nevertheless, there have been cases of delayed pericardial tamponade after cardiac surgery from PCIS [62]; however, the presence of anticoagulants does not seem to play a role in its development. More importantly, PCIS has been implicated in many cases of late constrictive pericarditis after CABG [63]. Whether PCIS plays a role in the development of trapped lung after CABG or graft failure is uncertain. Although tamponade, constrictive pericarditis, and graft failure are uncommon, they can result in morbidity and be life-threatening. Therefore, patients with PCIS effusions should be followed closely during the course of the illness and periodically after resolution.

Late postcoronary artery bypass grafting pleural effusions

There are four distinct effusions that occur 2 to 12 months after CABG, the so-called "late" effusions. They include (1) PCIS-related effusions, (2) lymphocytic effusions of uncertain etiology, (3) effusions attributable to constrictive pericarditis, and (4) effusions from lung entrapment. The distinguishing characteristics of these effusions are shown in Table 3. PCIS effusions have previously been discussed. The incidence of pleural effusions 3 months after CABG was reported in a series of 200 patients at 20%; however, thoracentesis was required in only 1.5% [16]. In patients with large pleural effusions, who do not have congestive heart failure, management options include observation, serial thoracenteses, chest tube drainage, fibrinolytics, pleurodesis, pericardial stripping, or decortication depending on

the cause of the effusion, morbidity to the patient, and complexity of the affected pleural space.

Lymphocytic exudative effusions of uncertain cause

Lymphocytic exudative effusions of uncertain cause can persist after CABG or appear months later. Possible causes of these effusions include persistent lymphatic damage related to surgery [17] and immune mechanisms, such as the PCIS syndrome [17,64]. Unlike typical PCIS effusions and the perioperative pleural effusions that likely occur from pleural injury with IMA harvesting, these effusions are not hemorrhagic. The resolution of these effusions is slower than the resolution of those attributable to direct pleural injury [17]; they can persist and require definitive therapy. Lee and colleagues [27] reviewed all cases of post-CABG effusion over a 2-year period that required operative intervention. There were eight such effusions, four with PF analysis. PF analysis revealed lymphocyte-predominant exudates, one of which was hemorrhagic. All patients required at least two therapeutic thoracenteses for relief of symptoms. In those patients who had surgery within the previous 6 months, the pleural histologic findings revealed active lymphocytic inflammation without fibrosis [27]. It is our opinion that most of these post-CABG lymphocytic effusions of uncertain etiology represent a chronic form of PCIS with minimal symptomatology. In general, management should be conservative, including therapeutic thoracentesis for symptom relief and a trial of steroids, with thoracoscopic pleurodesis reserved for those with persistent symptoms that affect the quality of life.

Constrictive pericarditis effusions

Constrictive pericarditis is an uncommon cause of late pleural effusions after CABG. The reported incidence ranges from 0.2% [65] to 2.3% [66]. Presenting clinical features include dyspnea with exertion, abdominal swelling, and peripheral edema. The physical examination typically reveals jugular venous distention, deep X and Y descents, hepatomegaly, and a Kussmaul sign. Bilateral pleural effusions commonly occur. Thoracentesis reveals a transudate unless there is early effusive-constrictive pericarditis, from PCIS; in such a case, a bloody exudate may be present. The diagnosis of constrictive pericarditis is established at left and right heart catheterization with decreased cardiac output, equalization of pressures across the cardiac chambers during diastole, and a characteristic "dip and plateau" of right and left ventricular diastolic pressures indicative of early

Table 3
Late effusions after coronary artery bypass grafting (occurring 2–12 months after surgery)

	Clinical characteristics	Radiograph findings	Pleural fluid analysis	Proposed mechanism	Management	Sequelae
PCIS	See Table 2	See Table 2	See Table 2	See Table 2	See Table 2	See Table 2
Lymphocytic effusion of uncertain cause	Small to large effusion; usually apparent within days of CABG	Usually left-sided, small to large effusion	Exudative; non-hemorrhagic; lymphocyte predominant	May represent a chronic form of PCIS or persistent pleural injury from CABG;	Usually resolves with conservative management	Can progress to trapped lung requiring decortication
Constrictive pericarditis	Occurs months after CABG; dyspnea, edema, jugular venous distention, Kussmaul's sign	Bilateral effusions; may have calcified pericardium	Lymphocyte predominant transudate	persistent PCIS results in pericardial thickening with cardiac restriction and venous hypertension	Careful diuretic use if mild; if severe, pericardiectomy	
Entrapped lung	Small to large effusion; may have dyspnea	Usually left-sided, small to large effusion; may have ipsilateral volume loss	Exudative; nonbloody; lymphocyte predominant; pleural manometry bimodal elastance curve	Persistent inflammation results in exudative effusion with pleural restriction	May resolve with conservative management	Can progress to trapped lung requiring decortication

Abbreviations: CABG, coronary artery bypass grafting; PCIS, post-cardiac injury syndrome.

rapid ventricular filling followed by rapidly elevated pressure from the noncompliant pericardium. The primary risk factor for development of post-CABG constrictive pericarditis is pericardial effusion. In a series of 463 patients with CABG, 10 (91%) of 11 patients with constrictive pericarditis had evidence of antecedent pericardial effusion, although only 25% (41 of 463) of patients with postoperative pericardial effusion developed constrictive pericarditis [66]. It is likely that most patients who develop constrictive pericarditis have PCIS. In one series [63], 23 (62%) of 37 patients with constrictive pericarditis after CABG had PCIS. The pleural effusions from constrictive pericarditis resolve after pericardiectomy, which reduces pulmonary and systemic venous hypertension.

Effusions from lung entrapment

The incidence of pleural effusions from lung entrapment after CABG is unknown. Lung entrapment is defined as a process in which the lung is prevented from expanding to the chest wall, with a concomitant pleural inflammatory process. Restriction can result from a fibrin peel covering the visceral pleura that limits lung expansion, visceral pleural thickening, malignant encasement of the pleura, or severe parenchymal fibrosis. For a pleural effusion to form from an entrapped lung, the shape of the entrapped lung must be significantly different from that of the chest wall, such that the chest wall cannot conform to the unexpandable lung [67]. This creates a persistent negative intrapleural pressure that generates a chronic pleural effusion. In contrast to a trapped lung from remote inflammation or infection, however, there is still a persistent inflammatory or malignant process. As a result, there are two concomitant processes causing the pleural effusion. Malignancy is the most common cause of an entrapped lung, occurring in approximately 30% of patients with malignant pleural effusion presenting with dyspnea (unpublished data); however, it can occur with any persistent inflammatory process of the pleura, such as rheumatoid pleurisy, and likely represents a transition between the persistent lymphocytic exudative pleural effusion after CABG and a trapped lung. Thoracentesis typically reveals a lymphocyte-predominant exudate. Management of a patient with an entrapped lung from a persistent post-CABG effusion depends on the degree of symptoms. Because patients with an entrapped lung never attain complete pleurodesis, we routinely perform pleural manometry in evaluation of these patients so that they can be appropriately referred for

video-assisted thoracoscopic surgery (VATS) if they have significant dyspnea related to their effusion [67].

Persistent postcoronary artery bypass grafting pleural effusion

Trapped lung

Clinical features

Trapped lung is one of the few causes of a persistent benign effusion that develops after the resolution of an inflammatory process (Table 4). Dysfunctional healing leads to a fibrous peel on the lung surface, creating negative intrapleural pressure with the ultrafiltrate of the pleural capillaries filling the pleural space en vacuo. It is an uncommon complication of poorly treated empyema, tuberculous empyema, uremic pleuritis, rheumatoid pleurisy, and after cardiac surgery [67]. A trapped lung should be suspected in a patient with a persistent effusion that reaccumulates rapidly to the same volume as before thoracentesis. Radiographic characteristics include a small to moderate pleural effusion without contralateral and sometimes ipsilateral mediastinal shift indicative of a restrictive pleural space.

The incidence of trapped lung after CABG is unknown; however, in the study by Lee and colleagues [27], an analysis of 2 years of follow-up of patients who had CABG revealed eight patients with a persistent pleural effusion who required surgical intervention. Only four required decortication; these patients presumably had a trapped lung with restriction and clinically significant dyspnea. The patient with a trapped lung may not be symptomatic. Because a trapped lung represents an end-stage fibrotic process [67], it usually manifests several months to years after the pleural injury. Thus, a trapped lung should be considered when a patient presents with a persistent left-sided pleural effusion in the months to years after CABG.

Pathophysiology

The pathophysiology of a trapped lung explains why effusions occur and why the patient may or may not experience dyspnea. A trapped lung likely represents dysfunctional healing of the pleura during a significant inflammatory process. The pleural mesothelium has an active role in modulating the inflammatory response. The normal pleural mesothelial cells are flat, and their enzymatic reactions follow the pentose pathway [68]. During an inflammatory process like empyema or PCIS, the mesothelial cells become reactive and columnar, the number of micro-

Table 4
Persistent effusions after coronary artery bypass grafting (after 6 months after surgery)

	Clinical characteristics	Radiograph findings	Pleural fluid analysis	Proposed mechanism	Management	Sequelae
Trapped lung	Small to large effusion; may have dyspnea	Usually left-sided, small to large effusion; ipsilateral volume loss	Usually transudative; lymphocyte predominant; pleural manometry reveals elevated elastance	Remote inflammatory process with dysfunctional pleural healing results in visceral pleural peel that prevents expansion of lung to chest wall with resultant pleural effusion	Decortication if patient has significant dyspnea from restriction; if asymptomatic, observe	Rarely progresses to fibrothorax

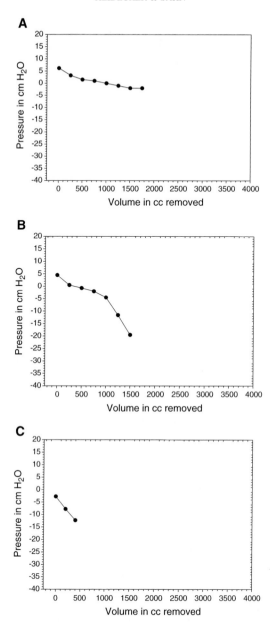

278 HEIDECKER & SAHN

Fig. 2. Elastance curves for patients with normal pleural elastance, entrapped lung, and trapped lung, respectively. In all figures, the *x* axis represents volume in milliliters removed, the *y* axis represents intrapleural pressure in centimeters of H_2O, and the elastance is the change in pressure divided by the change in volume in centimeters of H_2O per liter. (*A*) Normal elastance. Note that the pressure does not decrease as fluid is removed. (*B*) Entrapped lung. Note that the initial elastance is normal, followed by a rapid decrease in pressure indicating two separate intrapleural processes; the data points are the specific intrapleural pressures measured during removal of fluid. (*C*) Trapped lung. Note the initial negative intrapleural pressure and single curve with high elastance.

villi is increased, and oxidative capacity in enzymatic reactions is increased [69,70]. The mesothelial cells attempt to organize, contain, and remove inflammatory debris as well as to maintain the mesothelial lining and basement membrane [71,72]. In some pathologic states, the mesothelium is incapable of complete self-repair and removal of inflammatory debris. An extracellular neomatrix develops, which serves as a scaffolding for persistent inflammation and dysfunctional pleural repair [73]. This scaffolding most likely forms because of abnormal fibrin turnover and upregulation of profibrotic cytokines.

During pleural inflammation, there is increased fibrin generation from leakage of coagulation proteins into the pleural space [36] as well as impaired fibrinolysis. When stimulated by an inflammatory process, the mesothelium secretes vascular endothelial growth factor (VEGF). VEGF is a chemokine that not only causes angiogenesis but increases vascular permeability, both of which promote movement of coagulation proteins into the pleural space [74–76]. Tissue factor released from mesothelial cells results in conversion of fibrinogen to fibrin, which provides the scaffolding for the extracellular matrix. Simultaneously, plasminogen activator inhibitor-1 (PAI-1) expression is increased, which prevents fibrinolysis and maintains the integrity of the scaffold [77,78].

Understanding of the physiology of trapped lung has been enhanced by studying the mechanisms of fibrosis during pleurodesis. After talc instillation into the pleural space, there is increased expression of basic fibroblast growth factor (b-FGF) from mesothelial cells [79,80]. In addition, transforming growth factor-β (TGFβ) plays a role in creation of the visceral pleural peel [81,82]. During talc pleurodesis, TGFβ is upregulated intrapleurally [83] and is associated with increased pleural thickness [84]. TGFβ has been shown to induce pleural fibrosis in experimental models [85,86]. TGFβ also inhibits PAI-1, resulting in stabilization of the extracellular matrix scaffolding [82,87], and upregulates collagen formation, fibronectin synthesis, and matrix remodeling [73]. TGFβ seems to orchestrate many of the processes involved in development of pleural fibrosis and the visceral pleural peel.

Assuming that an inflammatory process like PCIS persists without the normal reparative mechanisms, a thick visceral pleural peel is likely to develop over months to years, resulting in restriction of lung expansion. In addition, the chest wall is unable to conform to this local geometry. The result is a persistently negative pleural space pressure. This space fills with fluid in an attempt to "normalize" the intrapleural pressure. It is important to note that with a trapped lung, dyspnea, if present, is caused by lung restriction and not by the pleural effusion per se. Therefore, thoracentesis is ineffective in alleviating the patient's dyspnea [67]. PF analysis of the fluid from a trapped lung reveals protein and LDH in the transudative range, because the effusion is attributable to hydrostatic pressure imbalance with normal pleura.

Diagnosis, treatment, and sequelae

The diagnosis of a trapped lung can be confirmed radiographically and physiologically. We routinely perform pleural manometry during therapeutic thoracentesis of any patient with a suspected trapped lung. During manometry, intrapleural pressures are monitored as fluid is drained in sequential aliquots [88]. Manometric characteristics of a trapped lung are an initial negative intrapleural pressure and a pleural elastance greater than 16 (a change in intrapleural pressure of >16 cm H_2O after removal of 1 L of fluid). These patients have a characteristic elastance curve that is diagnostic of trapped lung. The elastance curves of patients with normal elastance, entrapped lung, and trapped lung are shown in Fig. 2. When pleural manometry is compatible with trapped lung, we routinely allow air to enter the pleural space to relieve the chest pain induced by fluid removal and perform a CT scan to document pleural thickening as shown in Fig. 3. A postprocedure radiograph demon-

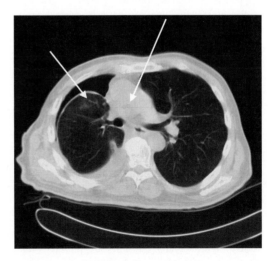

Fig. 3. CT scan of a patient with a trapped lung and pneumothorax after thoracentesis. Note the marked visceral pleural thickening limiting lung expansion to the chest wall resulting in a trapped lung (*open arrow*) and the presence of a marked ipsilateral mediastinal shift in the presence of pneumothorax suggestive of negative intrapleural pressure (*solid arrow*).

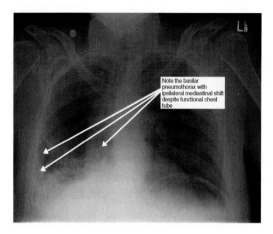

Note the basilar pneumothorax with ipsilateral mediastinal shift despite functional chest tube

Fig. 4. Chest radiograph of the same patient as in Fig. 3 with a trapped lung with characteristic basilar pneumothorax and ipsilateral mediastinal shift. Note the absence of lung expansion despite chest tube placement as well as the basilar pneumothorax (*open arrow*), small-bore chest tube (*closed arrow*), and presence of an ipsilateral mediastinal shift (*arrowhead*), respectively.

strates the pleural peel, volume loss, and a pneumothorax. Furthermore, a chest tube placed into the pleural space does not result in complete lung expansion (Fig. 4). An additional characteristic of a trapped lung is rapid recurrence of the effusion, usually over 48 to 72 hours. At thoracoscopy or thoracotomy, the trapped lung expands completely with decortication if the underlying lung is relatively normal up to 20 years after the initial pleural insult.

Pleural effusions are common after CABG. The timing of the effusion after CABG affects the etiology and clinical course of pleural effusion. Pleural effusions occurring in the immediate postoperative period are usually caused by diaphragm dysfunction and atelectasis or by IMA harvesting. Management is generally conservative, because these effusions are usually self-limited. Only large symptomatic effusions require thoracentesis. The early post-CABG pleural effusions that occur within the first month after CABG are likely usually attributable to the PCIS, with the patient presenting with chest pain, fever, and lymphocytic exudates on PF analysis. If symptoms are severe, corticosteroids are usually effective. When pleural effusions are present within 12 months of CABG (late effusions), they likely represent a variant of PCIS, constrictive pericarditis, or an entrapped lung. Persistent pleural effusions in the months after CABG surgery are usually attributable to a trapped lung. If significant pleural restriction is present, dyspnea can occur, which is only relieved with decortication. Management of pleural effusions

after CABG encompasses observation to thoracotomy with decortication. Proper diagnosis is critical to differentiate whether these patients with effusions should be observed, undergo therapeutic thoracentesis, receive corticosteroids, or undergo decortication.

References

[1] Light RW. Pleural effusions after coronary artery bypass graft surgery. Curr Opin Pulm Med 2002; 8(4):308–11.

[2] Peng MJ, Vargas FS, Cukier A, et al. Postoperative pleural changes after coronary revascularization. Comparison between saphenous vein and internal mammary artery grafting. Chest 1992;101(2):327–30.

[3] Daganou M, Dimopoulou I, Michalopoulos N, et al. Respiratory complications after coronary artery bypass surgery with unilateral or bilateral internal mammary artery grafting. Chest 1998;113(5):1285–9.

[4] Hurlbut D, Myers ML, Lefcoe M, et al. Pleuropulmonary morbidity: internal thoracic artery versus saphenous vein graft. Ann Thorac Surg 1990;50(6): 959–64.

[5] Vargas FS, Cukier A, Terra-Filho M, et al. Relationship between pleural changes after myocardial revascularization and pulmonary mechanics. Chest 1992;102(5): 1333–6.

[6] Vargas FS, Uezumi KK, Janete FB, et al. Acute pleuropulmonary complications detected by computed tomography following myocardial revascularization. Rev Hosp Clin Fac Med Sao Paulo 2002;57(4):135–42.

[7] Hagl C, Harringer W, Gohrbandt B, et al. Site of pleural drain insertion and early postoperative pulmonary function following coronary artery bypass grafting with internal mammary artery. Chest 1999;115(3): 757–61.

[8] Fedullo AJ, Lerner RM, Gibson J, et al. Sonographic measurement of diaphragmatic motion after coronary artery bypass surgery. Chest 1992;102(6):1683–6.

[9] Benjamin JJ, Cascade PN, Rubenfire M, et al. Left lower lobe atelectasis and consolidation following cardiac surgery: the effect of topical cooling on the phrenic nerve. Radiology 1982;142(1):11–4.

[10] Nikas DJ, Ramadan FM, Elefteriades JA. Topical hypothermia: ineffective and deleterious as adjunct to cardioplegia for myocardial protection. Ann Thorac Surg 1998;65(1):28–31.

[11] Marco JD, Hahn JW, Barner HB. Topical cardiac hypothermia and phrenic nerve injury. Ann Thorac Surg 1977;23(3):235–7.

[12] Canbaz S, Turgut N, Halici U, et al. Electrophysiological evaluation of phrenic nerve injury during cardiac surgerya prospective, controlled, clinical study. BMC Surg 2004;4(2):1–5.

[13] Mazzoni M, Solinas C, Sisillo E, et al. Intraoperative phrenic nerve monitoring in cardiac surgery. Chest 1996;109(6):1455–60.

[14] Landymore RW, Howell F. Pulmonary complications following myocardial revascularization with the internal mammary artery graft. Eur J Cardiothorac Surg 1990;4(3):156–61 [discussion: 161–2].

[15] Jain U, Rao TL, Kumar P, et al. Radiographic pulmonary abnormalities after different types of cardiac surgery. J Cardiothorac Vasc Anesth 1991;5(6):592–5.

[16] Aarnio P, Kettunen S, Harjula A. Pleural and pulmonary complications after bilateral internal mammary artery grafting. Scand J Thorac Cardiovasc Surg 1991; 25(3):175–8.

[17] Light RW, Rogers JT, Cheng D, et al. Large pleural effusions occurring after coronary artery bypass grafting. Ann Intern Med 1999;130(11):891–6.

[18] Light RW, Rogers JT, Moyers JP, et al. Prevalence and clinical course of pleural effusions at 30 days after coronary artery and cardiac surgery. Am J Respir Crit Care Med 2002;166(12 Pt 1):1567–71.

[19] Ali IM, Lau P, Kinley CE, et al. Opening the pleura during internal mammary artery harvesting: advantages and disadvantages. Can J Surg 1996;39(1):42–5.

[20] Noera G, Pensa PM, Guelfi P, et al. Extrapleural takedown of the internal mammary artery as a pedicle. Ann Thorac Surg 1991;52(6):1292–4.

[21] Bonacchi M, Prifti E, Giunti G, et al. Respiratory dysfunction after coronary artery bypass grafting employing bilateral internal mammary arteries: the influence of intact pleura. Eur J Cardiothorac Surg 2001;19(6): 827–33.

[22] Olearchyk AS, Magovern GJ. Internal mammary artery grafting. Clinical results, patency rates, and long-term survival in 833 patients. J Thorac Cardiovasc Surg 1986;92(6):1082–7.

[23] Sadikot RT, Rogers JT, Cheng DS, et al. Pleural fluid characteristics of patients with symptomatic pleural effusion after coronary artery bypass graft surgery. Arch Intern Med 2000;160(17):2665–8.

[24] Payne M, Magovern Jr GJ, Benckart DH, et al. Left pleural effusion after coronary artery bypass decreases with a supplemental pleural drain. Ann Thorac Surg 2002;73(1):149–52.

[25] Dunning J, Megahed M, Millner RW. The frequency of pleural effusions after Bellovac drainage following coronary bypass grafting. Cardiovasc Surg 2003;11(4): 309–12.

[26] Niva M, Biancari F, Valkama J, et al. Effects of diclofenac in the prevention of pericardial effusion after coronary artery bypass surgery. A prospective, randomized study. J Cardiovasc Surg (Torino) 2002; 43(4):449–53.

[27] Lee YC, Vaz MA, Ely KA, et al. Symptomatic persistent post-coronary artery bypass graft pleural effusions requiring operative treatment: clinical and histologic features. Chest 2001;119(3):795–800.

[28] Laine GA, Allen SJ. Left ventricular myocardial edema. Lymph flow, interstitial fibrosis, and cardiac function. Circ Res 1991;68(6):1713–21.

[29] Massoudy P, Zahler S, Becker BF, et al. Evidence for inflammatory responses of the lungs during coronary artery bypass grafting with cardiopulmonary bypass. Chest 2001;119(1):31–6.

[30] Asimakopoulos G, Smith PL, Ratnatunga CP, et al. Lung injury and acute respiratory distress syndrome after cardiopulmonary bypass. Ann Thorac Surg 1999; 68(3):1107–15.

[31] Aguilar MM, Battistella FD, Owings JT, et al. Posttraumatic empyema. Risk factor analysis. Arch Surg 1997;132(6):647–50 [discussion: 650–1].

[32] Smith JA, Mullerworth MH, Westlake GW, et al. Empyema thoracis: 14-year experience in a teaching center. Ann Thorac Surg 1991;51(1):39–42.

[33] Weissberg D, Refaely Y. Pleural empyema: 24-year experience. Ann Thorac Surg 1996;62(4):1026–9.

[34] Kollef MH, Schuster DP. Ventilator-associated pneumonia: clinical considerations. AJR Am J Roentgenol 1994;163(5):1031–5.

[35] Kollef MH. Ventilator-associated pneumonia. A multivariate analysis. JAMA 1993;270(16):1965–70.

[36] Sahn SA. The pathophysiology of pleural effusions. Annu Rev Med 1990;41:7–13.

[37] British Thoracic Society and Public Health Laboratory Service. Community-acquired pneumonia in adults in British hospitals in 1982–1983: a survey of aetiology, mortality, prognostic factors and outcome. The British Thoracic Society and the Public Health Laboratory Service. Q J Med 1987;62(239):195–220.

[38] Pego-Fernandes PM, Ebaid GX, Nouer GH, et al. Chylothorax after myocardial revascularization with the left internal thoracic artery. Arq Bras Cardiol 1999; 73(4):383–90.

[39] Dressler W. The post-myocardial-infarction syndrome: a report on forty-four cases. AMA Arch Intern Med 1959;103(1):28–42.

[40] Kaminsky ME, Rodan BA, Osborne DR, et al. Postpericardiotomy syndrome. AJR Am J Roentgenol 1982;138(3):503–8.

[41] Engle MA, Zabriskie JB, Senterfit LB, et al. Immunologic and virologic studies in the postpericardiotomy syndrome. J Pediatr 1975;87(6 Pt 2):1103–8.

[42] Loughlin V, Murphy A, Russel C. The postpericardiotomy syndrome and penetrating trauma of the chest. Br J Accidental Surg 1987;18:412–4.

[43] Soloff L, Zatuchni J, Janton D, et al. Reactivation of rheumatic fever following mitral commissurotomy. Circulation 1953;8:481–93.

[44] Stelzner TJ, King Jr TE, Antony VB, et al. The pleuropulmonary manifestations of the postcardiac injury syndrome. Chest 1983;84(4):383–7.

[45] Engle MA, McCabe JC, Ebert PA, et al. The postpericardiotomy syndrome and antiheart antibodies. Circulation 1974;49(3):401–6.

[46] Engle MA. Pericardiotomy and allied syndromes. In: Reddy PS, editor. Pericardial disease. New York: Raven Press; 1982. p. 313–23.

[47] De Scheerder I, De Buyzere M, Robbrecht J, et al. Postoperative immunological response against contractile proteins after coronary bypass surgery. Br Heart J 1986;56(5):440–4.

[48] Engle MA, Gay Jr WA, McCabe J, et al. Post-pericardiotomy syndrome in adults: incidence, auto-immunity and virology. Circulation 1981;64(2 Pt 2): II58–60.

[49] Engle MA, Zabriskie JB, Senterfit LB. Heart-reactive antibody, viral illness, and the postpericardiotomy syndrome. Correlates of a triple-blind, prospective study. Trans Am Clin Climatol Assoc 1976;87:147–60.

[50] De Scheerder I, Vandekerckhove J, Robbrecht J, et al. Post-cardiac injury syndrome and an increased humoral immune response against the major contractile proteins (actin and myosin). Am J Cardiol 1985;56(10): 631–3.

[51] Miller RH, Horneffer PJ, Gardner TJ, et al. The epidemiology of the postpericardiotomy syndrome: a common complication of cardiac surgery. Am Heart J 1988;116(5 Pt 1):1323–9.

[52] Maisch B, Schuff-Werner P, Berg PA, et al. Clinical significance of immunopathological findings in patients with post-pericardiotomy syndrome. II. The significance of serum inhibition and rosette inhibitory factors. Clin Exp Immunol 1979;38(2):198–203.

[53] Kim S, Sahn S. Postcardiac injury syndrome. An immunologic pleural fluid analysis. Chest 1996;109(2): 570–2.

[54] Shrivastava R, Venkatesh S, Pavlovich BB, et al. Immunological analysis of pleural fluid in post-cardiac injury syndrome. Postgrad Med J 2002;78(920):362–3.

[55] Morton KE, Gavaghan TP, Krilis SA, et al. Coronary artery bypass graft failure—an autoimmune phenomenon? Lancet 1986;2:1353–6.

[56] Urschel H, Razzuk M, Gardner M. Coronary artery bypass occlusion secondary to postcardiotomy syndrome. Ann Thorac Surg 1976;22(6):528–31.

[57] Khan AH. The postcardiac injury syndromes. Clin Cardiol 1992;15(2):67–72.

[58] Mukherjee D, Nissen SE, Topol EJ. Risk of cardio-vascular events associated with selective COX-2 inhibitors. JAMA 2001;286(8):954–9.

[59] Hammerman H, Kloner R, Schoen F, et al. Indo-methacin-induced scar thinning after experimental myocardial infarction. Circulation 1983;67:1290–5.

[60] Jugdutt B, Basualdo C. Myocardial infarct expansion during indomethacin or ibuprofen for symptomatic post-infarction pericarditis. Influence of other pharma-cologic agents during early remodeling. Can J Cardiol 1989;5:211–21.

[61] Engle MA, Gay Jr WA, Kaminsky ME, et al. The post-pericardiotomy syndrome then and now. Curr Probl Cardiol 1978;3(2):1–40.

[62] Ofori-Krakye S, Tyberg T, Geha A, et al. Late cardiac tamponade after open heart surgery: incidence, role of anticoagulants in its pathogenesis and its relationship to the postpericardiotomy syndrome. Circulation 1981; 63(6):1323–8.

[63] Killian DM, Furiasse JG, Scanlon PJ, et al. Constric-tive pericarditis after cardiac surgery. Am Heart J 1989; 118(3):563–8.

[64] Kim YK, Mohsenifar Z, Koerner SK. Lymphocytic pleural effusion in postpericardiotomy syndrome. Am Heart J 1988;115(5):1077–9.

[65] Fowler NO. Constrictive pericarditis: its history and current status. Clin Cardiol 1995;18(6):341–50.

[66] Matsuyama K, Matsumoto M, Sugita T, et al. Clinical characteristics of patients with constrictive pericarditis after coronary bypass surgery. Jpn Circ J 2001;65(6): 480–2.

[67] Doelken P, Sahn SA. Trapped lung. Semin Respir Crit Care Med 2001;22(6):631–5.

[68] Whitaker D, Papadimitriou JM, Walters MN. The mesothelium: a histochemical study of resting meso-thelial cells. J Pathol 1980;132(3):273–84.

[69] Whitaker D, Papadimitriou JM, Walters MN. The mesothelium: a cytochemical study of "activated" mesothelial cells. J Pathol 1982;136(3):169–79.

[70] Wang NS. The regional difference of pleural meso-thelial cells in rabbits. Am Rev Respir Dis 1974; 110(5):623–33.

[71] Ryan GB, Grobety J, Majno G. Mesothelial injury and recovery. Am J Pathol 1973;71(1):93–112.

[72] Shumko JZ, Feinberg RN, Shalvoy RM, et al. Re-sponses of rat pleural mesothelia to increased intra-thoracic pressure. Exp Lung Res 1993;19(3):283–97.

[73] Huggins JT, Sahn SA. Causes and management of pleural fibrosis. Respirology 2004;9(4):441–7.

[74] Yano S, Shinohara H, Herbst RS, et al. Production of experimental malignant pleural effusions is dependent on invasion of the pleura and expression of vascular endothelial growth factor/vascular permeability factor by human lung cancer cells. Am J Pathol 2000;157(6): 1893–903.

[75] Becker PM, Alcasabas A, Yu AY, et al. Oxygen-independent upregulation of vascular endothelial growth factor and vascular barrier dysfunction during ventilated pulmonary ischemia in isolated ferret lungs. Am J Respir Cell Mol Biol 2000;22(3):272–9.

[76] Thickett DR, Armstrong L, Millar AB. Vascular endothelial growth factor (VEGF) in inflammatory and malignant pleural effusions. Thorax 1999;54(8): 707–10.

[77] Idell S, Zwieb C, Kumar A, et al. Pathways of fibrin turnover of human pleural mesothelial cells in vitro. Am J Respir Cell Mol Biol 1992;7(4):414–26.

[78] Idell S, Girard W, Koenig KB, et al. Abnormalities of pathways of fibrin turnover in the human pleural space. Am Rev Respir Dis 1991;144(1):187–94.

[79] Antony VB, Nasreen N, Mohammed KA, et al. Talc pleurodesis: basic fibroblast growth factor mediates pleural fibrosis. Chest 2004;126(5):1522–8.

[80] Antony VB, Kamal M, Godbey S, et al. Talc-induced pleurodesis: role of basic fibroblast growth factor (bFGF). Eur Respir J 1997;10:403S.

[81] Idell S, Zwieb C, Boggaram J, et al. Mechanisms of fibrin formation and lysis by human lung fibroblasts: influence of TGF-beta and TNF-alpha. Am J Physiol 1992;263(4 Pt 1):L487–94.

[82] Idell S, Kumar A, Zwieb C, et al. Effects of TGF-beta and TNF-alpha on procoagulant and fibrinolytic path-

ways of human tracheal epithelial cells. Am J Physiol 1994;267(6 Pt 1):L693–703.

[83] Lee YC, Lane KB. Cytokines in pleural diseases. In: Light RW, Lee YC, editors. Textbook of pleural diseases. New York: Arnold; 2003. p. 63–89.

[84] Sasse SA, Jadus MR, Kukes GD. Pleural fluid transforming growth factor-beta1 correlates with pleural fibrosis in experimental empyema. Am J Respir Crit Care Med 2003;168(6):700–5.

[85] Lee YC, Devin CJ, Teixeira LR, et al. Transforming growth factor beta2 induced pleurodesis is not inhibited by corticosteroids. Thorax 2001;56(8):643–8.

[86] Light RW, Cheng DS, Lee YC, et al. A single intrapleural injection of transforming growth factor-beta(2) produces an excellent pleurodesis in rabbits. Am J Respir Crit Care Med 2000;162(1):98–104.

[87] Grande JP. Role of transforming growth factor-β in tissue injury and repair. Proc Soc Exp Biol Med 1997; 214:27–40.

[88] Doelken P, Huggins JT, Pastis NJ, et al. Pleural manometry: technique and clinical implications. Chest 2004;126(6):1764–9.

ELSEVIER
SAUNDERS

Clin Chest Med 27 (2006) 285 – 308

CLINICS
IN CHEST
MEDICINE

Pleural Effusions of Extravascular Origin

Steven A. Sahn, MD

Division of Pulmonary, Critical Care, Allergy, and Sleep Medicine, Medical University of South Carolina,
96 Jonathan Lucas Street, Suite 812-CSB, PO Box 250630, Charleston, SC 29425, USA

As pulmonologists are aware, there are a limited number of causes of transudative pleural effusions that are the result of imbalances in hydrostatic and oncotic pressures; in these instances, the pleura is normal. In contrast, the number of exudates exceeds transudates by at least 10-fold; these exudative effusions are caused by inflammation, infection, malignancy, and lymphatic abnormalities [1]. There are a small number of effusions, transudates and exudates, that develop from an extravascular origin (Table 1), however. Because these effusions tend to be uncommon or rare, the clinician often does not consider these diagnoses when confronted with an undiagnosed pleural effusion. The purpose of this article is to familiarize the clinician with these effusions of extravascular origin by discussing their frequency, pathogenesis, clinical presentation, radiographic appearance, pleural fluid analysis, diagnosis, and management.

Transudative effusions of extravascular origin

Peritoneal dialysis

Although the first reported successful long-term treatment with peritoneal dialysis was by Boen and colleagues in 1962 [2], it was not until the late 1970s when chronic ambulatory peritoneal dialysis (CAPD) was introduced by Popovich and coworkers [3] that a significant increase in the use of peritoneal dialysis for the management of patients with end-stage renal

disease began. A worrisome complication of peritoneal dialysis is bacterial infection, which can affect the exit site or cause peritonitis [4]. In addition, there is emerging evidence that chronic inflammation may increase the risk of atherosclerotic cardiovascular disease and mortality in patients on CAPD [5]. Other complications, the consequences of the increase in intra-abdominal pressure that accompanies the infusion of peritoneal dialysate, can also occur, however [6]. Although more than 70 cases of pleural effusion from peritoneal dialysis had been reported by the early 1990s, the precise incidence of this complication is unknown. Data from 161 centers performing CAPD found an incidence of pleural effusion of 1.6% occurring, on average, 1 day to 8 years after initiation of dialysis [7]. The consequences of a pleural effusion include tension hydrothorax, respiratory failure, ultrafiltration failure, and short-term or permanent discontinuation of peritoneal dialysis [8].

Pathogenesis

Clinical studies have demonstrated that although the empty peritoneal cavity has a pressure of approximately 0.5 to 2.2 cm H_2O, intra-abdominal pressure increases linearly in proportion to the volume of the dialysate that is instilled [9]. Intra-abdominal pressure ranges from 2 to 10 cm H_2O with the volume of dialysate used in clinical practice [9,10]. With a 3-L volume of dialysate exchanges, pressures of 12 cm H_2O have been measured [11]. Weight, abdominal girth, age, and body mass index, as well as walking and routine activities, can also increase intra-abdominal pressure. When patients cough or strain, pressure can exceed 300 cm H_2O [10]. Pressure and volume intra-abdominally can increase tension on the abdominal

---

E-mail address: sahnsa@musc.edu

Table 1
Pleural effusion of extravascular origin

Transudates	Exudates
Peritoneal dialysis	Chylothorax
Urinothorax	Pancreaticopleural fistula
Duropleural fistula	Esophageal rupture
EVM of CVC	EVM of CVC
(saline or glucose)	(TPN, hemorrhage)
Glycinothorax	Ventriculoperitoneal fistula
	Ventriculopleural fistula
	Biliopleural fistula
	Gastropleural fistula
	Enteral tube feedings

Abbreviations: CVC, central venous catheter; EVM, extravascular migration.

wall, with these increases putting stress on supporting structures of the abdomen and leading to leakage of dialysate out of the peritoneal cavity.

It is possible that peritoneal fluid moves into the pleural space through congenital diaphragmatic defects that are rendered patent by the increased peritoneal pressure [12,13]. Postmortem studies on patients with peritoneal dialysis who clinically had pleural effusions have demonstrated defects in the tendinous portion of the right hemidiaphragm [14,15]. At surgery, diaphragmatic blisters have been confirmed [14,16]. Stoppage of peritoneal dialysis results in disappearance of the pleural effusion because of bidirectional flow via the parietal pleural stoma, lymphatics, or both.

Clinical presentation

Patients undergoing peritoneal dialysis who develop a pleural effusion may be asymptomatic, and the effusion is discovered on a chest radiograph performed for other reasons; some patients may complain of dyspnea with exertion or at rest or may present acutely with respiratory failure [17]. Determining the cause of the pleural effusion may be delayed because the patient's dyspnea may be misinterpreted initially as volume overload; in this case scenario, prescribing increased hypertonic dialysis fluid may lead to an increase in peritoneal volume and pressure, and thus increase the pleural effusion [6]. Risk factors for development of pleural effusions in patients on peritoneal dialysis are multiparity and peritonitis [18].

Chest radiograph

The most common radiographic finding is a small right-sided pleural effusion without other abnormalities; effusions can occur bilaterally. An acute massive pleural effusion, virtually always on the right side,

occurs predominantly in women [19,20]; these effusions have been reported on the first day of dialysis and up to 2 years after the initiation of dialysis [19,20].

Pleural fluid analysis

The pleural fluid has been described as having a yellow tinge. The total protein level is consistently less than 1.0 g/dL (the lowest concentration report by most clinical laboratories), with a reported range of 0.07 to 0.50 g/dL. The range of lactate dehydrogenase (LDH) is 6 to 55 IU/L. The fluid has a paucity of mononuclear cells (<100 cells/μL). The glucose concentration has been reported to range from 200 to 2030 mg/dL, and, to my knowledge, the pH has not been reported (Table 2) [17,19–24].

Diagnosis

In the patient on CAPD, the diagnosis can be established by documenting the combination of a low pleural fluid total protein concentration (<0.5 g/dL) with an extremely high pleural fluid glucose level. The only other entity that could have similar pleural fluid findings is extravascular migration of a central venous catheter with glucose infusion [25]. The diagnosis can also be confirmed if a patient is being dialyzed with icodextrin because of ultrafiltration failure attributable to high peritoneal glucose transport. A "black line sign" can be demonstrated by the reaction between iodine and starches [24,26]. Icodextrin is a glucose polymer that bears major similarities to starch. In the patient receiving icodextrin, the laboratory should be requested to add povidone iodine to the pleural aspirate to confirm or refute a peritoneal-to-pleural leak. An additional method of confirming the peritoneal-pleural communication is with peritoneal instillation of technetium-99m (^{99m}Tc)-sulfur colloid via peritoneoscintigraphy [19,27]. The rapidity of the appearance and extent of the radiotracer in the thorax are findings that relate to the size of the diaphragmatic defects.

Management

Patients who develop an acute massive hydrothorax require immediate thoracentesis for relief of dyspnea and discontinuation of peritoneal dialysis; these patients virtually always require a change to hemodialysis. Some patients with smaller symptomatic effusions have spontaneous closure of a diaphragmatic defect with stoppage of peritoneal dialysis; however, most require an alternative form of therapy. There have been reports of patching the abnormal diaphragm at thoracotomy or thoracoscopy with successful return to peritoneal dialysis [28]. Talc

Table 2
Pleural fluid analysis: effusions from extravascular origin

Diagnosis	Appearance	Total protein (g/dL)	LDH (IU/L) or ratio[a]	Nucleated cells (/μL)	Glucose (mg/dL)	pH	Diagnostic test
Peritoneal dialysis	Yellow tinge	<1.0, range 0.07–0.5	6–55	1–100 mononuclear	200–2030	NR	TP <1.0 and PF/S glucose ratio >2; black line sign
Urinothorax	Clear yellow	<1.0, range 0.1–1.6	<0.3	23–1500 mononuclear	PF = S	6.80–8.00	PF/S creatinine ratio >1.0; range 1.01–15.7
Duropleural fistula (nontraumatic)	Water-like	<1.0, range 0.2–0.8	56–97	30–150 mononuclear	CSF/PF ratio <1.0 but >0.5	7.55	β_2-Transferrin present
Extravascular migration of CVC	TPN/lipid: milky Glucose/saline: clear	<1.0 <1.0	NR 37–98	Variable Variable	PF >S PF >S	>7.45 >7.45	Triglycerides >110 mg/dL PF >S glucose ratio >1.0; TP <1.0
Ventriculopleural shunt	Hemorrhage: bloody Water-like	Exudate <1.0	Exudate Low	PMN Mononuclear	Variable CSF/PF ratio <1.0 but >0.5	>7.45 7.55	Hematocrit PF/B and >0.5 β_2-Transferrin present
Glycinothorax	Blood-stained and clear	0.2	NR	NR	NR	NR	High PF/S glycine ratio
Chylothorax	Milky, turbid, clear hemorrhage	2.1–7.1	<268	400–6800; >80% lymphocytes	48–200, PF/S ratio <1.0	7.40–7.80	Triglycerides >110 mg/dL; chylomicons present
Pancreaticopleural fistula	Clear to turbid yellow	4.5	>1000	PMN predominance	P=S	7.30–7.35	Amylase >100,000 IU/L
Esophageal rupture							
Intact mediastinal pleura	Serous or turbid	>3.0	PF/S ratio >0.82	50–25,000 PMN predominant	P=S	>7.30	None
Medistinal pleura ruptured	Purulent	>3.0	>1000	200–100,000 PMN predominant	0 to <60	<7.00	Increased salivary amylase (200–1922 IU/L); pH 6.00–7.00; PF cytology=food particles, squamous epithelial cells
Biliopleural fistula	Greenish	Exudate	Exudate	PMN predominant	P=S	>7.30	Bilirubin PF/S ratio >1.0
Gastropleural fistula	Turbid	Exudate	Exudate; LDH may be >100	Variable PMN predominant	P=S	May be >7.30	Radiographs, endoscopy; PF cytology=food particles, squamous epithelial cells
Small-bore enteral feeding tube entering pleural space	Color of enteral feeding	—	—	—	—	—	Visualization of pleural aspirate

Abbreviations: CSF, cerebrospinal fluid; CVC, central venous catheter; NR, not reported; PF, pleural fluid; PF/B, pleural/blood; PMN, polymorphonuclear leukocytes; S, serum; TP, total protein; TPN, total parenteral nutrition.

[a] PF/LDH/upper limits of normal serum LDH.

pleurodesis at thoracoscopy has also been successful [22,23].

Urinothorax

Most cases of urinothorax are the result of obstructive uropathy [29]. Reported causes of an urinothorax include bladder and prostate cancer, posterior urethral valves, renal cysts, nephrolithiasis, surgical ureteral manipulation, blunt trauma to the kidney, renal transplantation, ileal conduit with ureteral obstruction, bladder laceration, and pregnancy [29–48]. There have been two cases of urinothorax reported during pregnancy, which is usually associated with a urinoma on the right side [35,39]. Another rare cause of a urinothorax is a congenital urinary tract anomaly combining posterior urethral valves, unilateral vesicoureteral reflux, and renal dysplasia (the VURD syndrome) [49]. Lallas and colleagues [48] reported on 375 patients who underwent supracostal percutaneous nephrolithotomy; 4 (1%) patients developed a urinothorax. At least 40 cases have been reported in the English language literature.

Pathogenesis

Obstructive uropathy leads to perirenal fluid accumulation or urinomas, with urine entering the mediastinum and the urinoma rupturing into the pleural space or direct retroperitoneal movement into the pleural space through a diaphragm hiatus or defect [29,30,34]. A urinothorax is typically ipsilateral to the obstructed kidney, although there are rare reports of contralateral involvement [29]. It seems that a urinothorax develops relatively rapidly after the obstruction is severe enough to cause a retroperitoneal urinoma and likewise resolves relatively quickly after relief of the obstruction [29,34].

The pathogenesis of the low pH (<7.30) in a urinothorax is most likely related to the low pH of the extravasated urine with back-diffusion of hydrogen ions as the fluid passes from the retroperitoneal into the pleural space [36]. Alkaline urine at the time of extravasation could result in a pH in the normal range (7.30–7.55) or even a pH approaching 8.00.

Clinical presentation

The most common presenting symptom of a urinothorax is dyspnea after surgery [29] or trauma [42,45,46]. Occasionally, a small asymptomatic urinothorax is found on a routine postoperative chest radiograph. Patients with malignancy and obstructive uropathy may present with the insidious onset of dyspnea with exertion. The interval between the precipitating event and the urinothorax has ranged from 8 hours to 2 months, with most diagnosed within 48 hours [29].

Chest radiograph

The chest radiograph typically shows a small to moderate pleural effusion ipsilateral to the obstructed kidney (Fig. 1). There are reports of bilateral [35,38] and contralateral effusions [29], however. In most instances, there is no other abnormality on the chest radiograph.

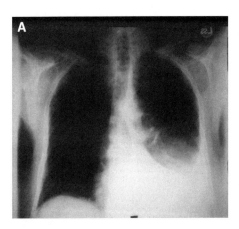
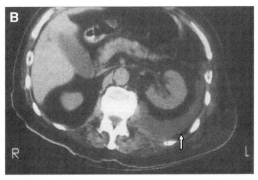

Fig. 1. A 66-year-old man with the recurrence of colon carcinoma presented with bilateral ureteral obstruction secondary to extrinsic compression by a tumor. Bilateral nephrostomy tubes were placed; however, the left nephrostomy tube became dislodged shortly after placement, and a left renal stent was placed by cystoscopy. At the time of cystoscopy, dye injection demonstrated extravasation of contrast into the left perirenal space. (*A*) Posteroanterior chest radiograph shows a moderate left pleural effusion. (*B*) Abdominal CT scan shows perirenal collection of urine (*arrow*) and left hydronephrosis. Thoracentesis revealed a clear yellow fluid with a pleural fluid–to-serum creatinine ratio greater than 1, diagnostic of a urinothorax.

Pleural fluid analysis

The pleural fluid is typically clear yellow with a total protein level of less than 1.0 g/dL, which may be greater than 1.0 g/dL in the trauma patient with a contribution from blood [29,34,36].The diagnosis is established by finding the pleural fluid creatinine to be greater than the serum creatinine. [34]The reported pleural fluid–to-serum creatinine difference ranges from 1.08 to 15.7. The pleural fluid glucose is similar to blood glucose, and the pH may be less than 7.30 or alkaline [29,36]. A urinothorax is the only single cause of a low pH transudative effusion (see Table 2) [36].

Management

The management of a urinothorax is straightforward and simply involves relief of the obstructive uropathy; when a urinothorax occurs in the setting of pregnancy, repair of the bladder injury and cesarean section also lead to resolution. The urinothorax resolves relatively quickly (within hours to a few days) after relief of the obstruction or repair of the bladder injury. Furthermore, the increased pleural fluid–to-serum creatinine difference tends to reverse rapidly as well [29,34]. Therefore, the timing of thoracentesis is critical in definitively establishing the diagnosis of a urinothorax. There is no pleural space sequela from a urinothorax.

Duropleural fistula

A duropleural fistula (DPF) or subarachnoid-pleural fistula represents a communication between the subarachnoid and pleural spaces. At least 30 cases have been reported in the English language literature [50–65]. DPF may be underreported because it seems to be a relatively common complication of spinal cord surgery that is often routinely repaired and not reported by neurosurgeons.

Pathogenesis

For a DPF to become established, there must be disruption of the dural and parietal pleural membranes, allowing a track to develop between the subarachnoid and pleural spaces. Once the fistula develops, a pressure gradient that allows cerebrospinal fluid (CSF) to flow from the positive-pressure subarachnoid space to the negative-pressure pleural space is established. Most cases of DPF are secondary to blunt or penetrating trauma [61]. A traumatic DFP can involve a missile traversing the pleural and subarachnoid spaces or a vertebral fracture that tears the dura and parietal pleura. A fistulous track usually occurs between the upper thoracic subarachnoid space and the pleural space. With blunt trauma, the disruption occurs from extreme extension of the spine, resulting in tearing of the relatively immobile nerve routes in the dura. Severe chest wall compression may perforate the pleura against the bony prominence of the spine [66]. Regardless of the cause, a DPF remains open because of the pressure gradient between the subarachnoid and pleural spaces. Although laminectomy is a common neurosurgical procedure to treat spinal injuries, there are only a few reports of DPF as a complication [50,57]; however, these cases may be underreported [50,57]. DPF has been documented as a complication of thoracotomy [61], thoracoscopy [58], and decompression of tumor [64].

Clinical presentation

A high degree of suspicion is necessary to establish the diagnosis of DPF. Symptoms that suggest a CSF leak include postural headaches, nausea, and vomiting. Often, symptoms related to the effusion, such as chest pain, dyspnea, or fever, may be minimal or overshadowed by concomitant injuries, often delaying the diagnosis [61]. In addition to the almost universal findings of severe spinal cord injury, other clues to the diagnosis may be pneumocephalus or meningitis.

Chest radiograph

The chest radiograph may initially be normal after trauma, with the effusion appearing days later. Pleural effusions range from small to massive [59,63] depending on the size and duration of the fistula (Fig. 2). Mediastinal widening may also be observed, and once aortic injury is excluded, a diagnosis of a subarachnoid-mediastinal or subarachnoid-pleural fistula should be considered.

Pleural fluid analysis

The pleural fluid in nontraumatic DPF is clear and "looks like water" [62]. The nucleated cell count is low. The glucose concentration is less than that of serum, but the pleural fluid-to-serum ratio is not less than 0.5 [61,62]. An important feature of this transudative effusion is a total protein level consistently less than 1.0 g/dL, with the LDH clearly in the transudative range [62]. Nevertheless, there are reports of exudates with a DPF; these exudative effusions are usually associated with trauma and pleural space hemorrhage or postoperative pneumonia [61]. In these scenarios, the pleural fluid analysis can be confounding. β_2-transferrin is produced by the action of neuraminidase on brain tissue; the only other location of this protein is in the perilymph of

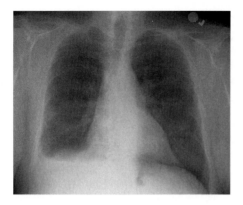

Fig. 2. An 81-year-old man was referred for evaluation of a chronic transudative effusion that required multiple thoracenteses over 11 months for relief of dyspnea. He had extensive lumbar disk surgery 2 years before the onset of dyspnea. Note the presence of a small right pleural effusion. Thoracentesis revealed a fluid that "looked like water," with a pH of 7.55, an LDH level of 92 IU/L, and total protein concentration of less than 1 g/dL. There were 150 nucleated cells, with 90% macrophages. β_2-transferrin was detected, confirming the diagnosis of a DPF.

the inner ear. β_2-transferrin is accepted as a sensitive and specific marker to identify CSF leaks into the pleural space after head or spinal trauma or spinal surgery [56,62–64]. Measurement of β_2-transferrin is available to practicing clinicians in most laboratories (see Table 2).

Management

Although the presence of β_2-transferrin in pleural fluid establishes the diagnosis of a DPF, definitive identification of the fistula requires radiographic visualization. Conventional and radionuclide myelography are most commonly used. Several authors have concluded that indium-111 diethylenetriaminepentaacetate (DPTA) myeloscintigraphy is more sensitive than conventional myelography [58,60,65,67]. There are reports of false-negative results using myelography alone in the setting of slow or intermittent leaks, however [67–71]. Therefore, CT scanning performed concomitantly with myelography aids in the delineation of the anatomic defect. In addition, the presence of contrast in the pleural space after myelography confirms the diagnosis in patients with slow CSF leaks.

Because of the limited number of reported cases, there is no strong consensus regarding management of DPF. Spontaneous resolution is rare, and most patients require surgical ligation or closed-tube drainage for management. Of the 19 posttraumatic DPFs reported in one series, 13 (68%) were treated defini-

tively with laminectomy or thoracotomy, 3 (16%) responded to chest tube drainage, 2 (11%) were treated with thoracentesis, and 1 (5%) was treated with "conservative" measures [54]. In 9 (82%) of the 11 patients who had a laminectomy performed, closure of the fistula was successful [54]. The appropriate timing of surgical intervention is unknown. Some surgeons advocate chest tube drainage for up to 2 weeks before surgical intervention, whereas others recommend early intervention, noting the low rate of spontaneous closure [66].

Extravascular migration of a central venous catheter (transudative or exudative effusion)

The percutaneous insertion of a central venous catheter is a common practice and is used to provide therapy for hospitalized and ambulatory patients. Although catheter design and techniques have been improved, complications are not uncommon. Well-recognized complications include pneumothorax, infection of the catheter, and thrombosis reported in up to 11% of cases [72–74]. A potentially more serious complication, often delayed in recognition, is abnormal migration of the central venous catheter with vascular erosion and perforation, which was highlighted mostly in single case reports in the 1970s and 1980s [75–95]. In 1992, Duntley and colleagues [25] reported on eight patients with vascular erosion from a central venous catheter and reviewed the literature.

Pathogenesis

Most reports of catheter erosion occur with placement on the left side, with the most common site being the left subclavian vein [25]. The predilection of left-sided catheters to perforate a vein is most likely attributable to the horizontal orientation of the left brachiocephalic vein compared with the right brachiocephalic vein. Left-sided catheters of insufficient length tend to contact the superior vena cava close to the perpendicular. This positioning increases the tendency to promote vascular erosion and perforation. The most precarious zone for left-sided catheters is the azygous recess of the proximal superior vena cava [85,96]. Erosions have also been reported in the right and left brachiocephalic veins, however [80]. When the vein is perforated, fluid may be infused into the pleural space or mediastinum.

Clinical presentation

If patients are neurologically alert, they usually manifest symptoms. The most common complaint is dyspnea (82%), followed by chest pain (46%) [25]. In lieu of chest pain, some patients may complain of epigastric discomfort. Rare manifestations of extravascular migration of the catheter include cough and Horner's syndrome [89].The literature reflects a delay in diagnosis, with a median of 2 days from catheter insertion and a range of 1 to 60 days [25].The slow onset of erosion, the nonspecific symptoms, and the confounding underlying surgical and medical conditions seem to contribute to the delayed diagnosis.

Chest radiograph

The chest radiograph typically demonstrates a pleural effusion, which may be bilateral or unilateral and ipsilateral or contralateral to the catheter insertion site (Fig. 3). The pleural fluid volume can be small to massive and, depending on the timing of the chest radiograph and migration of the catheter, can show mediastinal widening discernible on the chest radiograph. Mediastinal widening, however, may be the only early finding. Although the presence of the pleural effusion is nonspecific, its association with the abnormal location of the catheter tip suggests that perforation has occurred. Furthermore, curvature of the distal few centimeters of the catheter has been suggested as a possible sign of perforation [92]. It is rare that patients have progression of symptoms without obvious chest radiographic abnormalities [82].

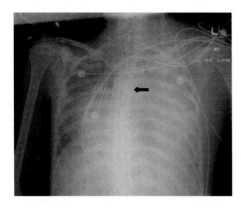

Fig. 3. A 19-year-old HIV-positive patient developed the acute onset of hypotension and oxygen desaturation after surgery and the placement of a left subclavian catheter. A supine chest radiograph showed a massive tension hydrothorax resulting from extravascular migration of the left subclavian catheter, with infusion of total parenteral nutrition with lipid into the mediastinum and the left pleural space. Note the abnormal position of the left subclavian catheter (*arrow*) and evidence of tension with a marked contralateral mediastinal shift to the right. Thoracentesis revealed a whitish fluid, confirming the diagnosis.

Pleural fluid analysis

If the patient is receiving total parenteral nutrition (TPN [which contains lipid]), the fluid appears milky. If a glucose solution is being infused, the pleural fluid–to-serum glucose ratio is substantially greater than 1.0 (absolute pleural fluid glucose range: 107–3000 mg/dL) [78,80,81,86,96]; however, the glucose concentration of the pleural fluid may not be as high as anticipated because of the rapid equilibration of pleural fluid and blood glucose [97]. If the infusion is saline or dextrose and water, the fluid is a transudate with a protein concentration of less than 1.0 g/dL. The protein concentration varies (reported range: 0.1–2.3 g/dL) depending on the protein content of the fluid that is being infused, the degree of pleural inflammation, the effect of hypertonic solutions, and pleural hemorrhage (see Table 2) [25,76,89,98].

Management

The best management is prevention of vascular erosion. This complication is less likely to occur if catheters are inserted from the right side. The catheter should be positioned parallel to the long axis of the superior vena cava, with the tip distal to the azygous recess. Clinicians should be cognizant of this complication and evaluate patients with a sense of urgency when clinical features are compatible with extravascular migration. New progressive cardiopulmonary symptoms, mediastinal widening, a new or enlarging pleural effusion, increased central venous pressure combined with systemic hypotension, and a curving or extravascular location of the distal catheter segment are all clues to the diagnosis. The inability to withdraw blood from the catheter supports the diagnosis, but free blood return does not exclude it. When the diagnosis is established, the catheter should be removed. If the effusion is small, observation is warranted. With a large effusion causing respiratory distress or a hemothorax, therapeutic thoracentesis or tube thoracostomy should be performed.

Ventriculopleural shunt

A ventriculoperitoneal shunt, a frequent operation performed in neurosurgical practice, is the safest route for CSF diversion [99]. Such conditions as adhesions, recent peritonitis, and abdominal cysts can affect the capability of the peritoneum to absorb CSF, however [99]. An alternate method of shunting CSF has been the ventriculovascular route; however, this methodology has been associated with significant complications. Ventriculoatrial shunts have been reported to have severe and even fatal complications, including shunt nephritis, pulmonary emboli, shunt infection during bacteremia, and the need for periodic catheter lengthening, which have resulted in decreased use over the past decade [99].

Compared with ventriculoperitoneal shunts, the ventriculopleural shunt (VPLS) has been used infrequently in the treatment of hydrocephalus. The use of a VPLS was initially reported in 1914 by Heile [100] as a temporary absorptive surface in managing shunt infections and in the decompression of acute hydrocephalus before tumor resection. Approximately 50 years ago, Ransohoff [101] reported a series of six patients with tumor-induced hydrocephalus who were treated with a VPLS and later reported a series of 85 children with hydrocephalus, 65% of whom were managed successfully with a VPLS [102]. The long-term results were less satisfactory, however, because most developed shunt obstruction by 3 years. It was hoped that differential pressure valves would reduce the incidence of pleural effusions. Despite the use of differential pressure valves, however, Venes and Shaw [103] reported six patients who developed large effusions.

In their review of 1500 patients, Hoffman and coworkers [104] analyzed 59 who had received a VPLS over a 10-year period. Twelve (20%) of the 59 patients became obstructed, 11 (17%) became infected, and 1 (2%) died, leaving 35 shunts that were patent. Twelve (34%) of the 35 patients with patent shunts developed symptomatic pleural effusions, with 9 (75%) of the 12 being 5 years of age or older. In 6 of the patients who were 5 years of age or older, antisiphon devices were placed and none developed symptomatic effusions, confirming the opinion of others that older children tended to tolerate these shunts without problems.

Pathogenesis

Intrathoracic complications of a ventriculoperitoneal shunt are rare. Approximately eight cases of pleural effusion from intrathoracic migration of a ventriculoperitoneal shunt have been reported [105]. The thoracic migration of peritoneal shunts can be classified into two types: supradiaphragmatic and transdiaphragmatic [106]. With supradiaphragmatic migration, the entry site into the chest is attributable to incorrect subcutaneous passage during distal tunneling. It is hypothesized that the shunt is unwittingly passed into and out of the pleural space, probably in the supraclavicular fascia, during the tunneling [107,108]. Negative inspiratory pressure and increased patient movement tend to draw the entire distal shunt catheter insidiously into the chest, with the tip entering the chest after the entire catheter has entered [106].

With transdiaphragmatic migration, the tip of the shunt does not seem to traverse a diaphragmatic hiatus but, instead, burrows through the diaphragm. Transdiaphragmatic migration seems to be possible, because local inflammation fixes the peritoneal catheter to the diaphragmatic surface, eventually leading to perforation [109]. Another plausible explanation is catheter movement through a congential defect in the diaphragm, as in the Morgagni or esophageal hiatus [110].

A small asymptomatic pleural effusion is typically visible on the chest radiograph, indicating that the VPLS is patent, but does not imply that the shunt in dysfunctional. A symptomatic pleural effusion can occur anytime as a result of a change in valve pressure or absorptive capacity of the parietal pleura. Tension hydrothorax has been reported by several authors [111–113].

Chest radiograph

The chest radiograph may be normal or show pleural effusions of varying sizes and, on occasion, evidence of tension. The presence of the VPLS or the tip of a ventriculoperitoneal shunt may be seen.

Pleural fluid analysis

The pleural fluid in the properly functioning VPLS is CSF, as seen with an uncomplicated DPF. The fluid is clear, with a paucity of mononuclear cells and low protein and LDH values. Only with infection is there a neutrophil leukocytosis. Pleural fluid eosinophilia was reported in three young children and was associated with peripheral eosinophilia in two of these patients [114]. The mechanism of eosinophilia in these cases remains obscure and may have been attributable to hemorrhage or infection. A rare case of empyema with *Staphylococcus aureus* and *Streptococcus mitis* was reported in a 62-year-old woman with an ipsilateral VPLS (see Table 2) [115].

Diagnosis

The diagnosis of VPLS obstruction in adults with hydrocephalus is often based on worsening clinical symptoms. The most common causes of shunt occlusion include accumulation of debris within the shunt catheter or adhesions and fibrous tissue blocking the distal catheter tip [116]. Most adults with shunt obstruction are ambulatory, and symptoms rarely become life threatening. A single patient has been reported with positive-pressure ventilation causing VPLS obstruction and coma [116]. It is postulated that the patient, who was receiving mechanical ventilation with a positive end-expiratory pressure (PEEP) of 5 cm H_2O and pressure support of 5 cm H_2O, developed increased pleural pressure; in conjunction with the patient's low intracranial pressure (ICP), this reversed the pressure gradient across the shunt and prevented CSF flow. This problem would not be anticipated in patients with a VPLS who need positive-pressure ventilation because their ICP is normally higher than the pleural pressure.

Management

Although the first option in the management of hydrocephalus should not be a VPLS, it seems to be a reasonable alternative to shunting into the peritoneal cavity in older children and adults, with the addition of an antisiphon device, which tends to prevent substantial CSF accumulation in the pleural space and is associated with a low infection rate comparable to that of peritoneal shunts. Carrion and colleagues [117] found that acetazolamide reduced CSF production, which led to tolerance of a VPLS. It seems that acetazolamide treatment of mechanically ventilated pediatric patients with hydrocephalus may improve tolerance of the VPLS and minimize respiratory compromise.

Glycinothorax

Glycinothorax is defined as having a high level of glycine in pleural fluid. Two elderly patients have been reported with a glycinothorax after a transurethral proctectomy for resection of a bladder tumor and for lithopexy for bladder stones [118,119]. Both patients had a 1.5% glycine solution used for irrigation of the bladder to optimize operating conditions and developed perforation of the bladder wall with leak of glycine into the peritoneal cavity. They subsequently developed right-sided effusions.

Pleural fluid analysis

The pleural fluid in the patient with the bladder tumor was clear and blood tinged, with a total protein level of 0.2 g/dL. The creatinine in the fluid was significantly less than the blood creatinine, excluding a urinothorax. The pleural fluid glycine level was 2.3 g/L (30,591 mmol/L). The normal range for blood glycine is 100 to 300 mmol/L. Presumably, a pleural fluid glycine level greater than the normal blood glycine concentration is diagnostic of a glycinothorax (see Table 2).

Pathogenesis

Irrigation fluid containing 15 g/L of glycine and 0.9% saline leaked from the bladder after an iatrogenic perforation of the wall and accumulated in the right pleural space. An extremely high pleural

fluid–to-blood glycine ratio of 300:1 confirmed the diagnosis. The authors speculated that the continued postoperative bladder irrigation with normal saline diluted the pleural glycine concentration from 15 to 2.3 g/L [118]. Normal pleural fluid glycine levels have not been measured but are assumed to be similar to blood concentrations. Presumably, the glycine-containing fluid moved retroperitoneally into the thorax as with a urinothorax. Both patients developed altered mental status, probably attributable to a combination of dilutional hyponatremia and elevated serum glycine levels.

Management

When the diagnosis is established, bladder irrigation should be discontinued and therapeutic thoracentesis performed if necessary.

Exudative effusions of extravascular origins

Chylothorax

Chylothorax, derived from the Latin terms *chylus* (juice) and *thorax* (breast plate), signifies the presence of chyle in the pleural space. A chylothorax is a relatively rare cause of a pleural effusion. The most common cause of chylothorax today is malignancy, especially non-Hodgkin's lymphoma [120,121]. Chylothorax has also been reported after cardiothoracic surgery, with esophagectomy and surgery for congenital heart disease being the most common causes [122,123]. The incidence of postoperative chylothorax remains low at less than 1%, however. Trauma, including innocuous hyperextension of the thoracic spine, has also been implicated. Of the miscellaneous causes of chylothorax, lymphangioleiomyomatosis (LAM) is the most frequent; approximately 25% of patients with LAM develop chylothorax during the course of their disease, and 9% develop it as a presenting manifestation (S.A.S., unpublished data, 2001). Other causes include any form of lymphangiectasia, cirrhosis, tuberculous lymphadenopathy, thrombosis of the left subclavian vein, filariasis, CABG surgery, chronic lymphocytic leukemia, Castleman's disease (angiocentric or giant lymph node hyperplasia), sarcoidosis, Kaposi's sarcoma, yellow nail syndrome, Noonan syndrome, multiple myeloma, Waldenström macroglobulinemia, after thoracic radiation, and goiter [120,121,124–126].

Pathogenesis

When the thoracic duct or one of its large tributaries ruptures, chyle flows into the surrounding tissues. If the mediastinal pleura remain intact, a few days elapse while chyle fills the mediastinum and forms a chyloma before rupturing into the pleural space, usually on the right at the base of the pulmonary ligament. The thoracic duct has its origin in the cisterna chyli, which are situated in the midline anterior to the first and second lumbar vertebrae [127]. The well-developed thoracic duct travels through the aortic hiatus of the diaphragm at the level of the 10th to 12th thoracic vertebrae to the right of the aorta. At the level of the fifth to sixth thoracic vertebrae, the duct enters the left posterior mediastinum and eventually joins the venous circulation, where the left subclavian and internal jugular veins merge. Therefore, disruption of the thoracic duct below T5 to T6 causes a right-sided chylothorax, whereas injury to the duct above this level results in a left chylothorax. Wide anatomic variation exists in the path of the thoracic duct in almost half of the population, however [127].

Chyle is normally transported from the intestine through the lymphatic system into the blood. Gastrointestinal lymph forms in the small intestine, which is the site of passage of fat into the lymphatic vessels. Long-chain triglycerides (containing ≥14 carbon units) in ingested fats are transformed into chylomicrons and low-density lipoproteins in the intestines and form chyle that enters intestinal lymphatic vessels. In contrast, medium-chain triglycerides (containing ≤12 carbon units) are directly absorbed into the portal vein without entering intestinal lymphatics. Approximately 60% of dietary fat enters the lymphatics, and 1500 to 2500 mL of chyle travels daily through these vessels. Lymph flow increases by 2- to 10-fold for 2 to 3 hours after ingestion of fat and by 20% after drinking water [127–129].

Clinical presentation

Patients with chylothorax may present with the subacute or insidious onset of dyspnea. The history, as stated previously, is typically a clue to its cause. A number of chylothoraces are termed *idiopathic*; these are most likely attributable to innocuous hyperextension of the spine or an occult malignancy. Fever or chest pain typically does not occur with a chylothorax, because chyle does not invoke an inflammatory response [130]. Chyle is bacteriostatic; therefore, empyema is rare. Infrequently, patients cough up chyle (chyloptysis) [131]. Sputum triglyceride concentrations have been reported to range from 662 to 2608 mg/dL, which is higher than the concurrent serum values; chylomicrons have also been documented in sputum [131].

Pleural fluid analysis

The color of chyle is typically white and opalescent if fat is present; however, it can be clear and yellow in the neonate who has not yet ingested milk, serous in the adult who has not eaten for 12 hours, or hemorrhagic if trauma has occurred. The supernatant of a chylothorax fails to clear after centrifugation. The primary cells in chyle are T lymphocytes [132], which typically represent greater than 80% of the cellular population. The total nucleated cell count ranges from 400 to 6800 cells/μL [127]. Pleural fluid protein has been reported from 2.2 to 5.9 g/dL [129]. In contrast to a cholesterol pleural effusion, the cholesterol levels in chyle are substantially lower and range from 65 to 220 mg/dL [133]. Electrolytes in chyle are similar to plasma. If the pleural fluid triglyceride level is greater than 110 mg/dL, there is a high likelihood that the patient has a chylothorax. Conversely, if the triglyceride level is less than 50 mg/dL, it is highly unlikely that a chylothorax is present [134]. If the patient has values between 50 and 110 mg/dL, lipoprotein electrophoresis should be performed; if chylomicrons are present, the diagnosis of chylothorax is definitively established [135]. Chylous fluid has been reported to have a pH ranging from 7.40 to 7.80 and a glucose concentration of 78 to 200 mg/dL. Measurement of the pleural fluid-to-serum glucose ratio assists in differentiating a chylous effusion (ratio <1.0) from pleural fluid attributable to the extravascular migration of a central venous catheter with glucose-containing parenteral nutrition with lipid into the pleural space (ratio >1.0) (see Table 2) [25].

Management

There are no prospective studies to guide management; however, there are two major principles that should be followed [135]. First, patients should be managed with a step-wise plan of care that starts with pleural space drainage if the patient is symptomatic and nutritional support with progression to pleural symphysis if necessary, which can be accomplished by various techniques. Second, prolonged drainage of a chylothorax should be avoided to prevent immunosuppression and malnutrition.

Patients who develop a traumatic chylothorax are typically managed with chest tube drainage, bowel rest, and parenteral nutrition to minimize the flow of chyle and maintenance of the fluid and electrolyte balance. Because most traumatic chylothoraces resolve within 10 to 14 days [136], protein loss and immunosuppression are usually minimal. If drainage is persistent at 2 weeks, drainage exceeds 1500 mL for 5 days, or the patient develops significant weight loss or progressive loss of protein despite nutritional therapy, surgical intervention is indicated. Repair of the defect is optimal; however, at times, the precise leak cannot be identified. Thoracic duct ligation, typically just above the right diaphragm, may have to be performed in some patients to stop the leak of chyle.

Postoperative chylothorax can result in a high mortality rate (up to 50%) [137]. Management includes chest tube drainage, parenteral nutrition, or orally supplemented medium-chain triglycerides. This regimen is continued for a variable period before surgical intervention is undertaken [138,139]. Patients with lymphoma or metastatic cancer may respond to chemotherapy or radiation [127]. Failure of these modalities usually leads to a pleurodesis procedure with the use of talc poudrage at thoracoscopy or talc slurry through a chest tube [140–143]. In some patients, a pleuroperitoneal or pleurovenous shunt [144] has been used to recirculate the chyle and avoid surgery.

There are recent reports of percutaneous catheterization and embolization of the thoracic duct in patients with traumatic chylothorax occurring after surgical procedures [145–147]. Somatostatin and octreotide, a somatostatin analogue, have been reported to decrease chyle production in postoperative chylothorax in experimental animals and in small case series [148–150].

Pancreaticopleural fistula

Pleural effusions are a well-known complication of pancreatitis. In acute pancreatitis, the patient may develop a small, self-limited, left-sided pleural effusion (3%–17% incidence), which resolves relatively rapidly once the pancreatitis subsides [151,152]. In contrast, pleural effusions from a pancreaticopleural fistula associated with chronic pancreatitis are less common, chronic, and typically recurrent [153–158]. Pancreaticopleural fistulas most commonly occur in patients with chronic alcoholism, who have predominantly pulmonary symptoms rather than abdominal complaints and may not have a previous history of pancreatic disease. Therefore, this diagnosis is often not considered by physicians as the cause of this chronic pleural effusion.

Pathogenesis

A pancreatic pseudocyst (not containing true walls) actually represents a collection of fluid and debris located within or juxtaposed to the pancreas that contains high concentrations of pancreatic enzymes [158,159]. A pseudocyst develops in ap-

proximately 10% of patients with acute pancreatitis, whereas only half of those with a pseudocyst develop pleural effusions [153]. The most likely cause of a large pleural effusion in pancreatic disease is a pancreaticopleural fistula, which has been delineated on endoscopic retrograde cholangiopancreatography (ERCP), sonography, CT, and magnetic resonance cholangiopancreatography. The fistulous track can enter the mediastinum, both pleural spaces, or the pericardial sac; fluid from the mediastinum can enter both pleural spaces [160–164].

Clinical presentation

The patient, who usually has a history of alcoholic pancreatitis, may only complain of dyspnea (42%) and chest discomfort (29%) from the large unilateral effusion and is less likely to have abdominal pain (28%) at the time of presentation.

Other less common symptoms include cough, malaise, weight loss, and fatigue [153,155]. The less frequent complaint of abdominal symptoms may be attributable to decompression of the pseudocyst by the pancreaticopleural fistula. The diagnosis should be considered in a chronically ill-appearing patient with an isolated, large, left pleural effusion or a history of pancreatic disease or abdominal trauma.

Chest radiograph

A large to massive left pleural effusion with a contralateral mediastinal shift is the most commonly observed radiographic finding (Fig. 4A). The effusion can occur on the right side or bilaterally, however (see Fig. 4A). No other abnormalities are usually noted [153,155] on the chest radiograph. Calcifications are often observed in the pancreas on an abdominal film, however (see Fig. 4B).

Pleural fluid analysis

The pleural fluid is a neutrophilic predominant exudate with an extremely high amylase level, usually greater than 100,000 IU/L. In contrast, the other causes of amylase-rich pleural effusions (ie, acute pancreatitis [pancreatic isoamylase], malignancy, esophageal rupture [salivary isoamylase]) have amylase levels several orders of magnitude lower (a few hundred or in the low thousands) [165,166]. The pH is usually between 7.32 and 7.50, and the glucose value is similar to serum values (see Table 2) [167].

Management

Conservative management consisting of therapeutic thoracentesis and TPN is effective in approximately 50% of patients. The theory behind this

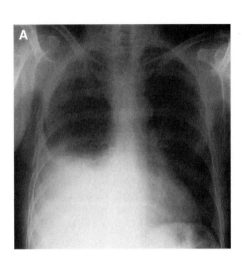
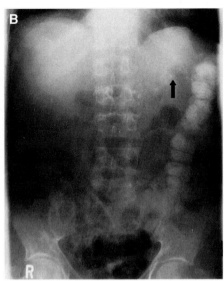

Fig. 4. (A) A 56-year-old alcoholic patient presented with the insidious onset of dyspnea with exertion and a moderate right pleural effusion. (B) Abdominal radiograph 10 months earlier demonstrates pancreatic calcifications (arrow). Thoracentesis revealed a turbid yellow fluid with an amylase level of 120,000 IU/L, confirming the diagnosis of a pancreaticopleural fistula.

nonsurgical approach is to minimize secretion of pancreatic enzymes and decrease the volume of fluid in the pseudocyst with eventual closure of the fistulous track. Some patients have had spontaneous closure of the fistula with somatostatin or its analogue, which inhibits pancreatic exocrine secretion [168,169]. If conservative therapy for 2 weeks is not effective, usually in those with severe pancreatic disease, surgical correction of the underlying pancreatic disease, including ductal decompression and drainage or resection of the pseudocyst, is indicated to prevent recurrence and to avoid the other complications of advanced chronic pancreatitis [170,171]. Most patients respond well to surgery, with a low mortality rate [153]. Percutaneous drainage is an alternative to surgery, with a success rate of approximately 75% [171].

Esophageal perforation

There are three distinct types of esophageal perforation, including traumatic (iatrogenic and barogenic), inflammatory, and neoplastic [172]. Iatrogenic causes account for most esophageal perforations, with the most common procedure being esophageal dilatation, which occurs 3 to 10 times more frequently than with diagnostic flexible fiberoptic esophagoscopy (the second most common cause) [173,174]. Less common causes of perforation include external

trauma, postthoracic surgical perforation, external tumor invasion, postinfectious causes, traumatic tears from endoesophageal tubes, and accidental pneumatic rupture [175–181].

Spontaneous esophageal rupture, more appropriately termed *barogenic rupture* (Boerhaave syndrome), is a rare occurrence that was first described in 1724 in a Dutch admiral [182]. Alcoholism associated with vigorous vomiting is frequently responsible. Mediastinitis and sepsis are responsible for the high morbidity and mortality in this syndrome [183,184].

Bladergroen and colleagues [185] retrospectively reviewed the 47-year experience with 127 patients who had an esophageal perforation. Iatrogenic perforation secondary to endoscopy or dilation occurred in 50 (39%) patients and was the most common cause. If those patients with a perforation resulting from other iatrogenic causes, such as nasogastric tubes and intraoperative esophageal injury, are included in this category, more than half of all perforations (55%) were iatrogenic. In 19 (15%) of the patients, spontaneous (barogenic) rupture was the cause. Other causes were a foreign body (14%) and traumatic perforations (10%). The distal esophagus was the most common location of injury (47%), followed by the cervical esophagus (29%) and midesophagus (24%). Underlying esophageal disease was documented in 63 (50%) of the patients, with benign esophageal stricture being most common (25% of 127 patients). Other esophageal lesions included paraesophageal hernias, esophageal webs and rings, carcinoma, achalasia, and lye-related injury.

Pathogenesis

In experimental studies of esophageal rupture, Macker [186] followed up on Mackenzie's experimental studies on esophageal rupture [187] and came to similar conclusions: (1) the esophageal tear always takes place longitudinally, (2) the tear always occurs in the lower half of the esophagus, (3) the rupture pressure is approximately 5 lb/sq in, and (4) the mucosa is the most resistant layer. The lower esophagus is believed to be more susceptible to rupture, because the upper esophagus is buttressed by striated and smooth muscle fibers, whereas the lower esophagus contains only smooth muscle that is unsupported. Duval [188] determined that the rate of pressure rise was more important than the peak. Because this syndrome is commonly associated with alcohol ingestion, the alcohol contributes to acute esophagitis and muscular incoordination of the esophagus. This syndrome can certainly occur in the absence of alcohol ingestion but not without vomiting or retching. As the esophagus deviates to the left to enter the esophageal hiatus, the left lateral wall is in direct contact with the mediastinal pleura. This explains why the left pleural space is predominantly involved. Bilateral empyema typically is found with extensive instrument trauma or with delayed diagnosis of a perforation. Perforation of the cervical esophagus usually does not involve the pleural space [187,189].

Clinical presentation

The most dramatic presentation of esophageal rupture is associated with barogenic perforation. It is seen most commonly in men in their fourth to sixth decades of life with a history of alcoholism, dietary indiscretion, and malnutrition who present with severe epigastric pain that is pleuritic and may be misdiagnosed as acute myocardial infarction, acute pancreatitis, perforated peptic ulcer, or empyema of the gallbladder [172,190,191]. The pain typically follows severe vomiting or retching and is persistent and severe in the epigastrium. Reflux spasm of the upper abdominal muscles may focus the clinician on a primary abdominal process. Fever, which is present in virtually all patients, occurs later than chest pain. Dysphagia is invariably present. Pneumomediastinum is a constant feature of esophageal rupture. With cervical perforation, crepitation may be palpated in the neck. After esophageal-mediastinal perforation, a "crunch" may be auscultated over the left heart synchronous with the cardiac cycle.

Chest radiograph

The presence or absence of some or all the chest radiographic findings depends on the time interval between the perforation and the initial radiographic examination, the site of the perforation, and the integrity of the mediastinal parietal pleura [192]. If the chest radiograph is performed within several minutes after an esophageal perforation, it is usually normal and, as such, would not exclude the diagnosis of perforation. Mediastinal widening at times with air-fluid levels indicates mediastinal infection and may take several hours to appear radiographically. Subcutaneous emphysema virtually never appears before 1 hour after perforation and never occurs in approximately 40% of patients [193]. Instrumental perforation of a normal esophagus takes place at one of three sites of normal narrowing. The most common site is in the neck, the second is just above the diaphragmatic hiatus, and the third is the midesophagus at the level of the left mainstem bronchus and the aortic arch [194]. With esophageal disease, the perforation typically occurs at the site of pathologic change. With perforation of the cervical esophagus, subcutaneous air in the cervical region is common. Mediastinal air is rarely seen. With intrathoracic esophageal perforation, mediastinal changes are more likely to occur [195]. The presence and timing of pleural changes are linked to the integrity of the mediastinal parietal pleura. Rupture of the mediastinal parietal pleura occurs in most patients, with the rapid development of a hydropneumothorax or pyopneumothorax. Most pleural lesions that are left-sided occur because 70% of barogenic esophageal ruptures develop in the left posterior lateral wall near the diaphragm [196]. When all causes of pleural perforation are considered, however, the proportion of left-sided mediastinal esophageal rupture is substantially less. Without pleural rupture, mediastinal and subcutaneous emphysema appear rapidly, and a small sympathetic pleural effusion attributable to mediastinitis develops insidiously in approximately 75% of patients.

Diagnosis

When esophageal rupture is suspected, a contrast study of the esophagus should be performed immediately. The choice of contrast is limited to a water-soluble iodinated compound and barium sulfate. Barium has the advantage of increased radiographic density and better mucosal adherence [197–199]. A disadvantage of barium is its ability to incite a foreign body reaction with development of pleural and mediastinal granulomas and possibly fibrosis [197–199]. Water-soluble contrast agents are rapidly absorbed and do not cause an inflammatory reaction [197–199]. The limitations of water-soluble compounds are related to hypertonicity, however. Therefore, aspiration of these compounds into the tracheobronchial tree can create significant inflammation and precipitate pulmonary edema. Furthermore, 25% to 50% of thoracic and esophageal perforations can be missed with the use of water-soluble compounds [197–199]. If a water-soluble compound is used initially for the detection of esophageal perforation and the results of the study are negative, a barium study should be done without delay. On chest CT, if air is found in the mediastinum in the appropriate clinical setting, an esophageal perforation is highly likely [200]. Thoracentesis can establish the diagnosis once the mediastinal pleura has ruptured, however.

Pleural fluid analysis

If mediastinitis alone is present without rupture into the pleural space, the pleural fluid is a predominantly neutrophilic exudate with a pH greater than 7.30, glucose level greater than 60 mg/dL, and amylase levels less than the upper limits of normal serum amylase. After mediastinal parietal pleural rupture, the patient develops an anaerobic empyema. The low pleural fluid pH and glucose are the result of enhanced glycolysis from neutrophil phagocytosis and bacterial metabolism causing increased carbon dioxide (CO_2) and lactic acid [201]. Therefore, finding a low pleural pH, typically between 5.00 and 7.00, in association with a high amylase level, which is salivary on isoenzyme analysis, establishes the diagnosis. The pleural fluid at this stage should show high protein and LDH levels (>1000 IU/L), and the glucose concentration should be less than 60 mg/dL and may be 0 mg/dL. In addition, pleural fluid cytologic analysis of high-speed cytocentrifugation concentrates may reveal undigested food particles that confirm the diagnosis [202], which may not be detectible on Gram stain and wet preparations. Squamous epithelial cells observed on cytologic examination also establish the diagnosis (see Table 2).

Management

The patient with a barogenic esophageal rupture represents an emergency. In their review of 127 patients with an esophageal perforation, Bladergroen and colleagues [185] reported that when primary closure was achieved within 24 hours of rupture, the outcome was excellent, with a 92% survival rate. After 24 hours, survival was substantially worse and no specific treatment was clearly superior. In addition, complications were frequent. The importance of early diagnosis has been reported by others [173,203,204]. Factors related to late diagnosis include delayed presentation by the patient, a lack of awareness of this rare entity by the treating physician, and uncertainty because of nonspecific symptoms mimicking other disease processes.

When the diagnosis of barogenic esophageal rupture is confirmed, immediate primary repair should be accomplished, with mediastinal and pleural space drainage as appropriate and prompt treatment with antibiotics that include anaerobic coverage. Conservative management has proven adequate in patients with small cervical ruptures that are virtually never attributable to barogenic causes [205–207]. Conservative treatment includes antibiotic therapy with anaerobic coverage, gastric suction, nothing by mouth, and TPN. Conservative treatment requires good judgment and careful observation of patients with small iatrogenic tears, however, as well as knowledge that the contents are contained in the mediastinum with drainage of the cavity back into the esophagus.

Biliopleural fistula

A bilious pleural effusion is a rare complication of pathologic change of the biliary tract. Causes of a biliopleural fistula include thoracoabdominal trauma [208,209], parasitic liver disease [210,211], suppurative complications of biliary tract obstruction, primary pyogenic liver abscess, syphilitic gummas [212], tuberculous liver abscess [213], radiofrequency ablation for liver metastasis [214], postoperative strictures [215], and percutaneous biliary drainage (PBD) from an obstructed biliary system [216]. PBD is a useful adjunct to the definitive surgical treatment of obstructive jaundice [217,218]. For those patients who cannot technically have an internal biliary stent placed, PBD is an effective method for palliation.

Like all procedures, however, PBD is not without complications, which include cholangitis, catheter dislodgment, obstruction, and leakage [216,219–221]. Also reported are peritonitis, hemobilia, arteriovenous malformation, hemorrhage, and subphrenic abscess.

Pleural complications are uncommon despite transgression of the pleural sulcus using the intercostal approach [222]. Hemothorax [223,224], pneumothorax [219,220], empyema [223], rib erosion [224], and malignant pleural seeding [225] have been noted. Fewer than 20 cases of biliothorax have been reported in the literature.

Pathogenesis

In 1988, we reported on three patients with a biliopleural fistula who manifested some common features that led to its development [216]. These features included complete biliary obstruction, catheter placement between the ninth and 10th ribs in the midaxillary line, and prolonged drainage of 7 days to 2 months. We speculated that prolonged drainage results in inflammation and a more defined fistulous track and that the development of a biliopleural fistula requires a dysfunctional PBD catheter. Empyema seems to occur with increased frequency in these patients. Possible risk factors for empyema include a direct track from the skin to the pleura, increasing the likelihood of pleural seeding with bacterial pathogens; cholangitis with complete obstruction of the biliary system; and a paucity of clinical symptoms, leading to delayed diagnosis. Therefore, when a biliopleural fistula is confirmed, the clinical suspicion for empyema should be high and evaluated appropriately. The diagnosis should always be considered in a patient with PBD who develops a right pleural effusion.

Clinical presentation

Common presenting symptoms are fever, dyspnea, right upper quadrant pain, and right lower chest pain. A rare manifestation is biliptysis, signifying a bronchobiliary fistula.

Chest radiograph

The chest radiograph typically shows a right pleural effusion, usually without other thoracic pathologic findings. An elevated right hemidiaphragm and an air-fluid level in the liver may be seen in some patients, however.

Pleural fluid analysis

The diagnosis is established when greenish fluid is aspirated in conjunction with a pleural fluid–to-serum total bilirubin ratio greater than 1.0 [216]. The pleural fluid is a neutrophil predominant exudate.

An experimental model suggests rapid clearance of bilirubin from the pleural space; therefore, a thoracentesis performed late in the course of a biliopleural fistula, after cessation of the leak, may provide false-negative results [216]. ^{99m}Tc–diisopropyl-iminodiacetic acid (DISIDA) hepobiliary scintigraphy can demonstrate bile leakage into the pleural space (see Table 2) [225,226].

Management

The most important component in the successful management of a biliopleural fistula is institution of drainage as soon as the diagnosis is established [216,227,228]. In a traumatic biliopleural fistula, it is clear that once an alternate route of biliary decompression is instituted, chest drainage dramatically decreases or ceases. Otherwise, re-establishing PBD can be problematic in the setting of biliary decompression into the chest. The benefits of biliary drainage by ERCP or PBD outweigh the risk of partially functioning catheters that leak around the track, however. Replacing the PBD catheter through a non-intercostal site is reasonable, such as with a subxiphoid approach [222]. Biliopleural fistulas are rare but serious complications of PBD. Early diagnosis with aggressive and expectant therapy should lead to a better outcome in this high-risk population.

Gastropleural fistula

A gastropleural fistula is a rare finding, because the diaphragm represents a relatively thick barrier. Approximately 25 cases have been reported to date [229–251].

Pathogenesis

A gastropleural fistula may occur with several pathologic conditions: (1) perforation of the intrathoracic portion of the stomach with an esophageal hiatal hernia, (2) trauma to the stomach with immediate formation of the fistula or a traumatic diaphragmatic hernia and delayed perforation of the intrathoracic portion of the stomach, and (3) perforation of the stomach contained entirely within the peritoneal cavity with secondary abscess formation and erosion through the diaphragm into the pleural space [251]. Intrathoracic gastric perforations seem to occur more frequently than when the stomach is in its normal location. Gastropleural fistulas may be classified by the perforated site of the stomach or by the pathologic causes. In the cases reported, the perforated site of the stomach was intrathoracic in 14 and intra-abdominal in 11 [229]. The pathologic cause was peptic ulcer in 11 cases, trauma in 7, empyema in 4, malignant lymphoma in 3, complications of surgery or radiation in 2, and gastric cancer in 1 [229]. Factors that may promote the formation of a gastropleural fistula include surgery, nonsteroidal anti-inflammatory drugs (NSAIDs), and corticosteroids.

Clinical presentation

Typical symptoms include fever, malaise, dyspnea, and left chest pain.

Chest radiograph

A large left pleural effusion with or without pneumothorax, which may demonstrate a contralateral mediastinal shift, is the most common finding.

Pleural fluid analysis

A paucity of data is available on the characteristics of the pleural fluid. The pleural fluid may be an empyema or may be nonpurulent. It is an exudate with a high LDH level. Pleural pH should be low because of the acidity of gastric secretions or the presence of an empyema (see Table 2).

Management

The possibility of a gastropleural fistula should be considered in patients with a pneumothorax or pyothorax that is resistant to standard therapy. When diagnosed, appropriate drainage and repair of the perforation should be accomplished without delay.

Misplacement of enteral feeding tubes

Enteral tube feeding of the chronically ill malnourished patient and those requiring short-term supplementation during an acute illness provides an attractive alternative to intravenous alimentation. Pulmonary and pleural [252–260] complications of enteral feeding tubes have been reported, however. There have been a number of complications associated with the large-bore stiff tubes (16–20 French), including patient discomfort; ischemia and necrosis of superficial tissues, esophagus, and stomach; tracheoesophageal fistula; and esophagotracheal fistula [261,262]. Subsequently, narrow-bore nasogastric tubes have replaced the large-bore tubes; these tubes range from 12 French (4–5 mm in external diameter) to 1 to 2 mm in external diameter and are soft, pliable, polyvinyl chloride–based tubes with weighted ends and stylets for use on insertion [263]. Although the stylet provides stiffness and strength to the tubing and allows easier advancement, it also provides stiffness to the tubing, which could perforate several structures if excessive pressure is applied with the distal tip deflected against an organ [263]. It is problematic to pass these tubes in patients who are uncooperative, obtunded, demented, critically ill, or on mechanical ventilation [252,263]. Such patients are unable to cooperate fully and are at increased risk for complications of tube placement. Review of the cases with complications have focused on attention to techniques of placement and a raised index of suspicion for adverse outcomes in patients with underlying risk factors, eg, depressed sensorium, a poor or absent gag reflex, recent endotracheal intubation, decreased laryngeal sensitivity, esophageal stricture, cardiomegaly, or neuromuscular blocking agents [252,263]. Complications arise from insertion of the feeding tube into the lung and pleural space, with subsequent infection, bleeding, or introduction of enteral feeding or air. Pneumomediastinum, subcutaneous emphysema, pneumothorax, pneumonitis, pulmonary hemorrhage, pleural effusions from enteral feeding, empyema, bronchopleural fistula, hemothorax, and perforation of the esophagus have all been reported [252–261].

Pathogenesis

Approximately 23 cases of pleuropulmonary complications of enteral feeding tubes have been reported. These include: (1) perforation of the esophagus into the pleural space; (2) perforation of the right mainstem bronchus into the pulmonary parenchyma; (3) passage of the feeding tube into the right lower lobe; (4) perforation of the right mainstem bronchus; (5) rupture of the left mainstem bronchus, with pulmonary hemorrhage and effusion; (6) perforation of the right mainstem bronchus; and (7) passage of the feeding tube around the tracheostomy tube, perforating a bronchus. In most of the patients, the enteral feeding was infused into the lung, esophagus, or pleural space.

Clinical presentation

The patients most likely to sustain complications from feeding tubes include those receiving mechanical ventilation through an endotracheal tube or tracheostomy tube, those with depressed sensorium, and those who are uncooperative. Symptoms depend on the location of the feeding tube and the patient's mental status. These include cough, dyspnea, fever, chest pain, and hemoptysis. Subcutaneous emphysema may be palpated and evidence of a pleural effusion suspected on chest examination.

Chest radiograph

The chest film should demonstrate an abnormal location of the small-bore catheter and a pleural effusion or hydropneumothorax. The mediastinum may be widened and contain air. A new alveolar infiltrate may be detected, representing tube feeding or blood.

Pleural fluid analysis

When the enteral feeding tube enters the pleural space directly or a tracheal or bronchial-esophageal fistula develops, thoracentesis returns the enteral feeding. If a hemothorax is present, however, it can mask the enteral tube feeding (see Table 2).

Management

The enteral feeding should be discontinued immediately on diagnosis, and the feeding tube should be removed. A chest tube should be inserted to drain tube feeding and air. There is usually no clinically significant pleural space sequela, and the patient generally recovers from the event if it is recognized relatively quickly.

For prevention of these potential hazards, only personnel familiar with placement of narrow-bore feeding tubes should be operators and traditional criteria need to be reassessed. The following guidelines should decrease the risk of these complications:

1. If any resistance is met with passage, the tube should be removed and repositioned.
2. Removal and reinsertion of the stylet should be avoided, because reinsertion can lead to the stylet exiting through a feeding port and puncturing any structure. Although modification of the distal end of the tube reportedly prevents the stylet from exiting through a feeding port, caution advises the absolute avoidance of this possibility.
3. Coughing or any evidence of respiratory distress should prompt removal of the tube.
4. It should be recognized that an endotracheal tube does not prohibit passage of a feeding tube into the lungs.
5. The feeding tube can be passed around a tracheostomy tube without eliciting symptoms from patients.

Once the feeding tube has been placed, traditional criteria for appropriate positioning should not be accepted. Before initiating feeding, placement of the tube should be verified radiographically. Inflation of air with sounds heard over the left upper quadrant should not be accepted as evidence of gastric placement, because: (1) small-bore tubes do not always allow sufficient passage of air; (2) vigorous peristalsis may be mistaken for insufflated air; (3) air bubbling in the pleural space, lung, pharynx, or esophagus may be transmitted below the diaphragm; (4) an inexperienced operator may misinterpret the sound [264]; (5) aspiration of fluid should not be interpreted as appropriate placement in the stomach, because the fluid may come from the pleural space or bronchial secretions [265]; and (6) if the tube passes the full 60 cm and the stylet is removed easily, the tube is straight and unlikely to be kinked or coiled up in the lung [257]; however, several reports refute this claim [256,260].

If it is difficult to pass a narrow-bore nasogastric tube, several options can be used: (1) the narrow-bore nasogastric tube can be coupled with a large-bore nasogastric tube with a gelatin capsule passed into the stomach, and the larger tube can be removed when the capsule dissolves [266]; (2) fluoroscopy may be used, because the tube is radiopaque; (3) direct passage with the use of an endoscope; and (4) direct visualization of the larynx with a laryngoscope in an optimally anesthetized patient with posterior passage of the tube.

A narrow-bore nasogastric tube offers an attractive and safe method to supply the caloric needs of the acute or chronically ill patient but is not without risk. The operator's familiarity, nonforceful insertion, careful observation for respiratory distress, and dependence on the chest radiograph after placement reduce the complications of this procedure. A high index of suspicion for complications in a compromised patient can prevent accidental infusion of enteral tube feeding into the lungs or pleural space. Finally, the presence of a cuffed tracheostomy tube does not prevent the advancement of an enteral feeding tube into the lungs or pleural space.

References

[1] Sahn S. State of the art. The pleura. Am Rev Respir Dis 1988;138:184–234.
[2] Boen S, Mulinari A, Dillard D, et al. Periodic peritoneal dialysis in the management of chronic uremia. Trans Am Soc Artif Int Organs 1962;8:256–65.
[3] Popovich R, Moncrif J, Decherd J, et al. The definition of a novel portable-wearable equilibrium dialysis technique [abstract]. Trans Am Soc Artif Int Organs 1976;5:64.
[4] Gokal R, Ramos J, Francis D, et al. Peritonitis and COPD. Lancet 1982;2:1388–91.
[5] Chung S, Heimbürger O, Lindholm B, et al. Chronic inflammation in PD patients. In: Ronoc C, Dell'Aquila R, Rodighiero M, editors. Peritoneal dialysis today. Basel: Karger; 2003. p. 104–11.
[6] Bargman J. Complications of peritoneal dialysis related to intra-abdominal pressure. Kidney Int 1993; 43(Suppl 40):s75–80.
[7] Nomoto Y, Suga T, Nakajima K, et al. Acute hydrothorax in continuous ambulatory peritoneal dialysis— a collaborative study of 161 centers. Am J Nephrol 1989;9:363–7.
[8] Winchester J, Kriger F. The fluid leaks: prevention and treatment. Perit Dial Int 1994;14(Suppl 3): S443–8.
[9] Gotloib L, Mine M, Garmiso L, et al. Hemodynamic effects of increasing intra-abdominal pressure in peritoneal dialysis. Perit Dial Bull 1981;1:41–3.

[10] Twardowski Z, Khanna R, Nolph K, et al. Intra-abdominal pressures during natural activities in patients treated with continuous ambulatory peritoneal dialysis. Nephron 1986;44:129–35.

[11] Twardowski Z, Nolph K, Prowant B, et al. High volume low frequency continuous ambulatory peritoneal dialysis. Kidney Int 1983;23:64–70.

[12] Johnston R, Loo R. Hepatic hydrothorax. Ann Intern Med 1964;61:385–401.

[13] Lieberman F, Hidemura R, Peters R, et al. Pathogenesis and treatment of hydrothorax complicating cirrhosis with ascites. Ann Intern Med 1966;64:341–51.

[14] Boeschoten E, Krediet R, Roos C, et al. Leakage of dialysate across the diaphragm: an important complication of continuous ambulatory peritoneal dialysis. Neth J Med 1986;29:242–6.

[15] Grefberg N, Danielson B, Benson L, et al. Right-sided hydrothorax complicating peritoneal dialysis. Nephron 1983;34:130–4.

[16] Pattison C, Rodger R, Adu D, et al. Surgical treatment of hydrothorax complicating continuous ambulatory peritoneal dialysis. Clin Nephrol 1984;21:191–3.

[17] Rudnick M, Coyle J, Beck L, et al. Acute massive hydrothorax complicating peritoneal dialysis, report of 2 cases and a review of the literature. Clin Nephrol 1979;12:38–44.

[18] Abraham G, Shokker A, Blake P, et al. Massive hydrothorax in patients on peritoneal dialysis: a literature review. In: Khanna R, Nolph K, Prowant B, et al, editors. Advances in continuous ambulatory peritoneal dialysis. Toronto (ON): Peritoneal Dialysis Bulletin, Inc.; 1988. p. 121–5.

[19] Lepage S, Bisson G, Verreault J, et al. Massive hydrothorax complicating peritoneal dialysis. Isotopic investigation (peritoneopleural scintigraphy). Clin Nucl Med 1993;18:498–501.

[20] Milutinovic J, Wuu-Shyong W, Lindholm D, et al. Acute massive unilateral hydrothorax: a rare complication of chronic peritoneal dialysis. South Med J 1980;73:827–8.

[21] Trust A, Rossoff L. Tension hydrothorax in a patient with renal failure. Chest 1990;97:1254–5.

[22] Jagasia M, Cole F, Stegman M, et al. Video-assisted talc pleurodesis in the management of pleural effusion secondary to continuous ambulatory peritoneal dialysis: a report of three cases. Am J Kidney Dis 1996;28:772–4.

[23] Kanaan N, Pietrs T, Jamar F, et al. Hydrothorax complicating continuous ambulatory peritoneal dialysis: successful management with talc pleurodesis under thoracoscopy. Nephrol Dial Transplant 1999;14:1590–2.

[24] Camilleri B, Glancey G, Pledger D, et al. The icodextrin black line sign to confirm a pleural leak in a patient on peritoneal dialysis. Perit Dial Int 2004;24:167.

[25] Duntley P, Siever J, Korwes M, et al. Vascular erosion by central venous catheters. Clinical features and outcome. Chest 1992;101:1633–8.

[26] Roberston S, Huxtable H, Blakemore C, et al. The icodextrin black line sign. Perit Dial Int 2001;21:621–3.

[27] Yen T, Lin K, Tzen K. Massive pleural effusion secondary to continuous ambulatory peritoneal dialysis, confirmed by Tc-99m sulfur colloid peritoneoscintigraphy. Clin Nucl Med 2000;25:62.

[28] Simmons L, Mir A. A review of management of pleuroperitoneal communication in five CAPD patients. Adv Perit Dial 1989;5:81–3.

[29] Salcedo J. Urinothorax: report of 4 cases and review of the literature. J Urol 1986;135:805–8.

[30] Corriere J, Miller W, Murphy J. Hydronephrosis as a cause of pleural effusion. Radiology 1968;90:79–84.

[31] Polsky M, Weber C, Ball Jr T. Infected pyelocaliceal diverticulum and sympathetic pleural effusion. J Urol 1965;114:301–3.

[32] Laforet E, Kornitzer G. Nephrogenic pleural effusion. J Urol 1977;117:118–9.

[33] Leung F, Williams A, Oill P. Pleural effusion associated with urinary tract obstruction: support for a hypothesis. Thorax 1981;36:632–3.

[34] Stark D, Shanes J, Baron R, et al. Biochemical features of urinothorax. Arch Intern Med 1982;142:1509–11.

[35] Weiss Z, Shalev E, Zuckerman H, et al. Obstructive renal failure and pleural effusion caused by the gravid uterus. Acta Obstet Gynecol Scand 1986;65:187–9.

[36] Miller K, Wooten S, Sahn S. Urinothorax: a cause of low pH transudative pleural effusions. Am J Med 1988;85:448–9.

[37] Fokaefs E, Melekos M. Pleural effusion associated with urinary extravasation due to renal colic. Br J Urol 1991;68:435.

[38] Williams J, Heaney J, Young W. Respiratory distress following cesarean section: cryptic presentation of bladder injury. Urology 1994;44:441–5.

[39] Hamoud K, Kaneti J, Smailowitz Z, et al. Spontaneous perinephric urinoma in pregnancy. Int Urol Nephrol 1994;26:643–6.

[40] Chanatry B, Gettinger A. Progressive respiratory insufficiency after cesarean section. Crit Care Med 1995;23:204–7.

[41] Kees-Folts D, Cole B. Ureteral urine leak presenting as a pleural effusion in a renal transplant recipient. Pediatr Nephrol 1998;12:666–7.

[42] Hase T, Kodama M, Domasu S, et al. A case of urothorax that manifested as posttraumatic pleural effusion after a motorcycle crash. J Trauma 1999;46:967–9.

[43] Kamble R, Bhat S, Joshi J. Urinothorax: a case report. Indian J Chest Dis Allied Sci 2000;42:189–90.

[44] Hendriks J, Michielsen D, Van Schil P, et al. Urinothorax: a rare pleural effusion. Acta Chir Belg 2002;102:274–5.

[45] Oguzulgen I, Oguzulgen A, Sinik Z, et al. An unusual cause of urinothorax. Respiration (Herrlisheim) 2002;69:273–4.

[46] Parvathy U, Saldanha R, Balakrishnan K. Blunt abdominal trauma resulting in urinothorax from a missed uretero-pelvic junction avulsion: case report. J Trauma 2003;54:187–9.

[47] Ray K, Rattan S, Yohannes T. Urinothorax: unexpected cause of a pleural effusion. Mayo Clin Proc 2003;78:1433–4.

[48] Lallas C, Delvecchio C, Evans B, et al. Management of nephropleural fistula after supracostal percutaneous nephrolithotomy. Urology 2004;64:241–5.

[49] Lee C, Fang C, Chou H, et al. Urinothorax associated with VURD syndrome. Pediatr Nephrol 2005;20: 543–6.

[50] Ozer H, Barki Y, Bertan V. Traumatic arachnoido-pleural fistula. Report of a case. J Can Assoc Radiol 1972;23:287–9.

[51] Rosen P, Chaudhuri T. Radioisotope myelography in the detection of pleural-dural communication as a source of recurrent meningitis. Clin Nucl Med 1983;8:28–30.

[52] Azambuja P, Fragaomeni L. Traumatic chylothorax associated with subarachnoid-pleural fistula. Thorax 1981;36:669–700.

[53] Singhi P, Nayak U, Ghai S, et al. Rapidly filling pleural effusion due to a subarachnoid-pleural fistula. Clin Pediatr 1987;26:416–8.

[54] Pollack I, Pang D, Hall W. Subarachnoid-pleural and subarachnoid-mediastinal fistulae. Neurosurgery 1990;26:519–24.

[55] Assietti R, Kibble M, Bakay R. Iatrogenic cerebrospinal fluid fistula to the pleural cavity: case report and literature review. Neurosurgery 1993;33:1104–8.

[56] Skedros D, Cass S, Hirsch B, et al. Beta-2 transferrin assay in clinical management of cerebral spinal fluid and perilymphatic fluid leaks. J Otolaryngol 1993; 22:341–4.

[57] Monla-Hassan J, Eichenhorn M, Spickler E, et al. Duropleural fistula manifested as a large pleural transudate: an unusual complication of transthoracic diskectomy. Chest 1998;114:1786–9.

[58] Fernadez P, Guyot M, Mangione P, et al. Subarachnoid-pleural fistula complicating thoracoscopy: value of In-111 DTPA myeloscintigraphy. Clin Nucl Med 1999;24:985–6.

[59] D'Souza R, Doshi A, Bhojraj S, et al. Massive pleural effusion as the presenting feature of a subarachnoid-pleural fistula. Respiration (Herrlisheim) 2002;69: 96–9.

[60] Spieth M, Kasner D. Traumatic thoracic thecal sac laceration, leak, and pleural effusion diagnosed by radionuclide cisternogram. Clin Nucl Med 2002;27: 830–1.

[61] Lloyd C, Sahn S. Subarachnoid pleural fistula due to penetrating trauma: case report and review of the literature. Chest 2002;122:2252–6.

[62] Huggins J, Sahn S. Duro-pleural fistula diagnosed by beta2-transferrin. Respiration (Herrlisheim) 2003;70: 423–5.

[63] Nyunoya T, Gross T, Rooney C, et al. Massive pleural

transudate following a vertebral fusion in a 49-year-old woman. Chest 2003;123:1280–3.

[64] Haft G, Mendoza S, Weinstein S, et al. Use of beta-2-transferrin to diagnose CSF leakage following spinal surgery: a case report. Iowa Orthop J 2004; 24:115–8.

[65] Maeda D, Kosuda S, Kusano S, et al. Pleural cerebrospinal fluid input and output kinetics dynamically demonstrated by In-111 DTPA myelography in a patient with pleural cerebrospinal fluid fistulae. Clin Nucl Med 2004;29:836–7.

[66] Sarwal V, Suri R, Shama O, et al. Traumatic subarachnoid-pleural fistula. Ann Thorac Surg 1996;62:1622–6.

[67] Hofstetter K, Bjelland J, Patton D, et al. Detection of bronchopleural-subarachnoid fistula by radionuclide myelography: case report. J Nucl Med 1977;18: 981–3.

[68] Peter J, Rode H. Traumatic subarachnoid-pleural fistula: case report and review of the literature. J Trauma 1993;34:303–4.

[69] Da Silva V, Shamji F, Reid R. Subarachnoid-pleural fistula complicating thoracotomy: case report and review of the literature. Neurosurgery 1987;20:802–5.

[70] Labadie E, Hamilton R, Lundel D, et al. Hypo-liquorreic headache and pneumocephalus caused by thoraco-subarachnoid fistula. Neurology 1977;27: 993–5.

[71] Lovaas M, Castillo R, Deutschman C. Traumatic subarachnoid-pleural fistula. Neurosurgery 1985;17: 650–2.

[72] Borja A, Masri Z, Shruck L, et al. Unusual and lethal complications of infraclavicular subclavian vein catheterization. Int Surg 1972;57:42–5.

[73] Herbst C. Indications, management, and complications of percutaneous subclavian catheters. An audit. Arch Surg 1978;113:1421–5.

[74] Feliciano D, Mattox K, Graham J, et al. Major complications of percutaneous subclavian vein catheters. Am J Surg 1979;138:864–74.

[75] Moorthy S, McCammon R, Deschner W, et al. Diagnosis and management of mediastinal migration of central venous pressure catheters. Heart Lung 1985; 14:80–3.

[76] Koch M. Bilateral "I.V. hydrothorax." N Engl J Med 1972;286:218.

[77] Holt S, Myerscough E. Pneumothorax and hydrothorax after subclavian vein cannulation. Postgrad Med J 1977;53:226–7.

[78] Oakes D, Wilson R. Malposition of a subclavian line. Resultant pleural effusions, interstitial pulmonary edema, and chest wall abscess during total parenteral nutrition. JAMA 1975;233:532–3.

[79] Rudge C, Bewick M, McColl I. Hydrothorax after central venous catheterization. BMJ 1973;3:23–5.

[80] Carvell J, Pearce D. Bilateral hydrothorax following internal jugular catheterization. Br J Surg 1976;63: 381–3.

[81] Reilly J, Cosimi B, Russell P. Delayed perforation of

the innominate vein during hyperalimentation. Arch Surg 1977;112:96.

[82] Usselman J, Seat S. Superior caval catheter displacement causing bilateral pleural effusions. AJR Am J Roentgenol 1979;133:738–9.

[83] Arbitman M, Kart B. Hydromediastinum after aberrant central venous catheter placement. Crit Care Med 1979;7:27–9.

[84] Barton B, Hermann G, Weil R. Cardiothoracic emergencies associated with subclavian hemodialysis catheters. JAMA 1983;250:2660–2.

[85] Iberti T, Katz L, Reiner M, et al. Hydrothorax as a late complication of central venous indwelling catheters. Surgery 1983;94:842–6.

[86] Armstrong C, Mayhall C. Contralateral hydrothorax following subclavian catheter replacement using a guidewire. Chest 1983;84:231–3.

[87] Macksood M, Setter M. Hydrothorax and hydromediastinum after use of an indwelling percutaneous catheter introducer. Crit Care Med 1983;11:957–8.

[88] Chute E, Cerra F. Late development of hydrothorax and hydromediastinum in patients with central venous catheters. Crit Care Med 1982;10:868–9.

[89] Milam M, Sahn S. Horner's syndrome secondary to hydromediastinum. A complication of extravascular migration of a central venous catheter. Chest 1988; 94:1093–4.

[90] Bardosi L, Mostafa S, Wilkes R, et al. Contralateral haemothorax: a late complication of subclavian vein cannulation. Br J Anaesth 1988;60:461–3.

[91] Barrowcliffe M. Catheter erosion of vessel walls. Br J Anaesth 1988;60:350–1.

[92] Au F, Badellino M. Significance of a curled central venous catheter tip. Chest 1988;93:890–1.

[93] Kozeny G, Bansal V, Vertuno L, et al. Contralateral hemothorax secondary to chronic subclavian dialysis catheter. Am J Nephrol 1984;4:312–4.

[94] Steiger M, Morgan A. Diagnostic aspiration of an iatrogenic hydrothorax following subclavian catheterization. Postgrad Med J 1990;66:672–3.

[95] Ellis L, Vogel S, Copeland E. Central venous catheter vascular erosions. Diagnosis and clinical course. Ann Surg 1989;209:475–8.

[96] Tocino I, Watanabe A. Impending catheter perforation of superior vena cava: radiographic recognition. AJR Am J Roentgenol 1986;146:487–90.

[97] Ball G, Whitefield C. Studies on rheumatoid disease pleural fluid. Arthritis Rheum 1966;9:846–50.

[98] Criado A, Mena A, Figueredo R, et al. Late perforation of superior vena cava and effusion caused by central venous catheter. Anaesth Intensive Care 1981; 9:286–8.

[99] Detwiler P, Porter R, Rekate H. Hydrocephalus—clinical features and management. In: Choux M, DiRocco C, Hockley A, et al, editors. Pediatric neurosurgery. London: Churchhill–Livingstone; 1999. p. 253–74.

[100] Heile A. Zur chirugischen Behandlung der Hydocehalus internus durch Ableitung der cerebrospinalfus-

sigkeit nach der bauchhohle und nach der Pleurakuppe [Surgical therapy of internal hydrocephalus with ventriculoperitoneal or ventriculopleural shunt.] Arch Rlin 1914;105:501–16 [in German].

[101] Ransohoff J. Ventriculo-pleural anastomosis in treatment of midline obstructional neoplasms. J Neurosurg 1954;44:295–8.

[102] Ransohoff J, Shulman K, Fishman R. Hydrocephalus: a review of etiology and treatment. J Pediatr 1960; 56:399–411.

[103] Venes J, Shaw R. Ventriculopleural shunting in the management of hydrocephalus. Childs Brain 1979;5:45–50.

[104] Hoffman H, Hendrick E, Humphreys R. Experience with ventriculo-pleural shunts. Childs Brain 1983;10: 404–13.

[105] Doh J-W, Bae J-G, Lee K-S, et al. Hydrothorax from intrathoracic migration of a ventriculoperitoneal shunt catheter. Surg Neurol 1995;43:340–3.

[106] Taub E, Lavyne M. Thoracic complications of ventriculoperitoneal shunts: case report and review of the literature. Neurosurgery 1994;37:181–4.

[107] Dickman C, Gilbertson D, Pittman H, et al. Tension hydrothorax from intrapleural migration of a ventriculoperitoneal shunt. Pediatr Neurosci 1989;15:313–6.

[108] Obeador S, Villarejo F. Hydrothorax: unusual complication of ventriculoperitoneal shunts. Acta Neurochir (Wien) 1977;39:167–72.

[109] Rubin R, Ghatak N, Visudhipan P. Asymptomatic perforated viscus and gram-negative ventriculitis as a complication of valve-regulated ventriculoperitoneal shunts. Report of two cases. J Neurosurg 1972;37:616–8.

[110] Van Trigt P. Diaphragm and diaphragmatic pacing. In: Sabiston D, Spencer F, editors. Surgery of the chest. 5th edition. Philadelphia: WB Saunders; 1990. p. 958–63.

[111] Arsalo A, Louhimo I, Santavuori P, et al. Subdural effusion: results after treatment with subdural-pleural shunts. Childs Brain 1977;3:79–86.

[112] Beach C, Manthey D. Tension hydrothorax due to ventriculopleural shunting. J Emerg Med 1998;16:33–6.

[113] Daviswon R, Zito J. Acute cerebrospinal fluid hydrothorax: a delayed complication of subdural-pleural shunting. Neurosurgery 1982;10:503–5.

[114] Venes J. Pleural fluid effusion and eosinophilia following ventriculo-pleural shunting. Dev Med Child Neurol 1976;16:72–6.

[115] Iosif G, Fleischman J, Chitkera R. Empyema due to ventriculopleural shunt. Chest 1991;99:1538–9.

[116] Chiang V, Torbey M, Rigamonti D, et al. Ventriculopleural shunt obstruction in positive-pressure ventilation. J Neurosurg 2001;95:116–8.

[117] Carrion E, Hertzog J, Medlock M, et al. Use of acetazolamide to decrease cerebrospinal fluid production in chronically ventilated patients with ventriculopleural shunts. Arch Dis Child 2001;84:68–71.

[118] Pittman J, Dirnhuber M. Glycinothorax: a new complication of transurethral surgery. Anaesthesia 2000; 55:155–7.

[119] Barker L. Glycinothorax revisited. Anaesthesia 2000;55:706–7.

[120] Valentine V, Raffin T. The management of chylothorax. Chest 1992;102:586–91.

[121] Doerr C, Allen M, Nichols FR, et al. Etiology of chylothorax in 203 patients. Mayo Clin Proc 2005; 80:867–70.

[122] Shimizu K, Yoshida J, Nishimura M, et al. Treatment strategy for chylothorax after pulmonary resection and lymph node dissection for lung cancer. J Thorac Cardiovasc Surg 2002;124:499–502.

[123] Terzi A, Furlan G, Magnanelli G, et al. Chylothorax after pleuro-pulmonary surgery: a rare but avoidable complication. Thorac Cardiovasc Surg 1994;42: 81–4.

[124] Hillerdal G. Chylothorax and pseudochylothorax. Eur Respir J 1997;10:1157–62.

[125] Doerr C, Miller D, Ryu J. Chylothorax. Semin Respir Crit Care Med 2001;22:617–26.

[126] Diaz-Guzman E, Culver D, Stoller J. Transudative chylothorax: report of two cases and review of the literature. Lung 2005;183:169–75.

[127] Miller JJ. Anatomy of the thoracic duct and chylothorax. In: Shields T, Locicero J, Ponn R, et al, editors. General thoracic surgery. 6th edition. Philadelphia: Lippincott, Williams & Wilkins; 2005. p. 879–88.

[128] Bessone L, Ferguson T, Burford T. Chylothorax. Ann Thorac Surg 1971;12:527–50.

[129] Roy T, Carr D, Payne W. The problem of chylothorax. Mayo Clin Proc 1967;42:457–67.

[130] Prakash U. Chylothorax and pseudochylothorax. Eur Respir Mon 2002;7:249.

[131] Lim K, Rosenow ER, Staats B, et al. Chyloptysis in adults: presentation, recognition, and differential diagnosis. Chest 2004;125:336–40.

[132] Hyde P, Jerky J, Gishen P. Traumatic chylothorax. S Afr J Surg 1974;12:57–9.

[133] Hamm H, Pfalzer B, Fable H. Lipoprotein analysis in a chyliform pleural effusion: implications for pathogenesis and diagnosis. Respiration (Herrlisheim) 1991;58:294–300.

[134] Staats B, Ellefson R, Budahn L, et al. The lipoprotein profile of chylous and nonchylous pleural effusions. Mayo Clin Proc 1980;55:700–4.

[135] Seriff N, Cohen M, Samuel P, et al. Chylothorax: diagnosis by lipoprotein electrophoresis of serum and pleural fluid. Thorax 1977;32:98–100.

[136] Browse N, Allen D, Wilson N. Management of chylothorax. Br J Surg 1997;84:1711–6.

[137] Robinson C. The management of chylothorax. Ann Thorac Surg 1985;39:90–5.

[138] Ferguson M, Little A, Skinner D. Current concepts in the management of postoperative chylothorax. Ann Thorac Surg 1985;40:542–5.

[139] Milsom J, Kron I, Rheuban K, et al. Chylothorax: an assessment of current surgical management. J Thorac Cardiovasc Surg 1985;89:221–7.

[140] Fahimi H, Casselman F, Mariani M, et al. Current management of postoperative chylothorax. Ann Thorac Surg 2001;71:448–50.

[141] Weissberg D, Ben-Zeev I. Talc pleurodesis. Experience with 360 patients. J Thorac Cardiovasc Surg 1993;106:689–95.

[142] Vargas F, Milanez J, Filomeno L, et al. Intrapleural talc for the prevention of recurrence in benign or undiagnosed pleural effusions. Chest 1994;106:1771–5.

[143] Mares D, Mathur P. Medical thoracoscopic talc pleurodesis for chylothorax due to lymphoma: a case series. Chest 1998;114:731–5.

[144] Tanaka E, Matsumoto K, Shindo T, et al. Implantation of a pleurovenous shunt for massive chylothorax in a patient with yellow nail syndrome. Thorax 2005;60:254–5.

[145] Cope C, Salem R, Kaiser L. Management of chylothorax by percutaneous catheterization and embolization of the thoracic duct: prospective trial. J Vasc Interv Radiol 1999;10:1248–54.

[146] Cope C. Management of chylothorax via percutaneous embolization. Curr Opin Pulm Med 2004;10: 311–4.

[147] Hoffer E, Bloch R, Mulligan M, et al. Treatment of chylothorax: percutaneous catheterization and embolization of the thoracic duct. AJR Am J Roentgenol 2001;176:1040–2.

[148] Kelly R, Shumway S. Conservative management of postoperative chylothorax using somatostatin. Ann Thorac Surg 2000;69:1944–5.

[149] Demos N, Kozel J, Scerbo J. Somatostatin in the treatment of chylothorax. Chest 2001;119:964–6.

[150] Markham K, Glover J, Welsh R, et al. Octreotide in the treatment of thoracic duct injuries. Am Surg 2000;66:1165–7.

[151] Kaye M. Pleural pulmonary complications of pancreatitis. Thorax 1968;23:297–306.

[152] Gumaste V, Singh V, Dave P. Significance of pleural effusion in patients with acute pancreatitis. Am J Gastroenterol 1992;87:871–4.

[153] Rockey D, Cello J. Pancreaticopleural fistula. Report of 7 patients and review of the literature. Medicine 1990;69:332–44.

[154] Anderson W, Skinner D, Zuidema G, et al. Chronic pancreatic pleural effusions. Surg Gynecol Obstet 1973;137:827–30.

[155] Uchiyama T, Suzuki T, Adachi A, et al. Pancreatic pleural effusion: case report and review of 113 cases in Japan. Am J Gastroenterol 1992;87:387–91.

[156] Miridjianian A, Ambruoso V, Derby B, et al. Massive bilateral hemorrhagic pleural effusions in chronic relapsing pancreatitis. Arch Surg 1969;98:62–6.

[157] Pottmeyer WR, Frey C, Matsuno S. Pancreaticopleural fistulas. Arch Surg 1987;122:648–54.

[158] Kaman L, Behera A, Singh R, et al. Internal pancreatic fistulas with pancreatic ascites and pancreatic pleural effusions: recognition and management. Aust NZ J Surg 2001;71:221–5.

[159] Shetty A. Pseudocysts of the pancreas: an overview. South Med J 1980;73:1239–42.

[160] Bronner M, Marsh W, Stanley J. Pancreaticopleural fistula: demonstration by computed tomography and endoscopic retrograde cholangiopancreatography. J Comput Tomogr 1986;10:167–70.

[161] Ito H, Matsubara N, Sakai T, et al. Two cases of thoracopancreatic fistula in alcoholic pancreatitis: clinical and CT findings. Radiat Med 2002;20:207–11.

[162] Kumar A, Upreti L, Bhargava S, et al. Sonographic demonstration of a pancreatopleural fistula. J Clin Ultrasound 2002;30:503–5.

[163] Mori Y, Iwai A, Inagaki T, et al. Pancreaticopleural fistula imaged with magnetic residence pancreatography. Pancreatology 2001;1:369–70.

[164] Akahane T, Kuriyama S, Matsumoto M, et al. Pancreatic pleural effusion with a pancreaticopleural fistula diagnosed by magnetic resonance cholangiopancreatography and cured by somatostatin analogue treatment. Abdom Imaging 2003;28:92–5.

[165] Joseph J, Viney S, Beck P, et al. A prospective study of amylase-rich pleural effusions with special reference to amylase isoenzyme analysis. Chest 1992;102: 1455–9.

[166] Villena V, Perez V, Pozo F, et al. Amylase levels in pleural effusions: a consecutive unselected series of 841 patients. Chest 2002;21:740–4.

[167] Good Jr J, Taryle D, Maulitz R, et al. The diagnostic value of pleural fluid pH. Chest 1980;78:55–9.

[168] Pederzoli P, Bassi C, Falconi M, et al. Conservative treatment of external pancreatic fistulas with parenteral nutrition alone or in combination with continuous intravenous infusion of somatostatin, glucagon or calcitonin. Surg Gynecol Obstet 1986;163:428–32.

[169] Parekh D, Segal I. Pancreatic ascites and effusion. Risk factors for failure of conservative therapy and the role of octreotide. Arch Surg 1992;127:707–12.

[170] da Cunha J, Machado M, Bacchella T, et al. Surgical treatment of pancreatic ascites and pancreatic pleural effusions. Hepatogastroenterology 1995;42:748–51.

[171] Lang E, Paolini RLE, Pottmeyer A. The efficacy of palliative and definitive percutaneous versus surgical drainage of pancreatic abscesses and pseudocysts: a prospective study of 85 patients. South Med J 1991;84:55–64.

[172] Ferguson T. Esopageal perforations and mediastinal sepsis in critical surgical illness. In: Hardy J, editor. 2nd edition. Philadelphia: WB Saunders; 1980. p. 270–89.

[173] Michel L, Grillo H, Malt R. Operative and non-operative management of esophageal perforations. Ann Surg 1981;194:57–63.

[174] Michel L, Grillo H, Malt R. Esophageal perforation. Ann Thorac Surg 1981;33:203–10.

[175] Brewster E. Traumatic perforation of the esophagus caused by self-catheterization with heavy electric wire: report of case with recovery by conservative treatment. Am J Surg 1957;93:1021–5.

[176] Gelfand E, Fisk R, Callaghan J. Accidental pneumatic rupture of the esophagus. J Thorac Cardiovasc Surg 1977;74:142–4.

[177] Gulbrandson R, Gaspard D. Steering wheel rupture of the pharyngoesophagus. A solitary injury. J Trauma 1977;17:74–6.

[178] Holaday W. Rupture of esophagus by compressed air. N Engl J Med 1959;261:1071–4.

[179] Lundy L, Mandal A, Lou M, et al. Experience in selective operations in the management of penetrating wounds of the neck. Surg Gynecol Obstet 1978; 174:845–8.

[180] Symbas P, Hatcher C, Vlasis S. Esophageal gunshot injuries. Ann Surg 1980;191:703–7.

[181] Worman L, Hurley J, Pemberton A, et al. Rupture of the esophagus from external blunt trauma. Arch Surg 1962;85:333–8.

[182] Boerhaave H. Atrocis, nec descripti prius, morbi historia. Secundum Medicae Artis Leges Conscripta. Lugduni Batavorum Boutestemiana, 1724. Bull Med Libr Assoc 1955;43:217–40.

[183] Samson P. Postemetic rupture of the esophagus. Surg Gynecol Obstet 1951;93:221–9.

[184] Campbell T, Andrews J, Neptune W. Spontaneous rupture of the esophagus (Boerhaave syndrome). Necessity of early diagnosis and treatment. JAMA 1976;235:526–8.

[185] Bladergroen M, Lowe J, Postlethwait R. Diagnosis and recommended management of esophageal perforation and rupture. Ann Thorac Surg 1986;42:235–9.

[186] Macker S. Spontaneous rupture of the esophagus; experimental and clinical study. Surg Gynecol Obstet 1952;95:345–56.

[187] Mackenzie M. A manual of diseases of the throat and neck including the pharynx, larynx, trachea, oesophagus, nasal cavities and neck. London: Churchhill Limited; 1884.

[188] Duval H. Bulletins et memoires de la societe medicale des hospitaux de Paris. Soc Med Paris 1921;47:450 [in French].

[189] Seybold W, Johnson MR, Leary W. Perforation of esophagus: analysis of 50 cases an account of experimental studies. Surg Clin North Am 1950;30: 1155–83.

[190] Campbell D, Cox W. Spontaneous rupture of the esophagus presenting as an acute abdominal catastrophe. Surgery 1969;66:304–8.

[191] Manour K, Teaford H. Atraumatic rupture of the esophagus into the pericardium simulating acute myocardial infarction. A case report. J Thorac Cardiovasc Surg 1973;65:458–61.

[192] Parkin G. The radiology of perforated oesophagus. Clin Radiol 1973;24:324–32.

[193] O'Connell N. Spontaneous rupture of the esophagus. AJR Am J Roentgenol 1967;99:186–203.

[194] Wichern WJ. Perforation of the esophagus. Am J Surg 1970;119:534–6.

[195] Loop F, Groves L. Esophageal perforations. Ann Thorac Surg 1970;10:571–87.

[196] Anderson R. Rupture of the esophagus. J Thorac Surg 1952;24:369–88.

[197] Dodds W, Stewart E, Vlymen W. Appropriate con-

trast media for evaluation of esophageal disruption. Radiology 1982;144:439–41.

[198] Foley M, Ghahremani G, Rogers L. Reappraisal of contrast media used to detect upper gastrointestinal perforations: comparison of ionic water-soluble media with barium sulfate. Radiology 1982;144:231–7.

[199] Wechsler R, Steiner R, Goodman L, et al. Iatrogenic esophageal-pleural fistula: subtlety of diagnosis in the absence of mediastinitis. Radiology 1982;144:239–43.

[200] Jaworski A, Fischer R, Lippmann M. Boerhaave's syndrome. Computed tomographic findings and diagnostic considerations. Arch Intern Med 1988;148(1):223–4.

[201] Good Jr J, Antony V, Reller L, et al. The pathogenesis of the low pleural fluid pH in esophageal rupture. Am Rev Respir Dis 1983;127:702–4.

[202] Drury M, Anderson W, Heffner J. Diagnostic value of pleural fluid cytology in occult Boerhaave's syndrome. Chest 1992;102:976–8.

[203] Skinner D, Little A, deMeester T. Management of esophageal perforation. Am J Surg 1980;139:760–4.

[204] Richardson J, Martin L, Borzotta A, et al. Unifying concepts in treatment of esophageal leaks. Am J Surg 1985;149:157–62.

[205] Lyons W, Seremetis M, deGuzman Jr V. Ruptures and perforations of the esophagus: the case for conservative supportive management. Ann Thorac Surg 1978;25:346–50.

[206] Mengoli L, Klassen K. Conservative management of esophageal management perforation. Arch Surg 1965;91:238–40.

[207] Sanderson R. Spontaneous of the esophagus: report of survival without surgical management. Am J Surg 1965;109:506–8.

[208] Rothberg M, Klingman R, Peetz D, et al. Traumatic thoracobiliary fistula. Ann Thorac Surg 1994;51:472–5.

[209] Anderson R. Traumatic bronchobiliary fistulae. Am Surg 1961;27:431–6.

[210] Amir-Jahed A, Sadrieh M, Farpour A, et al. Thoracobilia: a surgical complication of hepatic echinococcosis and amebiasis. Ann Thorac Surg 1972;14:198–205.

[211] Roy D, Ravindran P, Padmanabhan R. Bronchobiliary fistula secondary to amebic liver abscess. Chest 1972;62:523–4.

[212] Morton J, Phillips E. Bronchobiliary fistula: review of the recorded cases other than those due to echinococcus and amebic abscess. Arch Surg 1928;16:694–754.

[213] Flemma R, Anlyan W. Tuberculous bronchobiliary fistula. Report of an unusual case with demonstration of the fistulous tract by percutaneous transhepatic cholangiography. J Thorac Cardiovasc Surg 1965;49:198–201.

[214] Liberale G, Delhaye M, Ansay J, et al. Biliary pleural fistula as a complication of radiofrequency abla-

tion for liver metastasis. Acta Chir Belg 2004;104:448–50.

[215] Boyd D. Bronchobiliary and bronchopleural fistulas. Ann Thorac Surg 1977;24:281–7.

[216] Strange C, Allen M, Freedland P, et al. Biliopleural fistula as a complication of percutaneous biliary drainage: experimental evidence for pleural inflammation. Am Rev Respir Dis 1988;137:959–61.

[217] Denning D, Ellison E, Carey L. Preoperative percutaneous transhepatic biliary decompression lowers operative morbidity in patients with obstructive jaundice. Am J Surg 1981;141:61–5.

[218] Norlander A, Kalin B, Sundblad R. Effect of percutaneous transhepatic drainage upon liver function and postoperative mortality. Surg Gynecol Obstet 1982;155:161–6.

[219] Carrasco C, Zornoza J, Bechtel W. Malignant biliary obstruction: complications of percutaneous biliary drainage. Radiology 1984;152:343–6.

[220] Mueller P, van Sonnenberg E, Ferrucci JJ. Percutaneous biliary drainage: technical and catheter-related problems in 200 procedures. AJR Am J Roentgenol 1982;138:17–23.

[221] Hamlin J, Friedman M, Stein M, et al. Percutaneous biliary drainage: complications of 118 consecutive catheterizations. Radiology 1986;158:199–202.

[222] Neff C, Mueller P, Ferrucci JJ, et al. Serious complications following transgression of the pleural space in drainage procedures. Radiology 1984;152:335–41.

[223] Nichols D, Cooperberg P, Golding R, et al. The safe intercostal approach? Pleural complications and abdominal interventional radiology. AJR Am J Roentgenol 1984;142:1013–8.

[224] Severini A, Bellomi M, Cozzi G, et al. Rib erosion: late complication of long-standing biliary drainage catheters. Radiology 1984;150:666.

[225] Anschuetz S, Vogelzang R. Malignant pleural effusion: a complication of transhepatic biliary drainage. AJR Am J Roentgenol 1986;146:1165–6.

[226] Lee J. Tc-99m DISIDA hepatobiliary scintigraphy showing bile leakage into the thoracic cavity. Clin Nucl Med 2001;26:861–2.

[227] Oparah S, Mandal A. Traumatic thoracobiliary (pleurobiliary and bronchobiliary) fistulas: clinical and review study. J Trauma 1978;18:539–44.

[228] Ferguson T, Burford T. Pleurobiliary and bronchobiliary fistulas. Surgical management. Arch Surg 1967;95:380–6.

[229] Adachi Y, Sato Y, Yasui H, et al. Gastropleural fistula derived from malignant lymphoma. J Gastroenterol 2002;37:1052–6.

[230] Warburton C, Calverley P. Gastropleural fistula due to gastric lymphoma presenting as tension pneumothorax and empyema. Eur Respir J 1997;10(7):1678–9.

[231] Crucitti F. Traumatic hernia of the diaphragm and gastro-pleural fistula. Chir Ital 1966;18:346–66.

[232] MacArthur A, Wright J. Complications of intra-

thoracic gastric ulcer associated with hiatus hernia. A description of five cases. Br J Surg 1969;56:161–4.

[233] Kirkpatrick J, Allbritten FJ. A gastropleural fistula 12 years following gastric interposition for carcinoma of the esophagus. J Thorac Cardiovasc Surg 1969;58:769–72.

[234] Nigam B. Perforation of gastric ulcer into the pleural cavity: a case report. Indian J Chest Dis 1974;16:121–3.

[235] Melamed M, Barker W, Langston H. Unusual pleural fistulas. AJR Am J Roentgenol 1974;120:876–82.

[236] Lehmann L. Pleurogastral fistula as an unusual complication in unspecific pleural empyema. Chirurg 1974;45:554–5.

[237] Meredith H, Seymour E, Vujic I. Hiatal hernia complicated by gastric ulceration and perforation. Gastrointest Radiol 1980;5:229–31.

[238] Shevchuk V. [A case of perforated ulcer of the gastric fundus with the formation of a gastrodiaphragmatic-pleural fistula and pleural empyema]. Klin Khir 1981;4:69–70 [in Russian].

[239] Ennes FP, Biagini G, Arruda WO. [Pyopneumothorax and gastric pleural fistula caused by gastric carcinoma: report of a case and review of the literature]. AMB Rev Assoc Med Bras 1984;30(9–10):210–2 [in Portuguese].

[240] Rotstein O, Pruett T, Simmons R. Gastropleural fistula. Report of three cases and review of the literature. Am J Surg 1985;150:392–6.

[241] Malik S, Giacoia G. Candida tropicalis empyema associated with acquired gastropleural fistula in a newborn infant. Am J Perinatol 1989;6:347–8.

[242] Roberts C, Gelder C, Goldstraw P. Tension pneumothorax and empyema as a consequence of gastropleural fistulae. Respir Med 1990;84:253–4.

[243] Gaziano J, Gaziano D. Simultaneous gastropleural and gastrocolic fistulae in a quadriplegic male. WV Med J 1990;86:203–5.

[244] Cobo J, Gomez Cerezo J, Molina F, et al. [Gastropleural fistula: primary manifestation of gastric lymphoma]. Med Clin (Barc) 1990;94:757 [in Spanish].

[245] Schwab R, Jarvik J. Tension pneumothorax secondary to a gastropleural fistula in a traumatic diaphragmatic hernia. Chest 1991;99:247–9.

[246] O'Keefe P, Goldstraw P. Gastropleural fistula following pulmonary resection. Thorax 1993;48:1278–9.

[247] Hsieh H, Liu H, Lin P, et al. Gastro-pleural fistula related with penetrating stab injuries of the chest and abdomen: laparotomy or thoracotomy. Changgeng Yi Xue Za Zhi 1993;16(2):120–4.

[248] Anbari M, Levine M, Cohen R, et al. Delayed leaks and fistulas after esophagogastrectomy: radiologic evaluation. AJR Am J Roentgenol 1993;160:1217–20.

[249] Biswas I, Raghavan C, Sevcik L. Gastropleural fistula: an unusual cause of intractable postoperative nausea and vomiting. Anesth Analg 1996;83:186–8.

[250] Mussi A, Lucchi M, Davini F, et al. Gastropleural fistula as complication of postpneumonectomy empyema. J Cardiovasc Surg (Torino) 2000;41:147–9.

[251] Markowitz A, Herter F. Gastropleural fistula as a complication of esophageal hiatus hernia. Ann Surg 1960;152:129–34.

[252] Miller K, Tomlinson J, Sahn S. Pleural pulmonary complications of enteral tube feedings. Chest 1985;88:230–3.

[253] Biggart M, Choudhry P, Nickalls R. Dangers of placement of narrow-bore nasogastric feeding tubes. Ann R Coll Surg Engl 1987;69:119–21.

[254] Valentine R, Turner Jr W. Pleural complications of nasoenteric feeding tubes. JPEN J Parenter Enteral Nutr 1985;9:605–7.

[255] Hand R, Kempster M, Levy J, et al. Inadvertent transbronchial insertion of a narrow-bore feeding tube into the pleural space. JAMA 1984;251:2396–7.

[256] James H. An unusual complication of passing a narrow-bore nasogastric tube. Anesthesiology 1978;33:716–8.

[257] Vaughan E. Hazards associated with narrow-bore nasogastric tube feeding. Br J Oral Surg 1981;19:151–4.

[258] Culpepper J, Veremakis C, Guntupalli K, et al. Malpositioned nasogastric tube causing pneumothorax and bronchopleural fistula. Chest 1982;81:389.

[259] McDanal J, Wheeler D, Ebert J. A complication of nasogastric intubation: pulmonary hemorrhage. Anesthesiology 1983;59:856–8.

[260] Baloch G, Adler S, Vanderwoude J, et al. Pneumothorax as a complication of feeding tube placement. AJR Am J Roentgenol 1983;141:1275–7.

[261] Tucker A, Lewis J. Procedures in practice. Passing a nasogastric tube. BMJ 1980;281:1128–9.

[262] Spencer G. Tracheostomy and endotracheal intubation in the intensive care unit. 3rd edition. London: Butterworths; 1973.

[263] Marderstein E, Simmons R, Ochoa J. Patient safety: effect of institutional protocols on adverse events related to feeding tube placement in the critically ill. J Am Coll Surg 2004;199:39–47.

[264] Harvey P, Bull P, Harris D. Accidental entrapulmonary Clininfeed. Anesthesiology 1981;36:518–22.

[265] Fremstad J, Martin S. Lethal complication from insertion of nasogastric tube after severe basilar skull fracture. J Trauma 1978;18:820–2.

[266] Heymsfield S, Bethel R, Ansley J, et al. Enteral hyperalimentation: an alternative to central venous hyperalimentation. Ann Intern Med 1979;90:63–71.

ELSEVIER SAUNDERS

Clin Chest Med 27 (2006) 309–319

CLINICS IN CHEST MEDICINE

The Undiagnosed Pleural Effusion

Richard W. Light, MD

Vanderbilt University, T-1218 Medical Center North, Nashville, TN 37232–2659, USA

Frequently, the etiology of a pleural effusion is in question after the initial thoracentesis. In this article, I assume that the pleural effusion persists after the initial diagnostic workup, which includes measurement of a pleural fluid marker for tuberculosis, such as adenosine deaminase (ADA) or γ-interferon.

Diseases that cause undiagnosed persistent pleural effusions

When a patient with a persistent undiagnosed pleural effusion is encountered, the first step to be considered is the list of the diseases most likely to be associated with a persistent undiagnosed pleural effusion (Box 1). The first question to answer in a patient with a persistent undiagnosed pleural effusion is whether the effusion is a transudate or an exudate. For the past several decades, this differentiation has been made by measuring the levels of protein and lactate dehydrogenase (LDH) in the pleural fluid and in the serum (Light's criteria). If one or more of the following criteria are met, the patient has an exudative pleural effusion [1]:

1. Pleural fluid protein or serum protein > 0.5
2. Pleural fluid LDH or serum LDH > 0.6
3. Pleural fluid LDH > 0.67 the normal upper limit for serum

Light's criteria are sensitive at identifying exudates, but they also identify up to 25% of transudative pleural effusions as being exudative pleural effusions [2–4]. Usually, the transudates that are misclassified

E-mail address: rlight98@yahoo.com

only minimally meet the exudative criteria (eg, the protein ratio is 0.52 or the LDH ratio is 0.63). Moreover, the patients with transudates who are misclassified are usually receiving diuretics [4]. If the pleural fluid LDH is more than the upper limit for the serum LDH or if the protein level is more than 4.0 g/dL, the patient does not have a transudate. These transudates that are misclassified as exudates can be classified correctly if the difference or gradient between the protein levels in the serum and the pleural fluid is measured. If this gradient is greater than 3.1 g/dL, the exudative classification by Light's criteria can be ignored, because almost all such patients have a transudative pleural effusion [5,6]. The protein gradient alone should not be used to separate transudates from exudates because, by itself, it misidentifies approximately 13% of exudates as transudates [4,6].

Transudative pleural effusions

Congestive heart failure

Congestive heart failure is the most common cause of pleural effusion [7]. At times in patients with persistent pleural effusion, it is not obvious that the heart failure is the cause of the effusion. Certainly, symptoms of congestive heart failure, such as dyspnea on exertion, orthopnea, paroxysmal nocturnal dyspnea, and nocturia, should be sought when the history is taken. In addition, signs of congestive heart failure, such as basilar rales, S_3 gallop, distended neck veins, and pedal edema, should be sought during the physical examination. If the patient clinically has congestive heart failure but the initial pleural fluid analysis reveals an exudate that just

---

Box 1. List of diseases most likely to produce a persistent undiagnosed pleural effusion

Transudative pleural effusions

- Congestive heart failure
- Cirrhosis
- Nephrotic syndrome
- Urinothorax
- Myxedema
- Cerebrospinal fluid leaks to the pleura

Exudative pleural effusions

- Malignancy
- Pneumonia (especially anaerobic)
- Tuberculosis
- Pulmonary embolism
- Fungal infection
- Pancreatic pseudocyst
- Intra-abdominal abscess
- After coronary artery bypass graft surgery
- Postcardiac injury syndrome
- Pericardial disease
- Meigs' syndrome
- Ovarian hyperstimulation syndrome
- Rheumatoid pleuritis
- Lupus erythematosus
- Drug-induced pleural disease
- Asbestos pleural effusion
- Yellow nail syndrome
- Uremia
- Trapped lung
- Chylothorax
- Pseudochylothorax

---

barely meets Light's criteria, the difference between the pleural fluid and serum protein should be measured as detailed previously. If this gradient is greater than 3.1 g/dL, the effusion can be attributed to the congestive heart failure. If the patient has a transudative effusion but does not have obvious heart failure, further investigations of cardiac function, such as echocardiography, are indicated. It has recently been shown that measurement of the levels of pro-brain natriuretic peptide (BNP) in pleural fluid is useful in establishing the diagnosis of congestive heart failure. Patients with congestive heart failure have pleural fluid N terminal pro-BNP levels greater than 1500 pg/mL, whereas almost all other patients

have pleural fluid N terminal pro-BNP levels less than 1000 pg/mL [8,9].

Cirrhosis with hepatic hydrothorax

If the patient has overt cirrhosis and massive ascites, the diagnosis of hepatic hydrothorax is easy. If the patient does not have ascites, however, the diagnosis of hepatic hydrothorax may be difficult to establish. In 1998, Kakizaki and colleagues [10] reviewed the literature and were able to find 28 cases of hepatic hydrothorax without ascites. Of these 28 cases, 27 were on the right side. The only left-sided effusion occurred in a patient who had a tear in the left diaphragm as a result of a splenectomy. The mean serum albumin in these 28 cases was 2.7 g/dL, with a range of 1.9 to 3.6 g/dL [10]. The explanation for the pleural effusion in the absence of overt ascites is that the patients have defects in their diaphragm. When fluid is present in the peritoneal space, it flows immediately into the pleural space, because the pleural pressure is negative compared with the peritoneal pressure. This diagnosis can be established by demonstrating radioactivity in the thorax after the intra-peritoneal injection of technetium-99m (^{99m}Tc)-sulfur colloid [11].

Nephrotic syndrome

Another cause of a chronic transudative pleural effusion is the nephrotic syndrome. More than 20% of patients with the nephrotic syndrome have pleural effusions, which are usually bilateral [12]. Therefore, all patients with chronic transudative pleural effusions should be evaluated for proteinuria and hypoproteinemia. It should be remembered that the incidence of pulmonary emboli is high with the nephrotic syndrome [13], and this possibility should be considered in all patients with the nephrotic syndrome and a pleural effusion.

Urinothorax

A transudative pleural effusion can result when there is retroperitoneal urinary leakage secondary to urinary tract obstruction or trauma with subsequent dissection of the urine into the pleural space [14,15]. This diagnosis is easy if it is considered as the pleural fluid looks and smells like urine. Confirmation of the diagnosis can be made by demonstrating that the pleural fluid creatinine is greater than the serum creatinine [15,16]. The pleural fluid with urinothorax may also have a low glucose level and a low pH level. The only other instances in which a transudative pleural effusion has a low glucose or low pH level is when there is systemic hypoglycemia or acidosis, respectively [4].

Cerebrospinal fluid leak to the pleura

On rare occasions, cerebrospinal fluid (CSF) can collect in the pleural space and produce a pleural effusion. This most commonly occurs after ventriculopleural shunting [17] but can also occur after penetrating injuries and fractures of the thoracic spine as well as after thoracic spinal surgery [18,19]. The diagnosis should be suggested by the appearance of the pleural fluid, which appears to be CSF. The protein levels are usually very low. The diagnosis can be confirmed by radionuclide cisternography [19]. Another way to establish the diagnosis is by demonstrating the presence of β_2-transferrin in the pleural fluid [20]. This substance is normally present only in CSF [20].

Exudative pleural effusions

Malignant pleural effusion

There is no doubt that malignancy causes more persistent undiagnosed exudative pleural effusions than any other cause. It should be emphasized that there is no huge hurry to establish this diagnosis, however, because (1) the presence of the effusion indicates that the patient has metastases to the pleura and the malignancy cannot be cured surgically, (2) most malignant pleural effusions are attributable to tumors that cannot be cured with chemotherapy, and (3) there is no evidence that attempts to create a pleurodesis early improve the quality of the patient's life.

Most patients who have a pleural malignancy usually have other characteristics suggesting malignancy. For example, in the series of 211 patients reported by Poe and coworkers [21], the needle biopsy of the pleura was negative in 29 patients who were eventually proven to have malignant pleural effusions. All these patients were strongly suspected of having a malignant effusion by clinical criteria, such as weight loss, constitutional symptoms, or a history of a previous cancer, however [21]. Ferrer and coworkers [22] recently evaluated the characteristics of patients undergoing thoracoscopy who turned out to have a malignancy. They found four clinical characteristics that were suggestive of malignancy: symptoms for more than 1 month, absence of fever, blood-tinged pleural fluid, and chest CT scan findings

suggestive of malignancy [22]. All 28 patients who had all four characteristics had a malignancy, whereas none of the 21 patients with one criterion at most had a malignancy [22].

When patients with pleural effusions attributable to the most common types of tumors are analyzed, some interesting observations can be made. The tumor that causes the highest number of pleural effusions is lung cancer [7]. When patients with lung cancer are first evaluated, approximately 15% have a pleural effusion [23], but 50% of patients with disseminated lung cancer develop a pleural effusion [7]. The tumor that causes the second highest number of pleural effusions is breast cancer [7]. Patients with breast carcinoma rarely present with a pleural effusion. The mean interval between the diagnosis of the primary tumor and the appearance of a pleural effusion is 2 years [24]. Hematologic malignancies (lymphomas and leukemias) cause the third highest number of malignant pleural effusions [7]. Approximately 10% of patients with Hodgkin's lymphoma and 25% of patients with non-Hodgkin's lymphoma have pleural effusions at presentation. Those who do almost invariably have intrathoracic lymph node involvement [25]. If the patient has AIDS and cutaneous Kaposi's sarcoma, the likely diagnosis is a pleural effusion attributable to Kaposi's sarcoma. This diagnosis is usually established at bronchoscopy, which demonstrates erythematous or violaceous macules or papules in the respiratory tree [26].

There are several primary tumors of the pleura that should be considered if the patient has an undiagnosed pleural effusion. If the patient has a history of asbestos exposure, mesothelioma should be considered. Thoracoscopy or thoracotomy is usually necessary to make this diagnosis [7]. If the patient has AIDS and has a lymphocytic pleural effusion with a high LDH level, the diagnosis of a primary effusion lymphoma is likely [27]. This diagnosis can usually be established with pleural fluid cytology and flow cytometry [27]. If the patient had received an artificial pneumothorax many years previously, a likely diagnosis is pyothorax-associated lymphoma [28].

Parapneumonic effusion

The diagnosis of parapneumonic effusion is easy in the patient with an acute febrile illness, purulent sputum, and pulmonary infiltrates. On occasion, however, particularly with anaerobic infections, the patient may present with a chronic illness. In one study of 47 patients with anaerobic parapneumonic effusions, the median duration of symptoms before presentation was 10 days and 60% of the patients had substantial weight loss (mean of 29 lb) [29]. Therefore, if the patient has a chronic illness with predominantly neutrophils in the pleural fluid, it is imperative to obtain anaerobic cultures of the pleural fluid. Because patients with actinomycosis and nocardiosis sometimes have a chronic pleural effusion with predominantly neutrophils, cultures for these organisms should be obtained in patients with chronic neutrophilic pleural effusions.

Tuberculous pleural effusion

Throughout the world, tuberculosis remains one of the principal causes of pleural effusion. It is important to make this diagnosis, because if the patient has pleural tuberculosis and is not treated, the effusion resolves but the patient has a greater than 50% chance of developing active pulmonary or extrapulmonary tuberculosis over the next 5 years [30]. Therefore, all patients with a chronic undiagnosed pleural effusion should be evaluated for tuberculosis. The easiest way to do this is to measure the pleural fluid level of ADA or γ-interferon. If the level of ADA is less than 40 IU/L or the level of γ-interferon is less than 140 pg/mL, the diagnosis can be virtually excluded [31]. In one study, Ferrer and colleagues [32] followed 40 patients with a chronic undiagnosed pleural effusion and a pleural fluid ADA level less than 43 IU/L for a mean of 5 years, and none developed tuberculosis. Patients with lymphocytic pleural effusions because of other etiologies almost always have pleural fluid ADA levels less than 40 IU/L [33]. If the pleural fluid ADA level is greater than 40 IU/L or the level of γ-interferon exceeds 140 pg/mL and empyema and rheumatoid pleuritis are excluded, the patient probably has tuberculous pleuritis [31].

Pulmonary embolus

The diagnosis of a pulmonary embolism should be considered in every patient with an undiagnosed pleural effusion. Pleural effusions occur in at least 30% of patients with pulmonary emboli [34], and they are almost always exudative [35]. Most pleural effusions associated with pulmonary emboli are small, and it is uncommon for the effusion to occupy more than one third of the hemithorax [34]. Patients with undiagnosed pleural effusions should have the possibility of a pulmonary embolism investigated with a spiral CT scan [36]. The spiral CT scan not only identifies vascular filling defects, which are highly suggestive of pulmonary embolism, but dem-

onstrates concomitant parenchymal and pleural abnormalities and mediastinal lymphadenopathy.

Fungal pleural effusions

Fungal disease is responsible for a small percentage of pleural effusions [7]. At times, however, blastomycosis and coccidioidomycosis may cause a chronic lymphocytic pleural effusion [7]. Accordingly, cultures for fungi should be obtained in the patient with a chronic undiagnosed pleural effusion with predominantly lymphocytes in the pleural fluid. It is unknown whether the lymphocytic effusions attributable to fungal diseases have a high ADA level.

Chronic pancreatic pleural effusion

This is one diagnosis that should always be considered in a patient with a chronic undiagnosed pleural effusion. Some patients with a pancreatic pseudocyst develop a direct sinus tract between the pancreas and the pleural space [37]. The sinus tract decompresses the pancreas; therefore, the patient presents with symptoms usually referable only to the chest. The patient with a chronic pancreatic pleural effusion is usually chronically ill and looks like he or she has cancer. The diagnosis is virtually established if the level of amylase in the pleural fluid is greater than 1000 U/L [37]. It is important to consider this diagnosis, because the patient can be cured with appropriate surgery.

Intra-abdominal abscess

Subphrenic, intrahepatic, intrasplenic, and intrapancreatic abscesses are all associated with a pleural effusion in a large percentage of patients [7]. Patients with an intra-abdominal abscess are usually chronically ill with fever and weight loss. The pleural fluid is sterile and contains predominantly neutrophils. The diagnosis can be made with a CT or ultrasound scan of the abdomen.

Effusion after coronary artery bypass graft surgery

Approximately 10% of patients who undergo coronary artery bypass graft (CABG) surgery have a pleural effusion that occupies more than 25% of their hemithorax 28 days after surgery [38]. The primary symptom (if any) of a patient with a post-CABG pleural effusion is dyspnea; chest pain and fever are distinctly unusual [38]. The pleural fluid in these patients is an exudate characterized by a predominance of lymphocytes and an LDH level approximately equal to the upper limit of normal for serum [39]. Although the pleural fluid is similar to the pleural fluid in patients with tuberculous pleuritis, these two entities may be differentiated by the pleural fluid level of ADA; the ADA level is less than 40 U/L in patients with a post-CABG effusion [33]. The importance of these effusions is to know that they can persist for years on rare occasions [40] and not to be too aggressive in pursuing a diagnosis if the pleural fluid findings are as expected.

Postcardiac injury syndrome

Postcardiac injury syndrome (PCIS), also known as Dressler's syndrome, is characterized by the development of fever, pleuropericarditis, and parenchymal pulmonary infiltrates in the weeks after trauma to the pericardium or myocardium [41]. The PCIS has been reported after myocardial infarction, cardiac surgery, blunt chest trauma, percutaneous left ventricular puncture, pacemaker implantation, and angioplasty. The PCIS differs from the pleural effusion after CABG surgery, because fever and chest pain invariably occur with the PCIS and are rare after CABG surgery. After cardiac injury, symptoms usually develop between the first and third weeks but can develop any time between 3 days and 1 year [41]. The pleural fluid is frankly bloody in approximately 30% of patients, and the differential cell count may reveal predominantly neutrophils or mononuclear cells, depending on the acuteness of the process [42].

Pericardial disease

Approximately 25% of patients who have a pericardial effusion have a concomitant pleural effusion [43]. In patients with inflammatory pericarditis, most of the associated pleural effusions are unilateral and left-sided [43]. The characteristics of the pleural fluid seen in conjunction with pericardial disease are not well described [7]. The possibility of pericardial effusion should be evaluated in any patient with cardiomegaly and an isolated left pleural effusion.

Approximately 60% of patients with constrictive pericarditis have a concomitant pleural effusion [44]. The associated pleural effusion is bilateral and symmetric in most of these patients. In one report of four patients with constrictive pericarditis, the pleural fluid was transudative in one and exudative in three [44]. We recently reported one patient with constrictive pericarditis who had a pleural fluid protein level of 4.0 g/dL [45]. When a patient is seen with edema

and an exudative pleural effusion, the diagnosis of constrictive pericarditis should be considered. It is important to realize that the findings of echocardiography may be normal in the patient with constrictive pericarditis and that cardiac catheterization may be necessary to establish the diagnosis [45].

Meigs' syndrome

Meigs' syndrome is the constellation of a benign pelvic neoplasm associated with ascites and pleural effusion in which surgical extirpation of the tumor results in permanent disappearance of the ascites and pleural effusion [7]. The pleural fluid is an exudate with a relatively low cell count, which may sometimes have an elevated CA-125 level [46]. The importance of Meigs' syndrome is that not all patients with a pelvic mass, ascites, and a pleural effusion have metastatic disease.

Ovarian hyperstimulation syndrome

This syndrome is a serious complication of ovulation induction. The clinical picture is characterized by massive ovarian enlargement with multiple cysts, hemoconcentration, and the third space accumulation of fluid. Patients with the syndrome present within 2 to 3 weeks after receiving the human chorionic gonadotropin with abdominal pain and distention; a nonproductive cough; and dyspnea caused by the ascites, pleural effusion, or both. The pleural effusion is usually bilateral, and the pleural fluid is an exudate with predominantly neutrophils and a relatively low LDH level [7].

Rheumatoid pleuritis

Chronic pleural effusions may be a manifestation of rheumatoid pleuritis, and the diagnosis is usually straightforward. Classically, the effusion occurs in older men who have subcutaneous nodules. The pleural fluid is an exudate with low glucose, low pH, and high LDH levels. The first manifestation of rheumatoid disease is virtually never a pleural effusion [7].

Systemic lupus erythematosus

In contrast to rheumatoid pleuritis, patients with systemic lupus erythematosus (SLE) may present with a pleural effusion. The possibility of drug-induced lupus should always be considered in a patient with an undiagnosed pleural effusion. Drugs that are most commonly incriminated in drug-induced lupus are hydralazine, procainamide, isoniazid, phenytoin, and chlorpromazine [7]. The diagnosis of SLE with pleural involvement is based on the usual criteria for the diagnosis of lupus. Measurement of the pleural fluid antinuclear antibody (ANA) levels [47] or performance of lupus erythematosus preparations on the pleural fluid [7] do not assist in the diagnosis.

Drug-induced pleural disease

When a patient is evaluated with a chronic undiagnosed pleural effusion, the list of drugs that the patient is taking should be carefully reviewed, because the ingestion of certain drugs can lead to the development of a pleural effusion. The primary drugs associated with the development of a pleural effusion are nitrofurantoin (a urinary antiseptic), dantrolene (a muscle relaxant), and the ergot alkaloids, such as bromocriptine or pergolide, that are used to treat Parkinson's disease [7]. Other drugs that have been reported to induce pleural effusions include methysergide, amiodarone, procarbazine, methotrexate, clozapine, dapsone, metronidazole, mitomycin, isotretinoin, propylthiouracil, simvastatin, warfarin, and gliclazide [7,48]. Most patients who have drug-induced pleural effusions have peripheral eosinophilia. When the drug is discontinued, the effusion usually resolves rapidly [48].

Asbestos pleural effusion

Exposure to asbestos can lead to the development of an exudative pleural effusion. In one series of 1135 asymptomatic asbestos workers, the prevalence of pleural effusion was 3% [49]. In this series, all the patients developed effusions within 20 years of the initial exposure and many had done so within 5 years of the initial exposure [49]. The prevalence of pleural effusion was directly related to the total asbestos exposure. Patients with asbestos pleural effusions are usually asymptomatic [49,50]. The effusion tends to last several months and then clears, leaving no residual disease. The pleural fluid is an exudate and can contain predominantly neutrophils or mononuclear cells [50]. If a patient with a pleural effusion has a history of asbestos exposure and is asymptomatic, the patient can probably be observed to determine if the effusion disappears spontaneously.

Yellow nail syndrome

The yellow nail syndrome consists of the triad of deformed yellow nails, lymphedema, and pleural effusions [7]. The three separate entities may become manifest at widely varying times. The pleural effusions are bilateral in approximately 50% of patients and vary in size from small to massive [7]. Once a pleural effusion has occurred with this syndrome, it tends to persist and recur rapidly after a thoracentesis. The pleural fluid is usually a clear yellow exudate with a normal glucose level and predominantly lymphocytes in the pleural fluid differential. The pleural fluid LDH level tends to be low relative to the pleural fluid protein level.

Uremia

The prevalence of pleural effusions with uremia is approximately 3% [51]. As many as 50% of patients on long-term hemodialysis have a pleural effusion [52]. There is not a close relation between the degree of uremia and the occurrence of a pleural effusion [51]. More than 50% of the patients are symptomatic, with fever (50%), chest pain (30%), cough (35%), and dyspnea (20%) being the most common symptoms [51]. The pleural fluid is an exudate, and the differential usually reveals predominantly lymphocytes [51]. Tests of renal function should be obtained in every patient with an undiagnosed exudative effusion.

Trapped lung

When there is intense inflammation in the pleural space, a fibrous peel may form over the visceral pleura. This peel can prevent the underlying lung from expanding; therefore, the lung is said to be trapped [53]. The initial event producing the pleural inflammation is usually a pleural infection or a hemothorax, but it can be a spontaneous pneumothorax, thoracic operations (particularly CABG surgery) [40], uremia, or collagen vascular disease. The pleural fluid is usually clear yellow and is a borderline exudate with predominantly mononuclear cells. The diagnosis can be made by measuring the pleural pressure while fluid is withdrawn during a thoracentesis. If the initial pleural pressure is less than -10 cm H_2O or if the pleural pressure falls more than 20 cm H_2O per 1000 mL of fluid removed, the diagnosis is confirmed provided that the patient does not have a bronchial obstruction [53].

Chylothorax and pseudochylothorax

When pleural fluid is found to be milky or extremely turbid, the possibility of a chylothorax or a pseudochylothorax should be considered. When turbid fluid is found, the first step is to centrifuge the fluid. If the supernatant remains turbid, the turbidity is attributable to a high lipid content in the pleural fluid and the patient has a chylothorax or a pseudochylothorax.

A chylothorax is usually easy to differentiate from a pseudochylothorax on clinical grounds. Patients with a chylothorax have an acute illness, and their pleural surfaces are normal on CT. In contrast, patients with a pseudochylothorax usually have had a pleural effusion for more than 5 years, and their pleural surfaces are markedly thickened on CT. Measurement of the lipid levels in the pleural fluid is also useful in distinguishing these two conditions. Pleural fluid from a chylothorax has a triglyceride level greater than 110 mg/dL, and the ratio of the pleural fluid to serum cholesterol is less than 1.0. In contrast, fluid from a pseudochylothorax has cholesterol crystals or a cholesterol level greater than 200 mg/dL and higher than the simultaneous serum level [7].

Tests to consider for patients with persistent undiagnosed pleural effusion

History

There are certain points in the patient's history that should receive special attention if the patient has a persistent undiagnosed pleural effusion. If a patient has a transudative pleural effusion, particular attention should be paid to symptoms of congestive heart failure, such as dyspnea on exertion, orthopnea, paroxysmal nocturnal dyspnea, and nocturia. In addition, historical evidence of cirrhosis, alcoholism, or chronic hepatitis should be sought with the possibility of a hepatic hydrothorax in mind. A history of trauma or surgery to the thoracic spine should be sought with the diagnosis of a CSF leak in mind.

If the patient has an exudative pleural effusion, a history of malignancy should be sought. Malignant pleural effusions have been known to develop as long as 20 years after the primary tumor was diagnosed [54]. A history of exposure to asbestos should be sought, because this would suggest mesothelioma or an asbestos pleural effusion. A history of fever suggests a chronic anaerobic, tuberculous, or fungal infection or an intra-abdominal abscess. A history of alcoholism or previous pancreatic disease raises the possibility of a chronic pancreatic pleural effusion. A history of CABG surgery or myocardial trauma suggests a post-CABG surgery pleural effusion or the PCIS, respectively. A history of rheumatoid disease raises the possibility of rheumatoid pleuritis.

The patient should be questioned carefully regarding the medications he or she is taking to determine whether he or she is taking a medication that causes a pleural effusion or is associated with drug-induced lupus erythematosus. The patient should be questioned carefully about previous pleural problems, which raise the likelihood of a pseudochylothorax or a trapped lung.

Physical examination

In the patient with a chronic undiagnosed pleural effusion, it is worthwhile to repeat a careful physical examination. If the patient has a transudative pleural effusion, signs of congestive heart failure, such as basilar rales, an S_3 gallop, or distended neck veins, should be sought. In addition, evidence of ascites should be carefully sought. The presence of pedal edema suggests congestive heart failure, cirrhosis with hepatic hydrothorax, nephrotic syndrome, pericardial disease, or the yellow nail syndrome.

If the patient has an exudative effusion, a careful search for lymphadenopathy or other masses that would suggest malignancy is indicated. In women, a careful breast examination and a careful pelvic examination should be done to evaluate these locations for masses. Abdominal tenderness suggests an intra-abdominal abscess. Distant heart sounds, a pericardial friction rub, or Kussmaul's sign (increased jugular venous pressure that increases during inspiration) suggests pericardial disease. Ascites and a pelvic mass raise the possibility of Meigs' syndrome. Deformed joints and subcutaneous nodules make rheumatoid pleuritis likely. The presence of yellow nails establishes the diagnosis of the yellow nail syndrome.

Laboratory examinations

Several blood tests should be routinely obtained in patients with a persistent undiagnosed pleural effusion. The level of albumin and globulin should be measured to determine whether the patient has cirrhosis or the nephrotic syndrome, and liver function tests should be obtained to ascertain if there is chronic hepatitis. Additionally, I obtain a complete blood cell count with a differential. A serum ANA test should be obtained with the diagnosis of SLE in mind. Blood urea nitrogen (BUN) and creatinine levels should be obtained to evaluate the possibility of uremia, and a urinalysis should be obtained to detect proteinuria.

Several special tests on the pleural fluid are also indicated. The least expensive test is to smell the pleural fluid. If the pleural fluid smells like urine, the patient probably has an urinothorax, whereas if the pleural fluid smells feculent, the patient probably has an anaerobic pleural infection. As mentioned previously, the ADA or γ-interferon should be measured in the pleural fluid to assess whether the patient has pleural tuberculosis. Flow cytometry on the pleural fluid is indicated if lymphoma is suspected [55]. If the pleural fluid is milky or cloudy, it should be centrifuged, and if the supernatant remains milky or cloudy, the pleural fluid should be sent for measurement of cholesterol and triglycerides. Every time a thoracentesis is performed in a patient with a persistent undiagnosed pleural effusion, a pleural fluid LDH level should be determined. If this LDH level tends to decrease with time, the pleural process is resolving and one can be conservative in the approach to the patient. Alternatively, if the LDH level is increasing with time, the process is getting worse and one should be aggressive in pursuing a diagnosis [7].

Imaging procedures

Most patients with an undiagnosed persistent pleural effusion should have a spiral CT scan of the chest. With the spiral CT scan, the diagnosis of pulmonary emboli can be established [56]. In addition, parenchymal infiltrates and masses, pleural masses or thickening, and mediastinal lymphadenopathy can be identified. Finally, pericardial thickening and pericardial effusions can be identified on the CT scan. While the patient is receiving the CT scan, it is reasonable to obtain abdominal cuts also. These can demonstrate abdominal masses, lymphadenopathy, and ascites. An echocardiogram is indicated if congestive heart failure is suspected but is not definitely established and if a pericardial effusion is suspected. It is important to remember that the echocardiogram may not reveal any abnormality if the patient has constrictive pericarditis [45]. If constrictive pericarditis is suspected, the patient should undergo right heart catheterization.

Needle biopsy of the pleura

For the past 50 years, most cases of tuberculous pleuritis have been diagnosed with a needle biopsy of the pleura. In the past 10 years, however, it has been demonstrated that markers for tuberculosis obtained from the pleural fluid, such as the ADA or γ-interferon, are efficient at establishing this diagnosis. The other diagnosis that can be established with a needle biopsy of the pleura is pleural malignancy. In most series, however, cytology is much more sensitive in establishing the diagnosis. Moreover, if the cytology of the fluid is negative, the pleural biopsy is usually nondiagnostic. In one series of 118 patients from the Mayo Clinic who had a malignancy involving the pleura but negative pleural fluid cytology, the needle biopsy of the pleura was positive in only 20 (17%) patients [57]. Because thoracoscopy is diagnostic in more than 90% of patients with a pleural malignancy and negative cytology, it is the preferred diagnostic procedure in patients with a cytology-negative pleural effusion who are suspected of having a pleural malignancy. A needle biopsy of the pleura is indicated if the patient has an undiagnosed pleural effusion that is not improving and thoracoscopy is not available. A needle biopsy of the pleura is also indicated if pleural tuberculosis is suspected and a pleural fluid marker for tuberculosis is unavailable or equivocal [7]. If the patient has pleura thickening on contrast-enhanced CT, consideration should be given to performing an image-guided cutting needle biopsy of the pleura. In one report [58], the diagnosis of mesothelioma was established in 18 (86%) of 21 patients.

Thoracoscopy

When one is dealing with patients with pleural effusions, thoracoscopic procedures should be used only when less invasive diagnostic methods, such as thoracentesis with cytology and markers for tuberculosis, have not yielded a diagnosis. In the series of 620 patients reported by Kendall and coworkers [59], only 48 (8%) required thoracoscopy for a diagnosis. The final diagnoses in these 48 patients were a malignancy in 24, a parapneumonic effusion in 7, a rheumatoid pleural effusion in 4, congestive heart failure in 3, and pulmonary interstitial fibrosis in 2. In 8 patients, no diagnosis was established with the combination of the clinical presentation and thoracoscopy; 6 of these patients were subsequently diagnosed has having a malignancy (mesothelioma in 3 patients and adenocarcinoma in 3 patients) [59].

In general, if the patient has a malignancy, thoracoscopy establishes the diagnosis in approximately 90% of cases [60–62]. The diagnosis of tuberculous pleuritis can almost always be established with thoracoscopy [63]. It should be emphasized, however, that thoracoscopy rarely establishes the diagnosis of benign disease other than tuberculosis [64]. One advantage of thoracoscopy in the diagnosis of pleural disease is that pleurodesis can be performed at the time of the procedure. In general, thoracoscopy is indicated in the patient with an undiagnosed pleural effusion who is not improving spontaneously, provided that the patient has a significant likelihood of malignancy or tuberculosis.

Bronchoscopy

Bronchoscopy can be diagnostically useful in patients with a pleural effusion if the patient has one of the following four characteristics [65]; otherwise bronchoscopy is not indicated:

1. A pulmonary infiltrate is present on the chest radiograph or chest CT. If an infiltrate is present, particular attention should be paid to the area with the infiltrate at the time of bronchoscopy.
2. Hemoptysis is present. The presence of hemoptysis in the patient with a pleural effusion increases the likelihood of malignancy with an endobronchial lesion or pulmonary embolus. The former can be diagnosed with bronchoscopy.
3. The pleural effusion is massive. The most common cause of a massive pleural effusion is malignancy, particularly lung cancer, and this diagnosis can be established at bronchoscopy. The other two leading causes of massive pleural effusion are hepatic hydrothorax and tuberculous pleuritis; these diagnoses cannot be established with bronchoscopy.
4. The mediastinum is shifted toward the side of the effusion. With this finding, an obstructing endobronchial lesion is probably responsible, and this can be identified and biopsied at bronchoscopy.

Open biopsy

In many institutions, open thoracotomy with direct biopsy of the pleura has been replaced by video-assisted thoracoscopy. If both procedures are available, thoracoscopy is usually preferred because it is associated with less morbidity. The primary indication for an open pleural biopsy is progressive undiagnosed pleural disease in an institution where thoracoscopy is not available or when there is a contraindication for thoracoscopy, such as marked adhesions between the visceral and parietal pleura.

One should realize that even with an open biopsy of the pleura, a diagnosis is not always obtained. In one study, the experience at the Mayo Clinic between 1962 and 1972 with an open pleural biopsy for undiagnosed pleural effusion was reviewed. It was found that no diagnosis was established at open biopsy in 51 patients [66]. Thirty-one of the patients had no recurrence of their pleural effusion; however, 13 of these 51 patients were eventually found to have malignant disease (lymphoma in 6 patients, mesothelioma in 4 patients, and other malignancy in 3 patients). In another study of 21 patients subjected to open pleural biopsy for undiagnosed pleural effusion, no diagnosis was obtained in 7 (33%) [67].

Summary

When faced with a patient with an undiagnosed pleural effusion, the first question to be answered is whether the patient has a transudate or an exudate. This is most commonly done with Light's criteria. If it seems clinically that the patient has a transudative effusion but Light's exudative criteria are met, the demonstration of a serum pleural fluid protein gradient of greater than 3.1 g/dL indicates that the effusion is transudative. The diagnosis of congestive heart failure is strongly suggested if the pleural fluid BNP level is greater than 1500 pg/mL. Patients with undiagnosed exudative effusions should have a spiral CT scan to evaluate the possibility of a pulmonary embolism and to demonstrate parenchymal, pleural, or mediastinal disease. Patients with a malignant pleural effusion usually have the following characteristics: symptoms for more than 1 month, absence of fever, blood-tinged pleural fluid, and chest CT scan findings suggestive of malignancy.

References

[1] Light RW, MacGregor MI, Luchsinger PC, et al. Pleural effusions: the diagnostic separation of transudates and exudates. Ann Intern Med 1972;77:507–14.
[2] Romero S, Candela A, Martin C, et al. Evaluation of different criteria for the separation of pleural transudates from exudates. Chest 1993;104:399–404.
[3] Burgess LJ, Maritz FJ, Taljaard JJ. Comparative analysis of the biochemical parameters used to distinguish between pleural transudates and exudates. Chest 1995;107:1604–9.
[4] Romero-Candeira S, Hernandez L, Romero-Brufao S, et al. Is it meaningful to use biochemical parameters to discriminate between transudative and exudative pleural effusions? Chest 2002;122:1524–9.
[5] Romero-Candeira S, Fernandez C, Martin C, et al. Influence of diuretics on the concentration of proteins and other components of pleural transudates in patients with heart failure. Am J Med 2001;110:681–6.
[6] Romero-Candeira S, Hernandez L. The separation of transudates and exudates with particular reference to the protein gradient. Curr Opin Pulm Med 2004;10:294–8.

[7] Light RW. Pleural diseases. 4th edition. Baltimore: Lippincott, Williams & Wilkins; 2001.

[8] Porcel JM, Vives M, Cao G, et al. Measurement of pro-brain natriuretic peptide in pleural fluid for the diagnosis of pleural effusions due to heart failure. Am J Med 2004;15(116):417–20.

[9] Porcel JM. The use of probrain natriuretic peptide in pleural fluid for the diagnosis of pleural effusions resulting from heart failure. Curr Opin Pulm Med 2005;11:329–33.

[10] Kakizaki S, Katakai K, Yoshinaga T, et al. Hepatic hydrothorax in the absence of ascites. Liver 1998;18:216–20.

[11] Ajmi S, Hassine H, Guezguez M, et al. Isotopic exploration of hepatic hydrothorax: ten cases. Gastroenterol Clin Biol 2004;28:462–6.

[12] Cavina C, Vichi G. Radiological aspects of pleural effusions in medical nephropathy in children. Ann Radiol Diagn (Bologna) 1958;31:163–202.

[13] Llach F, Arieff AI, Massry SG. Renal vein thrombosis and nephrotic syndrome: a prospective study of 36 adult patients. Ann Intern Med 1975;83:8–14.

[14] Belie JA, Milan D. Pleural effusion secondary to ureteral obstruction. Urology 1979;14:27–9.

[15] Garcia-Pachon E, Padilla-Navas I. Urinothorax: case report and review of the literature with emphasis on biochemical diagnosis. Respiration (Herrlisheim) 2004;71:533–6.

[16] Stark D, Shades J, Baron RL, et al. Biochemical features of urinothorax. Arch Intern Med 1982;142:1509–11.

[17] Beach C, Manthey DE. Tension hydrothorax due to ventriculopleural shunting. J Emerg Med 1998;16:33–6.

[18] Monla-Hassan J, Eichenhorn M, Spickler E, et al. Duropleural fistula manifested as a large pleural transudate: an unusual complication of transthoracic diskectomy. Chest 1998;114:1786–9.

[19] Gupta SM, Frias J, Garg A, et al. Aberrant cerebrospinal fluid pathway. Detection by scintigraphy. Clin Nucl Med 1986;11:593–4.

[20] Huggins JT, Sahn SA. Duro-pleural fistula diagnosed by beta2-transferrin. Respiration (Herrlisheim) 2003;70:423–5.

[21] Poe RH, Israel RH, Utell MJ, et al. Sensitivity, specificity, and predictive values of closed pleural biopsy. Arch Intern Med 1984;144:325–8.

[22] Ferrer J, Roldan J, Teixidor J, et al. Predictors of pleural malignancy in patients with pleural effusion undergoing thoracoscopy. Chest 2005;127:1017–22.

[23] Naito T, Satoh H, Ishikawa H, et al. Pleural effusion as a significant prognostic factor in non-small cell lung cancer. Anticancer Res 1997;17:4743–6.

[24] Apffelstaedt JP, Van Zyl JA, Muller AG. Breast cancer complicated by pleural effusion: patient characteristics and results of surgical management. J Surg Oncol 1995;58:173–5.

[25] Romano M, Libshitz HI. Hodgkin disease and non-Hodgkin lymphoma: plain chest radiographs and chest computed tomography of thoracic involvement in previously untreated patients. Radiol Med (Torino) 1998;95:49–53.

[26] Huang L, Schnapp LM, Gruden JF, et al. Presentation of AIDS-related pulmonary Kaposi's sarcoma diagnosed by bronchoscopy. Am J Respir Crit Care Med 1996;153:1385–90.

[27] Ascoli V, Lo-Coco F. Body cavity lymphoma. Curr Opin Pulm Med 2002;8:317–22.

[28] Nakatsuka S, Yao M, Hoshida Y, et al. Pyothorax-associated lymphoma: a review of 106 cases. J Clin Oncol 2002;20:4255–60.

[29] Bartlett JG, Finegold SM. Anaerobic infections of the lung and pleural space. Am Rev Respir Dis 1974;110:56–77.

[30] Roper WH, Waring JJ. Primary serofibrinous pleural effusion in military personnel. Am Rev Respir Dis 1955;71:616–34.

[31] Perez-Rodriguez E, Jimenez Castro D, Light RW. Effusions from tuberculosis. In: Light RW, Lee YC, editors. Textbook of pleural diseases. London: Arnold Publishers; 2003. p. 329–44.

[32] Ferrer JS, Munoz XG, Orriols RM, et al. Evolution of idiopathic pleural effusion. A prospective, long-term follow-up study. Chest 1996;109:1508–13.

[33] Lee YC, Rogers JT, Rodriguez RM, et al. Adenosine deaminase (ADA) levels in non-tuberculous lymphocytic pleural effusions. Chest 2001;120:356–61.

[34] Stein PD, Henry JW. Clinical characteristics of patients with acute pulmonary embolism stratified according to their presenting syndromes. Chest 1997;112:974–9.

[35] Romero-Candeira S, Hernnadez Blasco L, Soler MJ, et al. Biochemical and cytologic characteristics of pleural effusions secondary to pulmonary embolism. Chest 2002;121:465–9.

[36] Coche E, Verschuren F, Keyeux A, et al. Diagnosis of acute pulmonary embolism in outpatients: comparison of thin-collimation multi-detector row spiral CT and planar ventilation-perfusion scintigraphy. Radiology 2003;229:757–65.

[37] Rockey DC, Cello JP. Pancreaticopleural fistula. Report of 7 patients and review of the literature. Medicine 1990;69:332–44.

[38] Light RW, Rogers JT, Moyers JP, et al. Prevalence and clinical course of pleural effusions at 30 days post coronary artery bypass surgery. Am J Respir Crit Care Med 2002;166:1563–6.

[39] Sadikot RT, Rogers JT, Cheng D-S, et al. Pleural fluid characteristics of patients with symptomatic pleural effusion after coronary artery bypass graft surgery. Arch Intern Med 2000;160:2665–8.

[40] Lee YC, Vaz MAC, Ely KA, et al. Symptomatic persistent post-coronary artery bypass graft pleural effusions requiring operative treatment. Clinical and histologic features. Chest 2001;119:795–800.

[41] Light RW. Pleural effusions following cardiac injury and coronary artery bypass graft surgery. Sem Respir Crit Care Med 2001;22:657–64.

[42] Stelzner TJ, King Jr TE, Antony VB, et al. The pleuropulmonary manifestations of the postcardiac injury syndrome. Chest 1983;84:383–7.

[43] Weiss JM, Spodick DH. Association of left pleural effusion with pericardial disease. N Engl J Med 1983; 308:696–7.

[44] Tomaselli G, Gamsu G, Stulbarg MS. Constrictive pericarditis presenting as pleural effusion of unknown origin. Arch Intern Med 1989;149:201–3.

[45] Sadikot RT, Fredi JL, Light RW. A 43-year-old man with a large recurrent right-sided pleural effusion. Chest 2000;117:1191–4.

[46] Timmerman D, Moerman P, Vergote I. Meigs' syndrome with elevated serum CA 125 levels: two case reports and review of the literature. Gynecol Oncol 1995;59:405–8.

[47] Wang DY, Yang PC, Yu WL, et al. Serial antinuclear antibodies titre in pleural and pericardial fluid. Eur Respir J 2000;15:1106–10.

[48] Kalomenidis IT. Effusions due to drugs. In: Light RW, Lee YC, editors. Textbook of pleural diseases. London: Arnold Publishing; 2001. p. 382–93.

[49] Epler GR, McLoud TC, Gaensler EA. Prevalence and incidence of benign asbestos pleural effusion in a working population. JAMA 1982;247:617–22.

[50] Hillerdal G, Ozesmi M. Benign asbestos pleural effusion: 73 exudates in 60 patients. Eur J Respir Dis 1987;71:113–21.

[51] Berger HW, Rammohan G, Neff MS, et al. Uremic pleural effusion: a study in 14 patients on chronic dialysis. Ann Intern Med 1975;82:362–4.

[52] Coskun M, Boyvat F, Bozkurt B, et al. Thoracic CT findings in long-term hemodialysis patients. Acta Radiol 1998;40:181–6.

[53] Light RW, Jenkinson SG, Minh V, et al. Observations on pleural pressures as fluid is withdrawn during thoracentesis. Am Rev Respir Dis 1980;121:799–804.

[54] Fentiman IS, Millis R, Sexton S, et al. Pleural effusion in breast cancer: a review of 105 cases. Cancer 1981;47:2087–92.

[55] Moriarty AT, Wiersema L, Snyder W, et al. Immunophenotyping of cytologic specimens by flow cytometry. Diag Cytopathol 1993;9:252–8.

[56] Goodman PC. Spiral CT for pulmonary embolism. Semin Respir Crit Care Med 2000;21:503–10.

[57] Prakash URS, Reiman HM. Comparison of needle biopsy with cytologic analysis for the evaluation of pleural effusion: analysis of 414 cases. Mayo Clin Proc 1985;60:158–64.

[58] Adams RF, Gray W, Davies RJ, et al. Percutaneous image-guided cutting needle biopsy of the pleura in the diagnosis of malignant mesothelioma. Chest 2001; 120:1798–802.

[59] Kendall SW, Bryan AJ, Large SR, et al. Pleural effusions: is thoracoscopy a reliable investigation? A retrospective review. Respir Med 1992;86:437–40.

[60] Hucker J, Bhatnagar NK, al-Jilaihawi AN, et al. Thoracoscopy in the diagnosis and management of recurrent pleural effusions. Ann Thorac Surg 1991;52: 1145–7.

[61] Menzies R, Charbonneau M. Thoracoscopy for the diagnosis of pleural disease. Ann Intern Med 1991; 114:271–6.

[62] Hansen M, Faurschou P, Clementsen P. Medical thoracoscopy, results and complications in 146 patients: a retrospective study. Respir Med 1998;92:228–32.

[63] Diacon AH, Van de Wal BW, Wyser C, et al. Diagnostic tools in tuberculous pleurisy: a direct comparative study. Eur Respir J 2003;22:589–91.

[64] Daniel TM. Diagnostic thoracoscopy for pleural disease. Ann Thorac Surg 1993;56:639–40.

[65] Chang S-C, Perng RP. The role of fiberoptic bronchoscopy in evaluating the causes of pleural effusions. Arch Intern Med 1989;149:855–7.

[66] Ryan CJ, Rodgers RF, Unni KK, et al. The outcome of patients with pleural effusion of indeterminate cause at thoracotomy. Mayo Clin Proc 1981;56:145–9.

[67] Douglass BE, Carr DT, Bernatz PE. Diagnostic thoracotomy in the study of "idiopathic" pleural effusion. Am Rev Tuberc 1956;74:954–7.

ELSEVIER
SAUNDERS

Clin Chest Med 27 (2006) 321 – 334

CLINICS
IN CHEST
MEDICINE

Staphylococcal Superantigens of the Enterotoxin Gene Cluster (*egc*) for Treatment of Stage IIIb Non–Small Cell Lung Cancer with Pleural Effusion

David S. Terman, MD[a],*, Gregory Bohach, PhD[b],
Francois Vandenesch, MD, PhD[c], Jerome Etienne, MD, PhD[c],
Gerard Lina, MD, PhD[c], Steven A. Sahn, MD[d]

[a]*Jenomic, Inc., Carmel, CA, USA*
[b]*Department of Microbiology, Molecular Biology, and Biochemistry, University of Idaho, Moscow, ID, USA*
[c]*Centre Nationales de Reference des Staphylococcques, INSERM E0230, IFR62, Faculte de Medecine Laennec, Lyon, France*
[d]*Division of Pulmonary, Critical Care, Allergy, and Sleep Medicine, Medical University of South Carolina, Charleston, SC, USA*

More than 200,000 new cases of malignant pleural effusion (MPE) are diagnosed annually in the United States with approximately 40% from lung cancer and 25% from breast cancer. When first evaluated, about 15% of lung cancer patients exhibit a pleural effusion; however, 50% of patients with disseminated lung cancer may develop an MPE during the course of their disease [1–6]. MPE is the initial presenting manifestation in 40% to 60% of patients with non–small cell lung cancer (NSCLC) [7,8]. Most of these patients are symptomatic or disabled from the MPE and require prompt treatment. Although chemotherapy is the first option in MPE from small cell carcinoma of the lung, breast carcinoma, or lymphoma, symptomatic patients with MPE from NSCLC usually are offered palliative therapy initially to control the MPE using chemical pleurodesis or indwelling catheters. Even after successful pleurodesis or drainage, most of these patients exhibit poor performance (Eastern Cooperative Oncology Group [ECOG] ≤ 2 or Karnofsky Performance Score [KPS] ≤ 70) and still are not eligible for systemic chemotherapy [1–6]. The presence of MPE in NSCLC

signals a poor prognosis with a median survival of only 2 to 3 months [1,9–13].

Chemical pleurodesis commonly is performed with talc, bleomycin, or doxycycline through a chest tube, which is usually in place for several days. Variable response rates (range 50–93%) and late recurrences have been observed [3–6,14]. Talc poudrage at thoracoscopy has similar success to talc slurry through a chest tube, but also requires hospitalization and a period of tube drainage. An indwelling pleural catheter for drainage or injection of a pleurodesis agent provides an additional option [9,10]; however, intermittent drainage of the effusion at home by the patient or a caregiver is required. All of these latter modalities for control of MPE require chest tube insertion or thoracoscopy, and none has any demonstrable survival benefit [3–6,14]. Numerous intrapleurally administered chemotherapeutic agents, such as cisplatin, doxorubicin, etoposide, fluorouracil, and mitomycin, generally have proved ineffective in controlling MPE [3], and thoracentesis or chest tube drainage alone results in recurrence rates of 98% or 85% within 30 days [3–6,14].

Numerous biologic agents, such as *Corynebacterium parvum,* interleukin (IL)-2, tumor necrosis factor (TNF)-α, interferon (IFN)-α, IFN-β, and IFN-γ, had fair-to-poor success in the control of MPE and showed no significant effect on survival [3,7,8].

---

* Corresponding author. 3183 Palmero Way, Pebble Beach, CA 93953.
E-mail address: dst@sbcglobal.net (D.S. Terman).

None has been approved for this indication by the US Food and Drug Administration. However, A report describing the use of a family of new staphylococcal enterotoxin (SE) superantigens induced resolution of MPE from NSCLC, and a survival benefit in 14 patients with poor performance has generated new interest in immunotherapy as a potential treatment for patients with MPE from NSCLC [15]. This article focuses on this new family of superantigens and progress in understanding their mechanism, harnessing their potency, and adapting them for therapeutic use.

Superantigens

Background

The first bacterial superantigen was isolated in the late 1960s by Bergdoll's group [16] as a secreted toxin of *S aureus* and was named *staphylococcal enterotoxin A* (SEA) for its potent enterotoxin properties. Several additional SEs subsequently identified were found to be the causative agent in staphylococcal food poisoning associated with vomiting and diarrhea within 1 to 2 hours after ingestion. The mitogenic activity of SEs was discovered many years later, but the term *superantigen* was not associated with these toxins until 1989, when Marrack and Kappler [17] found that the mitogenic activity was a result of massive expansion of T cells that all shared the same T cell receptor (TCR) Vβ chain domains. Several members of the SE superantigen family, including the *S aureus* toxic shock syndrome toxin (TSST), have been found to be the causative agent of a toxic shock syndrome in humans and animals [17].

A prototypical feature of SE superantigens is the ability of very small quantities to stimulate T cells. In concentrations of 10^{-13} to 10^{-16} M, several SE superantigens induce proliferation (measured as DNA synthesis) of a high proportion of resting $CD4^+$ and $CD8^+$ T cells to proliferate (measured as DNA synthesis), differentiate into cytotoxic T cells, and release various cytokines, several of which are tumoricidal. Cells of the natural killer, NKT (natural killer T), and γ/δ T cell lineages also are activated by SE superantigens in these dose ranges. These bacterial superantigen enterotoxins (SE) are the most powerful stimulators of cytotoxic T lymphocytes known, evoking strong polyclonal proliferative responses at concentrations about 10^3-fold lower than any other known T cell mitogen [17–22].

The best characterized members of the superantigen family are evolutionarily related pyrogenic toxin molecules, which include the *S aureus* enterotoxins A to P, TSST-1, exfoliative toxins, and streptococcal pyrogenic exotoxins (SPE) A through C and F and M proteins from *Streptococcus pyogenes*. With few exceptions, most of these superantigens are globular proteins consisting of single polypeptide chains that have molecular weights ranging from approximately 20,000 to 30,000 kd. Based on their primary sequence homology, superantigens from *S aureus* and *S pyogenes* are clustered into four groups. The first group includes SEA, SED, and SEE, which share 53% to 81% homology. SEB, SEC1-3, SpeA, and SSA, which share approximately 50% to greater than 90% identity, form a second group. The third group consists of superantigens that have less than 40% identity to each other or to the other toxins. The latter group includes TSST-1, which has less than 30% homology to most superantigens. SpeA and SSA are highly homologous to SEB at the protein level; SSA is more related to SEB and SEC (60% identity) than it is to SPEA (49% identity) or to SPEC (22% identity). Several chains have a characteristic and functionally important disulfide loop near the middle of the chain. Despite differences in their sequences, there are remarkable similarities in their overall folded structures. For each superantigen studied so far, the molecule folds to generate two tightly packed domains, an amino-terminal hydrophobic β-barrel domain and a carboxy-terminal β-grasp domain, with one or more α helices spanning the center of the molecule suggesting a common ancestral origin [17–23]. The staphylococcal and streptococcal superantigens share common physicochemical properties of relative heat stability, trypsin resistance, and solubility in water and salt solutions. All have similar sedimentation coefficients, diffusion constants, partial specific volumes, and extinction coefficients [17–22].

An essential feature of superantigens is that they simultaneously bind and cross-link the TCR and MHC class II (MHCII) molecules. Despite its polymorphism, MHCII is the principal cell receptor for all superantigens. A schematic of the binding scheme of superantigens to the MHCII and the TCR is shown in Fig. 1. The cross-linking of MHC molecules and TCR by superantigens triggers proliferation of T cells and their differentiation into cytotoxic T cells and production of inflammatory cytokines. There are major differences between superantigens in the mode by which they interact with their receptors on the surface of T cells and antigen presenting cells (APCs). These differences influence the magnitude of immune stimulation by the superantigens and account for their observed variation in biologic activity. The affinity of

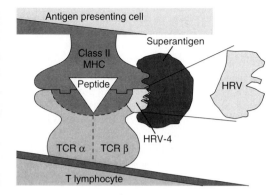

Antigen presenting cell

Superantigen

Class II MHC

Peptide

HRV

HRV-4

TCR α | TCR β

T lymphocyte

Fig. 1. Schematic representation of the mechanism by which superantigens bind to the MHC class II receptor and the T cell Vβ receptor. See text for details and comparison with the binding of conventional antigen peptides.

SE for MHCII and TCR varies with each superantigen and is a major determinant of T cell stimulating potency [17–21].

Superantigens have developed different modes by which they can interact with these receptors. In general, they have a common, relatively low-affinity amino-terminal site for binding to the α chain of the class II molecule (the SEB-like site), and several have one or more relatively high-affinity carboxy-terminal Zn-dependent sites, shared by SEA, SED, and SPEC, for binding to the β chain of the class II molecule. Some superantigens bind to either the α or the β chain, whereas others are bivalent, binding to both MHC chains. SEA and SEE are examples of bivalent homodimers that bind and cross-link two adjacent MHCII molecules on APCs (using at least one high-affinity Zn^{++}-dependent site) to evoke powerful signals from the APC for T cell stimulation [17–22,24]. Such cross-linking of MHCII molecules on monocytes leads to upregulation of Toll-like receptor 4 expression and production of TNF-α, IL-1, IL-6, and IFN-β when exposed to its natural lipopolysaccharide ligand. [25]. Likewise, superantigens can bind to CD-1 receptors on monocytes, which can support T cell proliferation in a Vβ-dependent fashion [26].

Superantigens versus conventional antigens

Superantigens are differentiated from conventional antigens primarily by the structural interaction formed with MHCII and TCR and the sheer magnitude of the response produced by this interaction. Superantigens engage the V region of the TCR β chain (Vβ region) on an exposed face of the

β pleated sheet. They also bind to the "sides" of the MHCII molecule rather than engaging the groove between the MHCII α and β chains as do conventional antigens (see Fig. 1) [17–22,24]. Conventional antigens are processed within APCs into peptides and are transported to the MHCII molecules on the cell surface in the groove between the α and β chains. From here, peptides are presented to the TCR α/β hypervariable loops on T cells, which have differentiated specifically in response to peptide recognition [17–22]. In contrast, superantigens do not require processing in the APC for recognition by the TCR. They simply bind in unprocessed form, as intact molecules to invariant regions of the MHCII expressed on APCs outside the peptide-binding groove. Although peptide antigen recognition by the TCR requires generation of diversity elements in the T cell, superantigen recognition by T cells via the TCR Vβ region is independent of other TCR components and does not require the T cell generation of diversity elements. When bound to the MHCII molecule, superantigens sequentially bind the TCR via the variable region of the TCR β chain. Each superantigen generally binds at least two subsets of TCR Vβ domains, resulting in activation of 20% of naive T cells compared with 0.01% to 0.0001% activation in response to conventional peptide antigens. The fundamental differences in the properties of conventional antigens and superantigens are shown in Table 1.

The distinctive binding characteristics of SEs and other superantigens that bypass the highly variable parts of the MHCII and TCR molecules endow them with the ability to activate a high frequency of T cells

Table 1
Superantigens versus classic antigens

Property	Superantigens	Classic antigens
Frequency of responding T cells	40% of resting T cells	0.001% of resting T cells
No. molecules required to activate T cells	10^{-15} M	10^{-3} M
Activate T cells via Vβ region of TCR	Yes	No
Activate tumoricidal cytokines	Yes	No
Processing required by antigen presenting cells and T cells	No	Yes
T cells of many specificities respond	Yes	No

and cause proliferation, cytokine induction, and cytotoxic T cell generation. Because the normal cytotoxic lymphocyte response in tumor-bearing hosts in response to tumor antigens is insufficient to interfere with tumor growth, superantigens, with their capacity to recruit and activate numerous tumor-specific cytotoxic lymphocytes, are particularly well suited for cancer treatment [17–22,27].

*Enterotoxin gene cluster (*egc*) staphylococcal enterotoxins*

SEs G and I were identified in two separate strains of *S aureus* [27a]. It subsequently was shown that the corresponding genes *seg* and *sei* are present in *S aureus* in tandem orientation, on a 3.2-kb DNA fragment. Sequence analysis of *seg-sei* intergenic DNA and flanking regions revealed three enterotoxin-like open reading frames related to *seg* and *sei,* designated *sem, sen,* and *seo,* and two pseudogenes, *ψent1* and *ψent2.* Reverse transcriptase polymerase chain reaction analysis showed that all these genes, including *seg* and *sei,* belong to an *S aureus* operon, designated the enterotoxin gene cluster (*egc*). Phylogenetic analysis of all known enterotoxin genes

indicated that they all are potentially derived from the *egc* SE, identifying *egc* as a putative nursery of enterotoxin genes [28]. Functionally, each recombinant SEG, SEI, SEM, SEN, and SEO showed superantigenic T cell proliferative activity with a specific Vβ profile. SE-producing strains of *S aureus* express genes encoding several SEs, and the *egc* SE genes were present in about 75% of all SE-producing *S aureus* strains usually in association with one or more classic SEs. Only a rare strain produced *egc* SEs alone [29]. *egc* expression was more likely associated with milder suppurative and cutaneous clinical manifestations of *S aureus* infection rather than septic shock or toxic shock [30]. Neutralizing antibodies against the *egc* SEs were found in a relatively small percentage of human sera compared with the classic SEs [31]. Fundamental properties of the *egc* superantigens are summarized in Box 1.

Tumoricidal effects of superantigens

Native superantigens

In the course of studies using *S aureus* protein A preparations to treat dogs with spontaneous mammary cancers, trace quantities of the SEs A, B, and C were identified in the protein A preparations. Initial in vivo investigations using purified native SEB in established canine melanoma and rabbit VX-2 carcinoma showed that these agents induced tumoricidal activity [32–37]. Subsequently, various superantigens in native form were used for treatment of tumors in a wide variety of animal tumor models of carcinoma, sarcoma, and lymphoma [38–41]. Administration of SEB produced antitumor effects against established tumors, such as canine mammary carcinoma [33], rabbit VX-2 carcinoma [37], murine A/20 lymphoma [38], murine CL62 melanomas [39], murine PRO4L fibrosarcoma [40], and human colon carcinoma [41]. Unmodified superantigens also showed antitumor activity when used as vaccines. Irradiated melanoma cells (dead vaccine) were administered to mice, followed 3 days later by administration of SEA and SEB. When subsequently challenged with live melanoma cells, a large proportion of mice were able to destroy the malignant cells, and survival of treated mice was increased substantially. Of mice that survived more than 150 days, 75% remained tumor-free after rechallenge with viable melanoma cells [42]. Strong immunologic memory developed after vaccination with irradiated cancer cells suggesting that prophylactic vaccination against

---

Box 1. General properties of *egc* staphylococcal enterotoxins

- Mobile pathogenicity island (operon) present in 60% of all SEs producing *S aureus*
- Five SEs, G, I, M, N, and O, and two pseudo-SEs 6500 bps
- Share 30–50% amino acid homology to classic SEs
- *egc* genes present in frame sequence on the operon
- In contrast to classic SEs, *egc* SEs weakly transcribed, but secreted in small quantities generally as multiple *egc* SE proteins
- Strongly mitogenic for T cells in range of classic superantigens
- Each *egc* SE shows TCR Vβ specificity (Vβ profile) characteristic of superantigens
- Induce T cell cytokines IFN-γ, TNF-α, and IL-2

cancer using superantigens as adjuvant-like agents is a realistic possibility.

The toxicity and efficacy of SEB dissolved in 0.9% sodium chloride administered intravesically once weekly for 6 weeks in a rat bladder cancer model were evaluated. In the intravesically SEB-treated animals (10 μg/mL), only 3 tumors remained versus 15 persisting tumors in the control group. The remaining tumors of the therapy group showed a significant amount of apoptosis and granulocytes, mainly in the urothelium, whereas no relevant apoptosis or infiltration of the bladder with lymphocytes or macrophages was found in the control group. These preclinical findings suggest that SEB is a candidate for further clinical evaluation [43].

Superantigen gene therapy

SEB transfected murine mammary carcinoma cells, which expressed and secreted SEB, were effective in reducing pulmonary metastases in a post-mastectomy metastatic breast cancer model [44]. Potent antitumor effects were elicited by superantigens, linked genetically or biochemically to tumor cells alone or additionally transduced with heat-shock protein 70 and IL-18 genes, when used as vaccines or against established tumors [45,46]. A transmembrane sequence from a *c-erb-B2* gene derived from human ovarian cancer cell line HO-8910 was fused to SEA to produce a transmembrane-SEA fusion protein that associated spontaneously with tumor cell membranes and stimulated the proliferation of human peripheral blood lymphocytes and splenocytes derived from C57BL/6 (H-2b) mice in vitro [47–50]. In addition, chimeric nucleic acid constructs consisting of EI or E7 papilloma viral DNA fused to SEB conferred protection against challenge with live papillomavirus in mouse and rabbit models of papillomavirus-induced squamous cell carcinoma. Vaccinations given once weekly for 3 weeks to rabbits induced freedom from papilloma outgrowth for more than 420 days [51].

The safety and efficacy of intratumoral injections of SEB DNA with a cytokine gene were evaluated in dogs with malignant melanoma, a spontaneous and highly malignant canine tumor. Twenty-six dogs with stage III melanoma were treated with lipid-complexed plasmid DNA encoding SEB and either granulocyte-macrophage colony-stimulating factor or IL-2 directly into the tumor. The overall response rate (complete or partial remissions) for all 26 dogs was 46% (12 of 26) and was highest in dogs with smaller tumors. Toxicity was minimal or absent. Tumors treated with injections developed marked infiltrates of CD4+ and CD8+ T cells and macrophages, and tumor regression was associated with development of high levels of antitumor cytotoxic lymphocyte activity in peripheral blood lymphocytes. Survival times of animals in stage III melanomas treated by intratumoral gene therapy were prolonged significantly compared with animals treated with surgical tumor excision only. Local tumor transfection with SEs and cytokine genes was capable of inducing local and systemic antitumor immunity in an outbred animal with a spontaneously developing malignant tumor [52].

Intralesional lipid-complexed immunogene therapy with constructs encoding SEA and canine IL-2 (L-SEA/cIL-2) was given weekly in escalating doses for 12 weeks to dogs with histologically confirmed soft tissue sarcomas. The overall response rate was 25%, consisting of three complete responses and one partial response. Diffuse lymphoplasmacytic inflammation was observed in all tumors from dogs experiencing a complete response or partial response, whereas these changes were not evident in tumors from nonresponders. The infiltrate was composed primarily of CD3+ cells at 48 hours from the single-injection study and was composed of CD3+ and CD79a+ cells at 12 weeks in responding dogs from the multiple-injection study. Overall, treatments were well tolerated, with no dose-limiting toxicities encountered [53].

Superantigens used ex vivo

Ex vivo application of superantigens to stimulate T cells was undertaken to avoid administering the SE in vivo with its attendant toxicity. SEB and SEC1 were employed ex vivo to stimulate a population of T cells pre-exposed to tumor, which, on reinfusion into host animals with established pulmonary metastases, induced a striking resolution of established metastases [54]. Twelve consecutive patients with newly diagnosed gliomas were treated with adoptive transfer of T lymphocytes derived from their own lymph nodes draining autologous tumors. Briefly, patients were injected intradermally with short-term cultured autologous irradiated tumor cells, admixed with granulocyte-macrophage colony-stimulating factor, to stimulate draining lymph node cells. The lymph nodes were surgically extracted and stimulated ex vivo with SEA for 48 hours, expanded by IL-2 for 6 to 8 days, then harvested and reinjected intravenously to the patients. The median dose of T cells infused was 1.1×10^{10}, most of which were CD4+

cells (mean 71%). The entire treatment was done as outpatient therapy. The toxicity consisted mainly of fever, nausea, and myalgias during the first 24 hours, which was of grade 2 or less. Four patients showed partial regression of residual tumor. The ex vivo culture system did not include key cytokines to prevent SEA-driven T cell death. With the addition of T cell–sparing agents IL-15, IL-7, and IL-23 and the use of a library of superantigens (eg, *egc* SEs) with a broader T cell Vβ stimulation repertoire, future clinical trials should produce even better results. Nevertheless, this phase I clinical trial of adoptive immunotherapy in patients with newly diagnosed malignant gliomas showed feasibility, lack of long-term toxicity, and several objective clinical responses [55]. Studies have used anti-CD3 monoclonal antibody in place of SE as the T cell stimulant ex vivo. Anti-CD3 is a weaker T cell mitogen than SEs, however, and induces a more restricted T cell Vβ activation than that noted with a library of SEs such as the *egc* SEs.

Staphylococcal enterotoxin–tumor-specific antibody conjugates

Promising results in animal tumor models also were obtained using SEA fused to a tumor-specific monoclonal antibody. Common findings include greater than 80% inhibition of tumor growth and substantially increased survival rates in a murine B16 melanoma model [56–58]. Fusion proteins consisting of SEA and fragments of bispecific antibodies ("diabodies") with specificity for a tumor-specific and a T cell–specific antigen showed complete disappearance of tumor mass in 50% of treated mice with the other 50% showing marked reduction in tumor growth [59].

Human clinical trials with superantigens

Toxicity in humans treated with native classic staphylococcal enterotoxins

Superantigens in native or conjugated form are currently under investigation as therapeutic agents in cancer immunotherapy, particularly in an attempt to treat cancers with a high mortality (e.g., lung cancer, gastrointestinal malignancies, and metastatic breast cancer). In early studies, SEB and SEA were used systemically to treat humans with metastatic breast cancer [34,60]. Severe toxicity manifested as hypotension, tachycardia, acute respiratory distress syn-

drome with hypoxemia, and prerenal azotemia was observed [61]. All five patients survived, but dopamine/metaraminol infusions were required to support blood pressure and avert acute renal failure. Prospective hemodynamic studies showed an acute increase in cardiac output and stroke volume followed by a decline in peripheral vascular resistance. The hypoxemia was worse in a patient with preexisting metastatic lung tumor who also developed severe bronchospasm and a large pleural effusion requiring repeated thoracenteses. Slowing the infusion rate from 5 mL/min to 2 mL/min attenuated the hypotension and respiratory distress [34,60,61]. Likewise, SEB administered to primates resulted in noncardiogenic pulmonary edema with localization of SEB and injury to the pulmonary vascular endothelial cells [62].

Initial studies using native SEA bound to a tumor-specific monoclonal antibody (to improve the ability of native SEs to localize to a tumor site in vivo) resulted in toxicity similar to that with native SEB [63,64]. By introducing a point mutation in SEA at its high-affinity, Zn^{++}-dependent MHCII binding site (which reduced its cytokine-inducing activity), cytokine-mediated toxicity of SEA was reduced 100 to 1000 fold [55]. Although reduction of MHCII binding activity attenuated the toxicity, the number of activated Vβ T cell clones also was reduced, and there was only a marginal improvement in efficacy [65,66].

The major impediment to efficacy of these native modified SEA preparations was the presence in patient sera of neutralizing antibodies to SEA, which was noted frequently. Their identification correlated with severe toxicity [63,67,68]. As a consequence, native and modified SEA molecules, rather than localizing to tumors, were more likely to be redirected to reticuloendothelial tissues, where they are degraded and eliminated. Attempts to overcome this problem by delivering amounts of SEA conjugate that exceeded the SEA-antibody neutralizing capacity only induced greater toxicity and higher levels of SEA-specific antibodies [67]. Further attempts to reduce toxicity and improve efficacy by "deimmunizing" the SEA molecule via substitution mutations of SEA epitopes recognized by neutralizing antibodies with SEE epitopes are presently under investigation [69]. Even these extensively modified SEA preparations still appear to retain binding to neutralizing antibodies, however [69]. None of these studies in humans has shown the localization in vivo of the native or genetically modified SE-antibody conjugates to tumor cells, suggesting that any therapeutic effect is not related to the tumor targeting of the SE by the antibody portion of the conjugate.

Phase 1 trial of superantigens in stage IIIb non–small cell lung cancer with pleural effusion with egc *staphylococcal enterotoxins*

A clinical trial was performed with a preparation[1] containing native *egc* SEs to which humans rarely make neutralizing antibodies. The *egc* SE preparation was given to 14 unselected, consecutive patients with stage IIIb NSCLC with a pleural effusion and poor performance status (KPS 30–60 or ECOG 3) who were not candidates for systemic chemotherapy. The *egc* SE preparation was administered intrapleurally immediately after partial drainage of the pleural effusion by thoracentesis [15].

These 14 patients with MPE from NSCLC and a median pretreatment KPS of 40 (range 10–60) received pleural instillation of *egc* SE, 100 to 400 pg, once or twice weekly (3.7 ± 1.3, mean ± SD treatments) until the pleural effusions resolved. Patients were evaluated for drug toxicity, resolution and duration of MPE, and survival. Other than mild fever (maximum grade 2), toxicity of *egc* superantigen treatment was trivial and devoid of respiratory distress or hypotension. Of patients, 11 had a complete response, and 3 had a partial response of their MPE. In 12 patients, the response endured for more than 90 days with a median time to recurrence of 5 months (range 3–23 months). The median survival for the *egc* SE–treated group was 7.9 months (range 2–36 months; 95% confidence interval [CI] 5.9–11.4 months) compared with a median survival of 2.5 months (range 0.1–57 months; 95% CI 1.3–3.4 months) for 18 consecutive, unselected patients with MPE from NSCLC (stage IIIb) treated with talc poudrage (P=.044). Survival duration of all 14 *egc* SE–treated cases and 13 talc poudrage–treated patients matched for pretreatment KPS range (10–60) was 7.9 months (95% CI 5.9–11.4 months) and 2 months (95% CI 0.4–2.9 months; P=.0023). Although none of the 13 talc-treated patients survived more than 6 months, 9 of 14 patients treated with *egc* SE survived more than 6 months, 4 survived more than 9 months, and 3 survived more than 350 days.

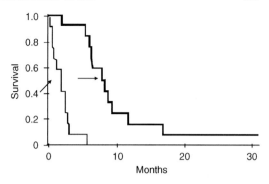

Fig. 2. Kaplan-Meier survival curve comparing 14 patients who received SE superantigens intrapleurally with 13 patients who received talc poudrage for treatment of MPE from NSCLC who had similar pretreatment KPS scores (range 10–60; medians 40 and 30) and distribution. The patients who received SE superantigens had a significantly increased median survival of 7.9 months compared with 2 months for the patients who received talc pleurodesis (P=.0023).

One of the patients in the complete response group has survived 45 months (Fig. 2) [15]. Native *egc* SEs administered directly into the pleural space resulted in partial or complete resolutions of MPE in 14 consecutive and unselected patients with MPE from NSCLC with minimal toxicity and a significant survival benefit compared with controls who received palliative treatment.

In multicenter trials conducted from 1994–1996 led by investigators at M.D. Anderson Cancer Center, groups of 61 and 35 patients with MPE from NSCLC treated with indwelling catheter drainage and doxycycline pleurodesis had median survivals of 2 months [9] and 3 months [10]. A meta-analysis of 156 patients with MPE from lung cancer showed a median survival of 3 months [11]. Compared with current populations treated with the best available palliative measures (talc, doxycycline, and indwelling catheter drainage), *egc* SE–treated patients had a 2.4 to 3 fold greater survival (Table 2) [1,9–13].

The median survival of 7.9 months for the 14 *egc* SE–treated patients was surprising in view of the low median pretreatment KPS of 40 or ECOG of 3 (disabled, bedridden >50% waking hours) for this group. Nine patients with KPS of 40 and less had a median survival of 8.6 months. Cisplatin-based chemotherapy generally is not recommended for patients with KPS of 70 or less (ECOG ≥2) because it induces a greater level of toxicity compared with patients with KPS of 70 or greater (ECOG 0–1). Chemotherapeutic regimens used in stage IIIb patients (with pleural effusion) selected for ECOG

---

[1] The preparation was prepared from a partially purified supernatant of an *S aureus* strain containing no other superantigen genes than *egc*. The preparation possesses superantigenic activity and its Vβ pattern matches that obtained when combining the five *egc* proteins. Finally, mass spectrometry analysis did not reveal the presence of proteins with potential biological activities against tumor cells. Henceforth, in the rest of this article the term *egc* preparation will be used to describe the product administrated in the phase I clinical trial.

Table 2
Other treatments of malignant pleural effusion from non–small cell lung cancer

Number	Survival (mo)[a]	Site	Reference
21 TALC	2 (median)	San Diego	[13]
61 PLEURX	2 (median)	MD Anderson	[9]
35 DOXY	3 (median)	MD Anderson	[10]
14 EGC SAg	7.9 (median)	China	[15]

[a] Survival measured from from date of first treatment.

0 to 1, KPS 70 or greater have shown an improved median survival of approximately 8 months comparable to the survival reported for *egc* SE–treated patients with a median KPS of 40 (ECOG 3) [70,71]. As a single treatment, *egc* SE seemed to be capable of inducing an MPE response rate exceeding talc with less morbidity and a survival duration in a group with poor performance status (KPS 40) comparable to cisplatin-based chemotherapy in patients with better performance (KPS ≥70). *egc* SE treatment may be useful in stage IIIb patients with MPE (KPS 40 or ECOG 3) who are not eligible for chemotherapy. Pretreatment KPS less than 70 (range 30–60) in eight patients improved to a KPS of 70 or greater (ECOG 2) after a single course of *egc* SE treatment, suggesting that patients considered ineligible for chemotherapy might become eligible after *egc* SE therapy.

The only toxicity of *egc* SE treatment was fever, which never exceeded grade 2 and was managed easily with conventional antipyretics. There was no grade 3 or 4 toxicity, and all patients were discharged from the hospital within 24 hours after the procedure. Acute respiratory distress syndrome, which was observed after talc insufflation or instillation [72], and hypotension, noncardiogenic pulmonary edema, and prerenal azotemia, which were reported after treatment of cancer patients with preparations containing SE superantigens A and B [60,61,63,64,67], were absent. In addition to the lack of significant toxicity, *egc* SE therapy may be performed in an outpatient setting. It may offer potential advantages over approved palliative agents used for MPE that require hospitalization, while avoiding thoracoscopy, chest tube insertion, and prolonged chest tube drainage, which often are required for chemical pleurodesis.

Although the classic SEs (alone or part of a fusion protein with tumor-specific antibodies) require genetic modification of antibody binding epitopes and MHCII binding sites to reduce their toxicity in humans [67–69], *egc* SEs in native form given intrapleurally and intravenously induced minimal toxicity [15]. The presence of naturally occurring neutralizing antibodies in patient sera inhibited SEA-induced T cell proliferation and abrogated the antitumor effects of native or modified SEA-antibody fusion proteins when used for tumor therapy. These blocking antibodies were associated with significant host toxicity; each successive SEA fusion protein treatment resulted in a progressively increased titer of SE-associated antibodies and more frequent toxicity [64,67,68]. In contrast, neutralizing antibodies against the *egc* SEs are rarely found in human sera despite the high prevalence of the *egc* locus in natural populations of *S aureus* [31]. The absence of neutralizing antibodies against *egc* SE may account for its minimal toxicity and enhanced therapeutic effect compared with native or modified SEA in humans. Although measurement of SEA-specific antibodies in patient's sera was required before each treatment to determine an effective dose [68], this was not required for *egc* SE treatment to be effective. Table 3 compares the properties of *egc* SE with the classic superantigens SEA and SEB as they have been used to date to treat human carcinoma.

Although the individual toxicity of SEA and other classic SEs precluded the use of more than one at a time, the *egc* SEs could be used as a group of five separate SEs without significant toxicity [15] with the advantage that *egc* SEs collectively are capable of activating 13 Vβ-specific T cell clones with potential antitumor activity compared with 5 for genetically modified SEA [66]. The absence of neutralizing antibodies coupled with the broad Vβ T cell profile may account for the greater antitumor potency of the *egc* SE compared with native or modified SEA. The *egc* SEs were employed in native form, whereas the SEA molecule required extensive genetic mutation of the native SEA sequence to improve toxicity profile [64,67]. These mutations came at the cost of

Table 3
Clinical properties: *egc* versus classic superantigens

Property	Superantigens	
	egc	classic
Neutralizing antibodies present	Rare	Common
Human sera inhibit T cell proliferation	Rare	Common
Clinical toxicity	Mild	Significant
Require structural mutation to reduce toxicity	No (are used in native form)	Yes (MHC class II and neutralizing antibody epitope)
Used as plurality of superantigens	Yes	No
Dosing required to exceed antibody levels	No	Yes

a reduction in the T cell Vβ activating capacity of SEA [66], whereas the native (unmodified) *egc* SEs retained their complete T cell Vβ activation profile. Although the *egc* SEs induced a 300% increase in survival in patients with advanced NSCLC, SE monoclonal antibody preparations produced a negligible response rate against human colon and pancreatic carcinoma and only a modest prolongation of survival in patients with advanced NSCLC [63,67].

egc SE–treated patients with a median KPS of 40 (range 10–60) had a median survival that exceeded survival after talc poudrage and was comparable to survival after current systemic chemotherapy used in patients with KPS of 70 or greater [67,68]. *egc* SE treatment is simple to perform, is minimally invasive, and does not require hospitalization. This therapy may be an attractive alternative to existing palliative modalities for stage IIIb patients with MPE and poor performance who are not candidates for systemic chemotherapy.

Although the precise frequency and duration of response or antineoplastic efficacy cannot be determined from this phase I trial, the lack of toxicity, ease of administration, and relatively low cost, make this treatment suitable for extension to a larger cohort of patients. Critical phase II clinical trials are planned with recombinant *egc* SE in advanced lung cancer.

Mechanism of the tumor killing effect of superantigens

Superantigens derive their name from the shared property of activating a high proportion of T cells via binding to the TCR Vβ region. Each superantigen activates a unique cluster of Vβ on the TCRs of CD4[+] and CD8[+] T cells. The resolution of pleural effusions and prolonged survival of NSCLC patients with *egc* SE therapy may be ascribed in part to an *egc* SE–induced tumoricidal reaction in the pleura and pleural space. The tumor killing noted histologically in the pleural fluid obtained 6 to 24 hours after the first *egc* SE treatment supports this notion [15]. Superantigens are known to induce a population of CD4[+] and CD8[+] effector T cells expressing CD44 and CD62$_{low}$ capable of trafficking to tumor sites and killing tumor cells directly or via release of tumoricidal cytokines and chemokines (Fig. 3) [17,54,73–80].

Physiologically, it is recognized that intrapleurally administered proteins and particles traffic primarily to regional lymphatic lacunae via stoma and foramina in the macula cribriformis and ultimately drain into the parasternal, costal, bronchial, and mediastinal lymph nodes [81]. If *egc* SEs are processed in this fashion, they would activate centrally located effector and migratory T cells [73–75]. These same effector T cells are capable of translocating via the blood into the pleural space [73,75,78], where their cytotoxic effect is exerted on carcinoma cells with or without surface-bound superantigens [82,83]. Likewise, tumoricidal effector cells generated in the mediastinal lymphatics may limit the growth of parenchymal or hilar tumor to account for the stability of lung tumor masses noted in the staphylococcal superantigen–treated cases for a median of 4 months. The absence of neutralizing antibodies against *egc* SEs in most human sera permitted the use of the *egc* SEs as a plurality (SE G, I, M, N, O) and may explain why the

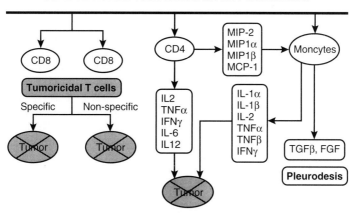

Fig. 3. Multiple mechanisms by which superantigen-activated T cells and monocytes induce tumor killing and pleurodesis are shown. Tumor cells contribute to this effect by expressing costimulants, chemokines, and proinflammatory cytokines constitutively or in response to superantigen-induced cytokines. See text for details.

Box 2. Proposed tumor-killing
mechanisms of *egc* superantigens

- Traffic directly to intercostals, bronchial, and mediastinal lymphatics
- Activate/induce naive and memory
  cytotoxic T cells (CD44$^+$, CD69$_{low}$),
  lymphokine-activated killer cells, and
  natural killer cells
- Induce T cell tumoricidal cytokines,
  IFN-γ, IL-1β, TNF-α, and perforins
- Induce T cell and mononuclear cell
  chemokine chemoattractants
- Induce mononuclear cell transforming growth factor-β and epidermal
  growth factor (pleurodesis)
- Bind to tumor cell superantigen or
  MHCII receptors and induce
  superantigen-dependent cytotoxicity
- Synergize with tumor cell constitutive
  or upregulated costimulants (eg, intercellular adhesion molecule-1)

egc SE family showed antitumor effects with minimal toxicity [15,31]. Box 2 summarizes the proposed tumor-killing mechanisms of the *egc* SE.

SEs also are known to bind to lung carcinoma cells by non-MHCII receptors [84,85] and induce tumor lysis by nonspecific cytotoxic lymphocyte [83,87,88]. In addition, superantigens are capable of costimulating T cells in the presence of constitutively expressed intercellular adhesion molecule-1 on tumor cells [86–89]. Superantigen-induced TNF-α and IFN-γ from T cells and mononuclear cells upregulate intercellular adhesion molecule-1 and other adhesion molecule expression on carcinoma, melanoma, and murine hepatoma cells, which are capable of costimulating T cells in the presence of additional superantigens [90–92]. Finally, SEB is known to induce chemokines, monocyte chemoattractant, and RANTES in tumor cells, which can promote further an inflammatory tumoricidal response [93]. If partial or complete pleurodesis results from intrapleural *egc* SE treatment, it may be a consequence of *egc* SE induction of transforming growth factor-β [94], which is known to induce pleurodesis in sheep [95].

Superantigens and chemotherapy

The initial suggestion that chemotherapy could potentiate or synergize with SEs in producing a tu-

moricidal response occurred in 1980–1981 when a preparation containing SEB and SEA was administered together with cytosine arabinoside to dogs and humans with advanced breast cancer [33,34,60]. Combined treatment resulted in objective tumoricidal responses that exceeded the effects of chemotherapy and SEs given individually [33,59]. More recently, a preparation containing the *egc* superantigens and soluble cisplatin (5 mg) given intratumorally once weekly for 3 weeks to a 67-year-old patient with a peripheral 21cm^2 lung adenocarcinoma mass induced a complete regression of the mass on chest radiograph and CT scan (Ren and Terman, in preparation, 2006). The mechanism underlying the synergy of SEs and chemotherapy may be related to dysfunction of the tumor cell membrane permeability barrier induced by systemic or locally administered *egc* superantigens with consequent passive diffusion of water-soluble cisplatin into tumor cells.

Summary

There has been progress in identifying naturally occurring and producing man-made superantigens that can induce tumor-killing effects in humans without severe toxicity. Recently discovered native *egc* SEs originating from an intact operon of *S aureus*, given as group of five SEs in low doses, intrapleurally induced resolution of pleural effusions and a survival benefit in patients with stage IIIb NSCLC and pleural effusion. The lack of toxicity of these agents makes them promising candidates for use not only against established tumors, but also as vaccines fused to tumor-specific antigens or antigenic groups. Protection against malignant papillomas has been produced in mice and rabbits by vaccination with a fusion gene consisting of an SE and a papilloma viral antigen. Superantigen-transfected tumor cells also have shown promise as a vaccine and against established metastatic tumor, as have superantigen-activated T cells used in adoptive immunotherapy against human glioblastoma multiforme. Several superantigens also have produced a synergy with chemotherapy. Additional clinical trials with more patients with purified recombinant *egc* proteins should shed further light on the mechanisms by which these potent agents induce tumoricidal effects.

References

[1] Chernow B, Sahn SA. Carcinomatous involvement of the pleura. Am J Med 1977;63:695–702.

[2] Sahn SA, Good JT. Pleural fluid pH in malignant effusions. Ann Intern Med 1988;108:345–9.

[3] Walker-Renard PB, Vaughan LM, Sahn SA. Chemical pleurodesis for malignant pleural effusions. Ann Intern Med 1994;120:56–64.

[4] Sahn SA. Malignancy metastatic to the pleura. Clin Chest Med 1998;19:351–61.

[5] Antony V, Loddenkemper R, Astoul P, et al. Management or malignant pleural effusions. Eur Respir J 2001;18:402–19.

[6] Light RW. Pleural diseases. 4th edition. Philadelphia: Lippincott Williams & Wilkins; 2001.

[7] Schrump DS, Nguyen DM. Malignant pleural and pericardial effusions. In: DeVita V, Hellman S, Rosenberg SA, editors. Cancer, principles and practice of oncology. Philadelphia: Lippincott Williams & Wilkins; 2001. p. 2729–44.

[8] Maghfoor I, Doll DC, Yarbro JW. Effusions in clinical oncology. In: Abeloff MD, Armitage JO, Lichter M, Niederhuber JE, editors. Clinical oncology. 2nd edition. New York: Churchill Livingstone; 2000. p. 922–49.

[9] Putnam Jr JB, Walsh GL, Swisher SG, et al. Outpatient management of malignant pleural effusion by chronic indwelling pleural catheter. Ann Thorac Surg 2000; 69:369–75.

[10] Putnam Jr JB, Light RW, Rodriguez RM, et al. A randomized comparison of indwelling pleural catheter and doxycycline pleurodesis in the management of malignant pleural effusions. Cancer 1999;86: 1992–9.

[11] Heffner JE, Nietert PJ, Barbieri C. Pleural fluid pH as predictor of survival for patients with malignant pleural effusions. Chest 2000;117:79–86.

[12] Swanson K, Jett JR, Sahn SA. Lung cancer with malignant pleural effusion: clinical and survival characteristics. Am J Respir Crit Care Med 2002; 165:A149.

[13] Burrows CM, Mathews WC, Colt HG. Predicting survival in patients with recurrent symptomatic malignant pleural effusion, an assessment of the prognostic values of physiologic, morphologic, and quality of life measures and extent of disease. Chest 2000; 117:73–8.

[14] Belani CP, Pajeau TS, Bennet CL. Treating malignant pleural effusions cost consciously. Chest 1998;113: 78S–85S.

[15] Ren S, Terman DS, Bohach G, et al. Intrapleural staphylococcal superantigen induces resolution of malignant pleural effusions and a survival benefit in non-small cell lung cancer. Chest 2004;126:1529–39.

[16] Chu FS, Thadhani K, Schantz EJ, Bergdoll MS. Purification and characterization of staphylococcal enterotoxin A. Biochemistry 1966;5:3281–9.

[17] Marrack P, Kappler J. The staphylococcal enterotoxins and their relatives. Science 1990;248:1066–72.

[18] Bohach GA, Fast DJ, Nelson RD, Schlievert PM. Staphylococcal and streptococcal pyrogenic toxins involved in toxic shock syndrome and related illnesses. Crit Rev Microbiol 1990;17:251–72.

[19] Proft T, Fraser JD. Bacterial superantigens. Clin Exp Immunol 2003;133:299–306.

[20] Papageorgiou AC, Acharya KR. Superantigens as immunomodulators: recent structural insights. Structure 1997;5:991–6.

[21] Kotb M. Superantigens of gram-positive bacteria: structure-function analyses and their implications for biological activity. Curr Opin Microbiol 1998;1:56–65.

[22] Petersson K, Forsberg G, Walse B. Interplay between superantigens and immunoreceptors. Scand J Immunol 2004;59:345–55.

[23] Betley MJ, Mekalanos JJ. Nucleotide sequence of the type A staphylococcal enterotoxin gene. J Bacteriol 1988;170:34–41.

[24] Fraser JD, Urban RG, Strominger JL, Robinson H. Zinc regulates the function of two superantigens. Proc Natl Acad Sci U S A 1992;89:5507–11.

[25] Hopkins PA, Fraser JD, Pridmore AC, et al. Superantigen recognition by HLA class II on monocytes up-regulates toll-like receptor 4 and enhances proinflammatory responses to endotoxin. Blood 2005;105: 3655–62.

[26] Gregory S, Zilber M, Charron D, Gelin C. Human CD1a molecule expressed on monocytes plays an accessory role in the superantigen-induced activation of T lymphocytes. Hum Immunol 2000;61:193–201.

[27] Dohlsten M, Sundstedt A, Bjorklund M, et al. Superantigen-induced cytokines suppress growth of human colon-carcinoma cells. Int J Cancer 1993;54: 482–8.

[27a] Munson SH, Tremaine MT, Betley MJ, et al. Identification and characterization of staphylococcal enterotoxin types G and I from *Staphylococcus aureus*. Infect Immun 1998;66:3337–48.

[28] Jarraud S, Peyrat MA, Lim A, et al. *egc*, a highly prevalent operon of enterotoxin gene, forms a putative nursery of superantigens in *Staphylococcus aureus*. J Immunol 2001;166:669–77.

[29] Becker K, Friedrich AW, Lubritz G, et al. Prevalence of genes encoding pyrogenic toxin superantigens and exfoliative toxins among strains of *Staphylococcus aureus* isolated from blood and nasal specimens. J Clin Microbiol 2003;41:1434–9.

[30] Ferry T, Thomas D, Genestier AL, et al. Comparative prevalence of superantigen genes in *Staphylococcus aureus* isolates causing sepsis with and without septic shock. Clin Infect Dis 2005;41:771–7.

[31] Holtfreter S, Bauer K, Thomas D, et al. *egc*-Encoded superantigens from *Staphylococcus aureus* are neutralized by human sera much less efficiently than are classical staphylococcal enterotoxins or toxic shock syndrome toxin. Infect Immun 2004;72:4061–71.

[32] Terman DS, Yamamoto T, Mattioli M, et al. Extensive necrosis of spontaneous canine mammary adenocarcinoma after extracorporeal perfusion over *Staphylococcus aureus* Cowans I. I. Description of acute tumoricidal response: morphologic, histologic, immunohistochemical, immunologic, and serologic findings. J Immunol 1980;124:795–805.

[33] Terman DS, Yamamoto T, Tillquist RL, et al. Tumoricidal response induced by cytosine arabinoside after plasma perfusion over protein A. Science 1980;209: 1257–9.

[34] Terman DS. Protein A and staphylococcal products in neoplastic disease. Crit Rev Oncol Hematol 1985;4: 103–24.

[35] Terman DS, Bertram JH. Antitumor effects of immobilized protein A and staphylococcal products: linkage between toxicity and efficacy, and identification of potential tumoricidal reagents. Eur J Cancer Clin Oncol 1985;21:1115–22.

[36] Terman DS. Preparation of protein A immobilized on collodion-coated charcoal and plasma perfusion system for treatment of cancer. Methods Enzymol 1988;137:496–515.

[37] Terman DS, Stone JS. Staphylococcal and streptococcal exotoxin (superantigen) induced regression of established tumor in vivo. Proceedings of International Workshop on Superantigens. New York: Cancer Research Institute; 1993. p. 12–4.

[38] Kalland T, Dohlsten M, Lind P, et al. Monoclonal antibodies and superantigen: a novel therapeutic approach. Med Oncol Tumor Pharmacother 1993; 10:37–47.

[39] Penna C, Dean PA, Nelson H. Antitumor X anti-CD3 bifunctional antibodies redirect T-cells activated in vivo with staphylococcal enterotoxin B to neutralize pulmonary metastases. Cancer Res 1994;54: 2738–43.

[40] Newell KA, Ellenhorn JD, Bruce DS, Bluestone JA. In vivo T-cell activation by staphylococcal enterotoxin B prevents outgrowth of a malignant tumor. Proc Natl Acad Sci U S A 1991;88:1074–8.

[41] Dohlsten M, Lando PA, Bjork P, et al. Immunotherapy of human colon cancer by antibody-targeted superantigens. Cancer Immunol Immunother 1995; 41:162–8.

[42] Kominsky SL, Torres BA, Hobeika AC, et al. Superantigen enhanced protection against a weak tumor-specific melanoma antigen: implications for prophylactic vaccination against cancer. Int J Cancer 2001;94: 834–41.

[43] Perabo FG, Willert PL, Wirger A, et al. Superantigen-activated mononuclear cells induce apoptosis in transitional cell carcinoma. Anticancer Res 2005;25: 3565–73.

[44] Pulaski BA, Terman DS, Khan S, et al. Cooperativity of Staphylococcal aureus enterotoxin B superantigen, major histocompatibility complex class II, and CD80 for immunotherapy of advanced spontaneous metastases in a clinically relevant postoperative mouse breast cancer model. Cancer Res 2000;60:2710–5.

[45] Huang C, Yu H, Wang Q, et al. Potent antitumor effect elicited by superantigen-linked tumor cells transduced with heat shock protein 70 gene. Cancer Sci 2004;95:160–7.

[46] Wang Q, Yu H, Zhang L, et al. Potent antitumor effects have been seen with linked tumor cells transduced with heat shock protein 70, IL-18: vaccination with IL-18 gene-modified, superantigen-coated tumor cells elicits potent antitumor immune response. J Cancer Res Clin Oncol 2001;127:718–26.

[47] Ma W, Yu H, Wang Q, et al. A novel approach for cancer immunotherapy: tumor cells with anchored superantigens SEA generate effective antitumor immunity. J Clin Immunol 2004;24:294–301.

[48] Wahlsten JL, Mills CD, Ramakrishnan S. Antitumor response elicited by a superantigen-transmembrane sequence fusion protein anchored onto tumor cells. J Immunol 1998;161:6761–7.

[49] Yi P, Yu H, Ma W, et al. Preparation of murine B7.1-glycosylphosphatidylinositol and transmembrane-anchored staphylococcal enterotoxin: a dual-anchored tumor cell vaccine and its antitumor effect. Cancer 2005;103:1519–28.

[50] Ma W, Yu H, Wang Q, et al. In vitro biological activities of transmembrane superantigen staphylococcal enterotoxin A fusion protein. Cancer Immunol Immunother 2004;53:118–24.

[51] Whang Z, Claden N, Terman DS, et al. Enhancement of DNA vaccine potency by administration of an antigen linked to SEB gene in mouse and rabbit models. International Symposium on Papilloma Viral Infection. Paris, France, October 4, 2002.

[52] Dow SW, Elmslie RE, Willson AP, et al. In vivo tumor transfection with superantigens plus cytokine genes induces tumor regression and prolongs survival in dogs with malignant melanoma. J Clin Invest 1998;101:2406–13.

[53] Thamm DH, Kurzman ID, Macewen EG, et al. Intralesional lipid-complexed cytokine/superantigens immunogene therapy for spontaneous canine tumors. Cancer Immunol Immunother 2003;52:473–80.

[54] Shu S, Krinock RA, Fox BA, et al. Stimulation of tumor-draining lymph node cells with superantigenic staphylococcal toxins leads to the generation of tumor-specific effector T cells. J Immunol 1994;152:1277–88.

[55] Plautz GE, Barnett GH, Miller DW, et al. Systemic T cell adoptive immunotherapy of malignant gliomas. J Neurosurg 1998;89:42–51.

[56] Hansson J, Ohlsson L, Persson R, et al. Genetically engineered superantigens as tolerable antitumor agents. Proc Natl Acad Sci U S A 1997;94:2489–94.

[57] Dohlsten M, Hedlund G, Akerblom E, et al. Monoclonal antibody-targeted superantigens: a different class of anti-tumor agents. Proc Natl Acad Sci U S A 1991;88:9287–91.

[58] Dohlsten M, Abrahmsen L, Bjork P, et al. Monoclonal antibody-superantigens fusion proteins: tumor-specific agents for T-cell-based tumor therapy. Proc Natl Acad Sci U S A 1994;91:8945–9.

[59] Takemura S, Kudo T, Asano R, et al. A mutated superantigen SEA D227A fusion diabody specific to MUC1 and CD3 in targeted cancer immunotherapy for bile duct carcinoma. Cancer Immunol Immunother 2002;51:33–44.

[60] Terman DS, Young JB, Shearer WT, et al. Preliminary observations of the effects on breast adenocarcinoma

of plasma perfused over immobilized protein A. N Engl J Med 1981;305:1195–200.

[61] Young JB, Ayus JC, Miller LK, et al. Cardiopulmonary toxicity in patients with breast carcinoma during plasma perfusion over immobilized protein A: pathophysiology of reaction and attenuating methods. Am J Med 1983;75:278–88.

[62] Finegold MJ. Interstitial pulmonary edema: an electron microscopic study of the pathology of staphylococcal enterotoxemia in Rhesus monkeys. Lab Invest 1967; 16:912–24.

[63] Giantonio BJ, Alpaugh RK, Schultz J, et al. Superantigen-based immunotherapy: a phase I trial of PNU-214565, a monoclonal antibody-staphylococcal enterotoxin A recombinant fusion protein, in advanced pancreatic and colorectal cancer. J Clin Oncol 1997; 15:1994–2007.

[64] Persson B, Persson R, Weiner LM, et al. Overview of clinical trials employing antibody-targeted superantigens. Adv Drug Deliv Rev 1998;31:143–52.

[65] Newton DW, Dohlsten M, Olsson C, et al. Mutations in the MHC class II binding domains of staphylococcal enterotoxin A differentially affect T cell receptor Vbeta specificity. J Immunol 1996;157:3988–94.

[66] Newton DW, Dohlsten M, Lando PA, et al. MHC class II-independent, Vbeta-specific activation of T cells by SAgsmutants fused to anti-tumor Fab fragments: implications for use in treatment of human colon carcinoma. Int J Mol Med 1998;1:157–62.

[67] Alpaugh RK, Schultz J, McAleer C, et al. Superantigen-targeted therapy: phase I escalating repeat dose trial of the fusion protein PNU-214565 in patients with advanced gastrointestinal malignancies. Clin Cancer Res 1998;4:1903–14.

[68] Cheng JD, Babb JS, Langer C, et al. Individualized patient dosing in phase I clinical trials: the role of escalation with overdose control in PNU-214936. J Clin Oncol 2004;22:602–9.

[69] Erlandsson E, Andersson K, Cavallin A, et al. Identification of the antigenic epitopes in staphylococcal enterotoxins A and E and design of a superantigen for human cancer therapy. J Mol Biol 2003; 333:893–905.

[70] Socinski MA, Morris DE, Masters GA, et al. Chemotherapeutic management of stage IV non-small cell lung cancer. Chest 2003;123:226S–43S.

[71] Bunn PA. Chemotherapy for advanced non-small cell lung cancer: who, what, when, why? J Clin Oncol 2002;20:23S–33S.

[72] Sahn SA. Talc should be used for pleurodesis. Am J Respir Crit Care Med 2000;162:2023–4.

[73] DeGrendele HC, Estess P, Siegelman MH. Requirement for CD44 in activated T cell extravasation into an inflammatory site. Science 1997;278:672–4.

[74] DeGrendele HC, Kosfiszer M, Estess P, et al. CD44 activation and associated primary adhesion is inducible via T cell receptor stimulation. J Immunol 1997;159: 2549–53.

[75] Siegleman MH, Stanescu D, Estess P. The CD44-initiated pathway of T cell extravasation uses VLA4 but not LFA-1 for firm adhesion. J Clin Invest 2000; 105:683–90.

[76] Miethke T, Wahl C, Holzmann B, et al. Bacterial superantigens induce rapid and T cell receptor V betaselective down-regulation of L-selectin (gp90Mel-14) in vivo. J Immunol 1993;151:6777–82.

[77] Kagamu H, Shu S. Purification of L-selectin (low) cells promotes the generation of highly potent CD4 antitumor effector T lymphocytes. J Immunol 1998;160: 3444–52.

[78] Von Andrian UH, Mackay CR. T cell function and migration. N Engl J Med 2000;343:1020–33.

[79] Tikhonov I, Moiz K, Wallance M, et al. Staphylococcal superantigens induce lymphotactin production by human CD4 + and CD8 + T-cells. Cytokine 2001;16: 73–8.

[80] Fujisawa N, Hayashi S, Kurdowska A, et al. Staphylococcal enterotoxin A-induced injury of human lung endothelial cells and IL-8 accumulation are mediated by TNFα. J Immunol 1998;161:5627–32.

[81] Miura T, Shimada T, Tanaka K, et al. Lymphatic drainage of carbon particles injected into the pleural cavity of the monkey as studied by video-assisted thoracoscopy and electron microscopy. J Thorac Cardiovasc Surg 2000;120:437–47.

[82] Dohlsten M, Hedlund G, Segren S, et al. Human major histocompatibility complex class II-negative colon carcinoma cells present staphylococcal superantigens to cytotoxic T lymphocytes: evidence for a novel enterotoxin receptor. Eur J Immunol 1991;21:1229–33.

[83] Haffner AC, Zepter K, Elmets CA. Major histocompatibility complex class I molecule serves as a ligand for presentation of the superantigen staphylococcal enterotoxin B to T cells. Proc Natl Acad Sci U S A 1996;93:3037–42.

[84] Lanne B, Jondal M, Karlsson KA. Gal alpha 4Galbinding antibodies: specificity and use for the mapping of glycolipids of Burkitt lymphoma and other human tumors. Glycobiology 1996;6:423–31.

[85] Chatterjee S, Khullar M, Shi WY. Digalactosylceramide is the receptor for staphylococcal enterotoxin-B in human kidney proximal tubular cells. Glycobiology 1995;5:327–33.

[86] Lamphear JG, Stevens KR, Rich RR. Intercellular adhesion molecule-1 and leukocyte function-associated antigen-3 provide costimulation for superantigeninduced T lymphocyte proliferation in the absence of a specific presenting molecule. J Immunol 1998;160: 615–23.

[87] Passlick B, Pantel K, Kubuschok B, et al. Expression of MHC molecules and ICAM-1 on non-small cell lung carcinomas: association with early lymphatic spread of tumour cells. Eur J Cancer 1996;32A:141–5.

[88] Vogetseder W, Feichtinger H, Schulz TF, et al. Expression of 7F7-antigen, a human adhesion molecule identical to intercellular adhesion molecule-1 (ICAM-1) in human carcinomas and their stromal fibroblasts. Int J Cancer 1989;43:768–73.

[89] Tomita Y, Nishiyama T, Watanabe H, et al. Expression of intercellular adhesion molecule-1 (ICAM-1) on renal-cell cancer: possible significance in host immune responses. Int J Cancer 1990;46:1001–6.

[90] Guo YJ, Che XY, Shen F, et al. Effective tumor vaccines generated by in vitro modification of tumor cells with cytokines and bispecific monoclonal antibodies. Nat Med 1997;3:451–5.

[91] Mortarini R, Belli F, Parmiani G, et al. Cytokine-mediated modulation of HLA-class II, ICAM-1, LFA-3 and tumor-associated antigen profile of melanoma cells: comparison with anti-proliferative activity by rIL1-beta, rTNF-alpha, rIFN-gamma, rIL4 and their combinations. Int J Cancer 1990;45:334–41.

[92] Kuppner MC, van Meir E, Hamou MF, et al. Cyto-kine regulation of intercellular adhesion molecule-1 (ICAM-1) expression on human glioblastoma cells. Clin Exp Immunol 1990;81:142–8.

[93] Jedrzkiewicz S, Kataeva G, Hogaboam CM, et al. Superantigen immune stimulation evokes epithelial monocyte chemoattractant protein 1 and RANTES production. Infect Immun 1999;67:6198–202.

[94] Nagelkerken L, Gollob KJ, Tielemans M, et al. Role of transforming growth factor-beta in the preferential induction of T helper cells of type 1 by staphylococcal enterotoxin B. Eur J Immunol 1993;23:2306–10.

[95] Lee YC, Lane KB, Parker RE, et al. Transforming growth factor beta(2) (TGF beta(2)) produces effective pleurodesis in sheep with no systemic complications. Thorax 2000;55:1058–62.

ELSEVIER
SAUNDERS

Clin Chest Med 27 (2006) 335 – 354

CLINICS
IN CHEST
MEDICINE

Management of Malignant Pleural Mesothelioma

Sophie D. West, MBChB, MRCP[a],
Y.C. Gary Lee, MBChB, PhD, FCCP, FRACP[a,b,]*

[a]Oxford Centre for Respiratory Medicine, Churchill Hospital, Oxford, UK
[b]Centre for Respiratory Research, University College London, London, UK

Malignant mesothelioma is an aggressive and universally fatal neoplasm. Mesothelioma is becoming a global epidemic with an exponential increase in incidence in many nations worldwide, owing to the late banning of asbestos use and the latency between asbestos exposure and disease development. Active research in mesothelioma has resulted in a large amount of published data in recent years. Many of the clinical reports were observation studies of early-stage data. Out of a desperate need for effective treatment for mesothelioma, researchers often began employing new approaches based on immature data, resulting in controversies and confusion in management of mesothelioma (eg, use of trimodality therapy). It is heartening to see the completion of more multicenter randomized clinical trials, such as that of pemetrexed—one of the largest clinical trials in pleural disease research. More large-scale clinical trials are under way, and exciting progress is expected in the near future. This article summarizes important advances in the management of mesothelioma, especially diagnostic and therapeutic aspects.

Mesothelioma: a global epidemic

Mesothelioma is characterized by a long latent period between exposure to the causative agent, usually asbestos, and subsequent tumor development:

96% have a latent period of more than 20 years [1]. This latency accounts for the delay in the peak incidence of mesothelioma deaths. The numbers of patients with mesothelioma are continuing to rise, despite the regulation of the use of asbestos in most developed countries since the 1980s.

In Europe, 5000 people die as a result of mesothelioma annually, and this is predicted to increase to 9000 in 2020 [2]. Over the next 3 decades, 250,000 deaths from mesothelioma are expected in Western Europe alone. Although data suggest the US epidemic already has reached its peak, an estimated 2200 deaths from mesothelioma still are expected annually in the United States [3]. Incidence of mesothelioma also has been increasing in many other parts of the world, from Australia and New Zealand to Egypt and Norway, leading to a truly global epidemic [4–8].

Active mining of chrysotile asbestos, although controversial, has continued (eg, in Canada and China), and the global consumption of asbestos is still increasing, especially in Asia and Latin America, often in countries with relatively little regulatory control on hazardous asbestos exposures [9,10]. It is likely that the global incidence of mesothelioma will continue to increase, especially in developing countries.

Etiology

Asbestos exposure

Greater than 80% of patients develop mesothelioma as a result of exposure to asbestos, which is

* Corresponding author. Centre for Respiratory Research, University College London, 5 University Street, London WC1E 6JJ, UK.
   E-mail address: ycgarylee@hotmail.com (Y.C.G. Lee).

usually occupational. Since the first report in 1960 from South Africa, numerous epidemiologic studies have confirmed the link between mesothelioma and asbestos exposure, and this knowledge has led to a ban in asbestos use in many countries [11]. Risk of mesothelioma is related to the duration and intensity of the exposure to asbestos (and the type of asbestos), with higher levels being associated with higher risk. No threshold of exposure is considered safe, however.

Asbestos is the commercial name for a hydrated magnesium silicate fiber, which is composed of two types: the serpentine and the amphibole [12]. Individuals involved in mining or processing asbestos were at high risks of asbestos-related diseases, including mesothelioma. Asbestos is a relatively cheap and effective insulation material and was used extensively in construction, manufacturing (eg, car brakes), and shipbuilding. Many of the patients presenting with mesothelioma today are "end-users" of asbestos products (eg, plumbers, builders). It is well recognized that the partners and children of asbestos workers have an increased risk of mesothelioma because they have been exposed to asbestos fibers on the clothes of the worker, typically during clothes washing. Most patients with mesothelioma are men, reflecting the demographics of the at-risk workforce, and most present in their 40s to 60s because of the latency between work exposure and disease onset.

Exactly how inhaled asbestos fibers reach the pleural surface is unknown. It traditionally is believed that inhaled fibers deposit in peripheral lung tissue, followed by translocation from the visceral pleura to the parietal membrane [13]. Other mechanisms of migration (eg, retrograde flow of fibers to the parietal lymphatics) have been proposed, but none have been proven.

The ability of asbestos to provoke carcinogenesis is related to its physical more than its chemical properties. Fibers of the amphibole type, which include crocidolite (blue asbestos), amosite (brown asbestos), anthophyllite, tremolite, and actinolite, are straight, long, and needle-shaped. They are eliminated slowly from the lungs, with a half-life of more than 7 years [14]. Crocidolite, mainly mined and exported from South Africa and Western Australia in the past, is the most potent subtype of fiber to induce mesothelioma.

Serpentine fibers, such as chrysotile (white asbestos), are pliable and curly and are cleared more rapidly from the lung because of their higher solubility and propensity to fragment [15]. Chrysotile accounts for greater than 90% of the global consumption of asbestos at present. Although not universally accepted, there is strong evidence that chrysotile

exposure is associated with development of mesothelioma in a dose-dependent manner, although the association is not as strong as that with amphiboles [16,17].

It is unclear whether asbestos fibers provoke neoplastic mesothelial changes by direct insult to the pleura or indirectly via mediators released from the lungs [18,19]. Contact between asbestos fibers and mesothelial cells is followed by a phagocytic process, with engulfment, fiber internalization, and degranulation of lysosymes in the phagocytic vacuole [20]. In vitro studies show that asbestos fibers exert cytotoxic and genotoxic effects, including DNA damage from reactive oxygen species possibly generated during the phagocytic process or by the oxido-reduction reactions at the surface of the fibers [21]. The current views on pathogenesis of mesothelioma have been summarized elsewhere [22].

Other exposures

Erionite, a naturally occurring nonasbestos zeolite mainly found in Turkey, can induce a similar spectrum of pleuropulmonary diseases. Erionite frequently is used as a building material in those regions and is as potent as crocidolite in inducing mesothelioma. Prior exposure to a radiologic contrast material, thorium dioxide (Thorotrast), also has been shown as a rare cause of mesothelioma. There is, however, no convincing evidence to link prior thoracic irradiation (eg, for Hodgkin's lymphoma) with subsequent mesothelioma. Smoking, although common in the workforce in asbestos-related industries, is not a risk factor for mesothelioma [23].

Genetic factors

Genetic susceptibility has been investigated to explain why some individuals exposed to asbestos develop mesothelioma and why some do not, even after adjustment for fiber exposure [24]. Observations in the village of Karain in Turkey have shown clusters of mesothelioma in families, where houses were built with erionite. In nearby villages, despite the fact the houses also were built with erionite, this clustering was not present. Familial clusters of mesotheliomas and a suggestion of an autosomal dominant pattern of inheritance was raised, although it remains unclear whether this reflects a genuine genetic predisposition or a result of shared environmental exposure [25].

Knowledge of the patterns of gene expression in mesothelioma is increasing with the use of global gene profiling technology. Transcriptional profiling from microarray experiments has revealed data that may help to differentiate mesothelioma from adenocarcinoma of the lung and may help predict treatment-related outcome in mesothelioma, by analyzing the expression of a selected panel of genes. Microarray studies also have revealed novel genes (eg, *Fra-1*) that are differentially regulated in mesothelioma. These genes potentially may enhance knowledge of the pathogenesis of mesothelioma and may present new diagnostic or therapeutic targets in the future [26–30]. The use of proteomics also has been applied to mesothelioma research and may enhance understanding of the disease mechanism further [31].

Controversy on simian virus 40

A potent DNA oncogenic virus, simian virus 40 (SV40), can induce pleural, peritoneal, and pericardial mesotheliomas when directly inoculated in experimental animals. This discovery led to the hypothesis that SV40 may be a direct causative factor, or a cofactor, in the development of mesothelioma. In many early studies, SV40 was reported as being present in human mesothelioma tissues, although there were conflicting reports. Data from two well-designed studies suggest, however, that previously published detection of SV40 in malignant mesothelioma tissue is the result of laboratory contamination, rather than genuine viral infection of the human tissue [32,33]. These studies showed that the polymerase chain reaction primers used to detect SV40 in many studies were targeting sequences within the SV40 genome that also are present in commonly used laboratory plasmids, leading to false-positive detection of SV40 detected in mesothelioma samples. Carefully designed laboratory experiments have confirmed that SV40 T antigen DNA was not present in any of the mesothelioma samples of a large cohort of 71 subjects [32]. Epidemiologic evidence also does not support a relationship between SV40 exposure (eg, via contaminated polio vaccines) and subsequent mesothelioma development. These laboratory and epidemiologic studies have seriously questioned the role (if any) of SV40 in the etiology of mesothelioma.

Pathology

The mesothelium consists of a monolayer of mesothelial cells, supported by submesothelial connective tissue [22]. In situ mesothelioma cells are 1 to 4 μm thick and are usually polygonal with a flattened appearance. There are tight gap junctions and des-

mosomes between mesothelial cells, and the cells seem to be able to synthesize and secrete inflammatory mediators and cytokines in response to stimuli. These are likely to have a key role in the modulation of inflammation in response to cell injury [34]. Mesothelioma results from the neoplastic transformation of mesothelial cells, associated with phenotypic modifications and genetic changes altering the cell-cell and cell-matrix interactions and regulation of cell proliferation and cell death. A proportion of pleural mesothelioma seems to develop through a preliminary mesothelioma in situ phase, with subsequent development of multiple small foci of invasive mesothelioma followed by diffuse spread along the pleura, with encasement of the underlying lung (Fig. 1) [35–37]. Mesothelioma spreads along the pleural surface in a "sheetlike" fashion and infiltrates underlying structures, such as the lung, mediastinum, contralateral lung, and chest wall, and later in the course of the disease, infiltrates the peritoneum. Macroscopically, round, gray, flat macules or nodules may be seen [38]. The gross appearance may be indistinguishable from pleural metastatic carcinoma. These tiny tumor foci coalesce to form larger nodules, which usually thicken and fuse the parietal and visceral pleurae, forming the characteristic rind that constricts the lung.

Asymptomatic spread to regional lymph nodes often occurs and was noted in 40% of patients undergoing extrapleural pneumonectomy with early Butchart stage I disease [39]. The proportion of patients with lymph node involvement in the setting

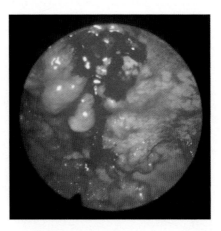

Fig. 1. Thoracoscopic view of the parietal pleura of a patient with malignant mesothelioma. (Courtesy of Dr. R.J.O. Davies, University of Oxford, United Kingdom. *From* Lee YC, Light RW. Management of malignant pleural effusions. Respirology 2004;9:150; with permission.)

of more extensive later stage disease is likely to be much higher. Lymph node involvement is an adverse prognostic factor.

Late distant metastases are a feature of mesothelioma, with 50% to 67% of patients having evidence of distant spread at autopsy [40,41], although most are unlikely to be clinically relevant in the context of advanced mesothelioma. Metastasis outside the ipsilateral hemithorax is common in patients who have had aggressive surgical resection and local irradiation [42].

Histologically, 60% of mesotheliomas are epithelioid in type, 10% are sarcomatoid, and the remainder are biphasic (ie, with epithelioid and sarcomatoid phenotypes) (Figs. 2 and 3) [43]. The modifications that cause the different subtypes to form are unknown. Histologic recognition of sarcomatoid mesothelioma can be more difficult than with epithelioid types. Epithelioid mesothelioma is associated with a significantly better survival, whereas sarcomatoid disease has the worst prognosis [15]. One series showed a median survival of 14 to 15 months for epithelioid type and 7 months for sarcomatoid type [44]. Rare histologic variants (eg, desmoplastic mesothelioma, deciduoid mesothelioma) can occur and can be difficult to diagnose [45].

Clinical picture

Mesothelioma symptoms are often insidious and nonspecific, which can lead to delay in presentation and in diagnosis. The mean time between symptom onset and diagnosis is 2 to 3 months, but 25% of patients may present more than 6 months after the onset of symptoms [46].

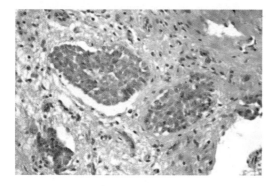

Fig. 2. Histology from a pleural biopsy specimen of a patient shows epithelioid mesothelioma.

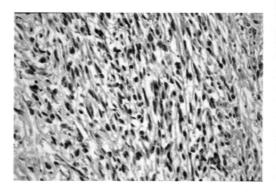

Fig. 3. Histology from a gastric biopsy specimen of the same patient in Fig. 2, 4 years later, shows a different histologic picture: that of sarcomatoid mesothelioma. (Courtesy of Dr. Colin Clelland, Oxford Radcliffe Hospital, United Kingdom. *From* Int Pleural Newsl 2003;2:7; with permission.)

Pleural mesothelioma

Greater than 90% of mesotheliomas are pleural in origin [47]. The most common symptoms a patient with pleural mesothelioma presents with are dyspnea, especially on exertion, and nonpleuritic chest pain. Chest pain is associated with a worse prognosis, probably secondary to the malignant infiltration of underlying tissue. Mesothelioma should be suspected in any person with an unexplained exudative pleural effusion, with or without radiologic signs of asbestos exposure. Patients may have a cough (10%), weight loss (30%), or fatigue [48]. Weight loss often becomes prominent with advanced disease. Examination often reveals only the signs of a pleural effusion.

Occasionally, patients present with symptoms or signs from involvement of other (mainly intrathoracic) structures, such as dysphagia, Horner's syndrome, spinal cord compression, superior vena cava obstruction, or pericardial effusions. Distant metastases (eg, cerebral involvement) have been reported, but are rare in initial presentation [48].

Peritoneal mesothelioma

Peritoneal mesothelioma accounts for about 7% of mesotheliomas [47]. It usually is related to heavy asbestos exposure, particularly to amphiboles (eg, amosite), with the latent period between exposure and mesothelioma being shorter than in pleural mesothelioma. It is postulated that swallowed asbestos fibers lead to development of peritoneal mesothelioma. Median survival figures are worse than for pleural mesothelioma (6 months versus 9 months) [48]. The incidence of peritoneal mesothelioma is becoming rarer because many patients with it have died. It tends to present with nonspecific abdominal symptoms, abdominal swelling, possible abdominal mass, fever, and ascites. Irregular or nodular peritoneal thickening is seen on CT, although CT findings are often nonspecific. There may be signs of asbestos exposure on radiologic examination of the thorax. A peritoneal biopsy is required for accurate diagnosis, although peritoneal fluid cytology may be diagnostic. An aggressive approach of local tumor excision, intraoperative peritoneal chemotherapy, and postoperative chemotherapy in one unselected uncontrolled study resulted in a median survival of 67 months [49].

Pericardial mesothelioma

There are about 150 cases of pericardial mesotheliomas reported in the literature. The diagnoses often were missed until surgery or autopsy [50]. Most often, the tumor invades the myocardium or the great vessels, and pericardial effusions with tamponade are common. Knowledge on its best management is limited [51]. Drainage of the pericardial effusion is important to relieve cardiac constriction. The roles of surgery and chemotherapy are not known.

Mesothelioma of tunica vaginalis testis

Mesothelioma of the tunica vaginalis of the testis is rare, with less than 100 cases reported [52]. It can occur at any age, with a median age of 60. There is an association with asbestos exposure in one third of men. The tumors are usually epithelioid, but also can be biphasic in type. The clinical picture is one of insidious scrotal enlargement, with local invasion including local lymph node spread being common. Ultrasound may be helpful in the investigation, but many cases are not diagnosed until surgery. Radical orchidectomy is recommended, and radiotherapy and chemotherapy have been attempted. Recurrence, usually associated with metastases, is common within 2 years of surgery. The median survival is 23 months.

Prognosis

The prognosis of mesothelioma is poor, with an untreated median survival of approximately 9 months, although figures vary depending on the patient's selection group and how survival is calculated. A small proportion of mesothelioma patients follow a more indolent course, and prolonged survival (eg, >10 years), although rare, has been reported [53]. The Cancer and Leukemia Group B prognostic index

identified poor performance status, age (>75 years old), chest pain, nonepithelioid histology, elevated serum lactate dehydrogenase, and elevated platelet counts as adverse prognostic indicators [54,55]; this was validated in a separate cohort [56]. The European Organization for Research and Treatment of Cancer identified similar prognostic markers [57]. Better performance status, early-stage disease, younger age, less than 5% weight loss, absence of chest pain, and shorter duration of symptoms before diagnosis all are associated with better prognosis in other studies [58–60]. Good performance status is probably at least as important prognostically as histologic subtype [61]. Epithelioid mesothelioma has a better prognosis than biphasic mesothelioma, which is better than sarcomatoid subtype. Patients with disease limited to the parietal pleura at thoracoscopy and patients with no macroscopic disease also have a better prognosis than patients with visceral involvement [62].

Diagnosis

Definitive diagnosis of malignant mesothelioma is made histologically or cytologically. Although radiology is helpful, diagnosis based on clinical picture or radiology alone is inadequate.

Pleural aspiration

Pleural fluid alone may give a cytologic diagnosis, but this depends on the experience of the cytologists, and the yield can be low (35–50%) [63]. Mesothelioma is not excluded even when fluid cytology is negative.

Pleural biopsy

Tissue samples for histology are obtained by sampling an area of affected pleura. To allow electron microscope examination, some of the biopsy tissue should be collected in gluteraldehyde preservative. An experienced pathologist is needed to distinguish mesothelioma from reactive mesothelial cells and other neoplastic conditions, particularly adenocarcinoma [64]. Blind pleural biopsies may not achieve a tissue diagnosis because of small sample size or sampling error, where the affected pleura is missed. Blind biopsies have been reported to yield a diagnosis in 39% to 60% [65]. Using contrast-enhanced CT, areas of abnormal pleural thickening can be identified better, and biopsy specimens can be obtained under image guidance. A randomized study confirmed a significantly higher diagnostic sensitivity for pleural malignancy with CT-guided biopsy than with blind (Abrams needle) pleural biopsy in the investigation of malignant pleural effusions (87% versus 47%) [66].

Alternatively, tissue samples can be obtained via thoracoscopy with a diagnostic sensitivity of 98% [62]. Medical thoracoscopy has been found to be as reliable as surgical thoracotomy to achieve diagnosis and pleurodesis. Pleurodesis also can be performed at the time of thoracoscopy if the diagnosis is confirmed (especially if an on-site pathologist is present to confirm the diagnosis).

Patients with pleural effusions requiring drainage and pleurodesis are probably best managed with a thoracoscopy; patients with pleural abnormalities but minimal pleural fluid are best managed with a CT-guided biopsy. Because there can be malignant seeding of tract sites in mesothelioma, it is best to avoid repeated diagnostic procedures and instead opt for the procedure most likely to give the tissue diagnosis. If several procedures are performed, ideally they all should be performed in the same area of the chest so that a radiotherapy field can encompass them all. Sites of previous procedures, particularly procedures performed with a small needle that leaves no scar, should be tattooed with India ink so that it can be ensured that all sites are treated with radiotherapy, to avoid tract metastasis.

Immunohistochemistry

The tissue diagnosis of mesothelioma is not straightforward. Morphologic examination is not reliable enough, and the definitive diagnosis often relies on immunohistochemistry. Differentiation of mesothelioma from reactive or normal mesothelia is not always easy; separating mesothelioma from metastatic carcinomas also can be troublesome. Numerous immunohistochemical markers have been tested, and no single molecule has adequate sensitivity and specificity to act as a solo marker. As a result, most laboratories rely on a panel of markers to separate benign mesothelial cells from malignant mesotheliomas and to distinguish the latter from carcinomas. The pros and cons of different panels of markers have been described elsewhere [67,68].

Blood markers of mesothelioma

In the United States alone, an estimated 8 million people have been exposed to asbestos and are potentially at risk of mesothelioma. As yet, no specific tumor markers have been identified to predict me-

sothelioma development in exposed individuals, and no serum markers are available to diagnose or follow the disease progress in mesothelioma.

The recent description of soluble mesothelin-related (SMR) proteins has attracted significant interest. SMR proteins, when assayed in patients with mesothelioma ($n = 48$), controls, and patients with other inflammatory or malignant lung and pleural diseases, showed a sensitivity of 83% and a specificity of 95% for mesothelioma [69]. Levels were significantly higher in patients with a higher tumor load (maximum tumor width >3 cm). The mesothelin gene encodes a precursor protein that is processed to yield the 40-kd protein, mesothelin. The biologic function of mesothelin is largely unknown, but its potential role as a therapeutic target in mesothelioma is being explored [70]. In the study by Robinson et al [69], four asbestos-exposed subjects with increased SMR levels without mesothelioma went on to develop mesothelioma or non–small cell lung cancer within the 5-year follow-up period, raising hope that SMR might be a predictor of disease development or a sensitive marker of early disease in some patients.

SMR proteins show promise as a diagnostic tool and are commercially available, but full clinical evaluation is awaited. Mesothelin is expressed by other tumors (eg, pancreatic and ovarian carcinomas), and its specificity as a marker for malignant mesothelioma may be lower than initially believed. The availability of a first blood test for mesothelioma is an exciting step, however, toward better methods of diagnosing mesothelioma and predicting disease development in at-risk populations. Osteopontin has also been studied as a serum marker: its levels were elevated in mesothelioma patients over control subjects. However, the ability of osteopontin to separate mesothelioma from metastatic carcinomas has not been evaluated [71].

Chest radiograph

Chest radiograph may show signs of pleural thickening, nodularity, and pleural effusion. Twenty percent of patients have signs of other radiologic evidence of asbestos exposure on chest radiograph, such as pleural plaques or interstitial fibrosis [72]. The absence of concurrent asbestos pleuropulmonary diseases on the radiograph (or CT scan) does not exclude mesothelioma.

Contrast-enhanced computed tomography

CT can be useful for diagnosis and assessment of tumor extent and progress. In one series, CT showed

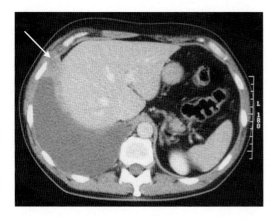

Fig. 4. Contrast-enhanced CT scan shows a right-sided pleural effusion and chest wall invasion by mesothelioma (*arrow*).

pleural thickening in 94% of patients, with a pleural effusion in 76% [73]. The pleural thickening may encase a portion of the lung [74]. It may be difficult to differentiate thin pleural tumor from pleural fluid, and CT cannot reliably differentiate mesothelioma from metastatic pleural malignancies [75,76]. CT is useful for assessing disease involvement of the chest wall or extension into neighboring structures, such as superior vena cava and spinal cord (Fig. 4).

CT commonly is used to measure tumor response in clinical trials. The validated, modified response evaluation in solid tumor criteria (RECIST) use unidimensional measurement of tumor thickness perpendicular to the mediastinum or chest wall, at two sites on three different levels on CT scan [77]. Transverse cuts used for measurement are at least 1 cm apart and related to anatomic landmarks in the thorax, preferably above the level of division of the main bronchi. Other lesions (eg, nodes and subcutaneous nodules) also are measured unidimensionally. The sum of these measurements is used to quantify tumor load and can be monitored at designated follow-up points. Partial response is defined as 30% or greater reduction of the sum, whereas 20% or greater increase defines disease progression [78].

Magnetic resonance imaging

MRI probably should be used for specific problem-solving issues in selected cases, particularly if surgery is being considered. T2-weighted images without fat suppression show fluid with increased signal intensity (white) compared with tumor with lower signal intensity (gray). There is a higher sensitivity for detecting fluid and tumor, which can be helpful in early-stage disease [79]. Similar to CT,

MRI is unable to distinguish mesothelioma from metastatic carcinomas reliably. Contrast-enhanced T1-weighted images are reliable for showing active enhancement of the tissues, particularly delineating tumor from normal tissues. CT and MRI achieve similar accuracies in staging most categories in the International Mesothelioma Interest Group staging system [80]. MRI is superior at assessing involvement of endothoracic fascia, chest wall, and diaphragmatic muscle, although demonstration of such involvement generally would not alter management.

MRI also can provide a more accurate assessment than CT of apical and diaphragmatic regions as a result of the additional coronal and sagittal images and mediastinal, chest wall, and spinal cord involvement [81]. MRI performed with different pulse sequences and gadolinium-based contrast material can improve the detection of tumor extension (eg, to the chest wall and diaphragm) [82]. Lymph node staging is difficult to assess accurately by CT and MRI because of low sensitivity and specificity [79].

Positron emission tomography

Positron emission tomography (PET) is used in the investigation of lung cancer to assess malignant involvement of mediastinal nodes and the presence of distant metastases. A few studies have investigated the role of PET in the staging of malignant mesothelioma. These studies indicate two roles for PET: One is the detection of extrathoracic disease and nodal disease in close proximity to the tumor, although the data on the efficacy of this are limited; the other is the correlation of tumors that have a high uptake of fluorodeoxyglucose giving high standard uptake values (SUV) with survival [83–85]. There is a near-linear correlation between increasing tumor SUV with poor survival. A steep dropoff in survival was seen with SUVs of 4 and greater. The median survival of patients with lesions with SUV of 4 and greater was 14 months compared with 24 months in patients with lesions with SUV of less than 4. Patients with epithelioid histology and low SUV had the best prognosis, whereas patients with high SUVs and nonepithelioid tumor histology had the worst prognosis. A high SUV in the primary tumor is more likely to be associated with mediastinal nodal metastases. Integrated PET/CT scanning may provide more precise morphologic and functional information to improve T and N staging and to provide information regarding tumor response to treatment more accurately than PET or CT alone [86]. The role of PET or PET/CT in routine clinical management of mesothelioma is limited at present.

Staging

Staging of mesothelioma is not easy to perform, and it is not justified or necessary in everyday clinical practice. Staging should be performed only if the patient is enrolled in clinical trials to categorize patients and to measure responses to treatment [48]. The necessary staging procedures should be governed by the study protocol.

Several staging classifications for mesothelioma have been suggested. The first, the Butchart classification, was devised in 1976, based on the experience of pleuropneumonectomy in 29 patients, with a correlation made between tumor stage, histologic type, and prognosis (Table 1) [87]. Survival was higher in patients with epithelial mesothelioma and with stage I tumors; significantly more patients with epithelial tumors survived 1 year or more ($P < .05$). This staging system has been widely used. Other investigators have noted there is a range of survival in patients with stage I disease, depending on the extent of their parietal pleural involvement [88]. These authors suggested dividing Butchart stage I patients into two subgroups: IA, in which only the parietal or diaphragmatic pleura is involved, and stage IB, in which the visceral pleura is invaded. Patients with IA stage at diagnosis have a better prognosis than patients with IB.

The International Mesothelioma Interest Group (IMIG) proposed another staging system, as did the Union Internationale Contre Cancer (UICC) [89]. These systems are tumor-nodal-metastasis (TNM) based. The UICC staging system is simpler, but not as widely used as the Butchart or IMIG systems. The IMIG staging system was developed at a consensus meeting of IMIG members involved in mesothelioma

Table 1
Clinicopathologic staging of diffuse malignant mesothelioma

Stage	Clinicopathologic staging
I	Tumor confined to homolateral pleura, lung and pericardium
II	Tumor invading chest wall or invading mediastinal structures, eg, esophagus, heart, opposite pleura
	Lymph node involvement within chest
III	Tumor penetrating diaphragm to involve peritoneum directly
	Lymph node involvement outside chest
IV	Distant bloodborne metastases

Data from Butchart EG, Ashcroft T, Barnsley WC, et al. Pleuropneumonectomy in the management of diffuse malignant mesothelioma of the pleura: experience with 29 patients. Thorax 1976;31:15–24.

research in 1994, based on surgical and pathologic findings (Table 2). It has tried to stage mesothelioma more precisely, building on previous staging systems and incorporating specific TNM descriptors. The T variable is imprecise, however, owing to the nature of mesothelioma, which invades beyond the limits of presumed tumor boundaries. It has been argued that this system is not refined enough for the increasing treatment options for mesothelioma, including chemotherapy and multimodality therapies, but no other consensus staging classification has been determined [90].

Treatment

To date, there is no cure for mesothelioma. Malignant mesothelioma is difficult to treat and different from other malignant tumors for several reasons. It spreads along the serosal surface and infiltrates the underlying vital structures early, so surgery is unable to eradicate the tumor. It often arises from multiple sites on the parietal pleura and involves the visceral pleura early. Patients tend to present late in the clinical course because the symptoms are nonspecific and of gradual onset. Patients are frequently older with associated comorbid conditions. Effective management for this incurable malignancy should aim to improve quality of life and prolong survival. Treatment needs to encompass the control of local disease and systemic spread.

Active symptom control and best supportive care

A multidisciplinary team approach involving professionals experienced in the care of mesothelioma patients is recommended because the clinical course of mesothelioma differs from other solitary tumors. The team should comprise chest physicians, palliative care specialists, nurses, social workers, dietitians, and psychologists working with the patient and family [48]. Age, comorbid disease, and poor performance status may prevent aggressive therapeutic options. Best supportive care aims to provide the maximum symptom relief with minimal adverse effects, preferably within the home. Patients may want to pursue legal claims for compensation—often a lengthy and stressful process—and may require appropriate legal guidance.

Analgesia
Most patients with mesothelioma eventually experience pain and dyspnea. Adequate analgesia is essential, to maintain pain control with minimal side

Table 2
International Mesothelioma Interest Group staging for mesothelioma

T1a	Tumor limited to ipsilateral parietal pleura, including mediastinal and diaphragmatic pleura
	No involvement of the visceral pleura
T1b	Tumor involving ipsilateral parietal pleura, including mediastinal and diaphragmatic pleura
	Scattered foci of tumor also involving the visceral pleura
T2	Tumor involving each of the ipsilateral pleural surfaces, with at least one of the following features:
	Involvement of diaphragm muscle
	Confluent visceral pleural tumor (including the fissures) or extension of tumor from the visceral pleura into the underlying pulmonary parenchyma
T3	Describes locally advanced but potentially resectable tumor
	Tumor involving all of the ipsilateral pleural surfaces, with at least one of the following features:
	Involvement of the endothoracic fascia
	Extension into mediastinal fat
	Solitary, completely resectable focus of tumor extending into the soft tissues of the chest wall
	Nontransmural involvement of the pericardium
T4	Describes locally advanced technically unresectable tumor
	Tumor involving all of the ipsilateral pleural surfaces with at least one of the following features:
	Diffuse extension or multifocal masses of tumor in the chest wall, with or without associated rib destruction
	Direct transdiaphragmatic extension of the tumor to the peritoneum
	Direct extension of tumor to the contralateral pleura
	Direct extension of tumor to one or more mediastinal organs
	Direct extension of tumor into the spine
	Tumor extending through to the internal surface of the pericardium with or without a pericardial effusion or tumor involving the myocardium
Nx	Regional lymph nodes cannot be assessed
N0	No regional lymph node metastases
N1	Metastases in the ipsilateral bronchopulmonary or hilar lymph nodes
N2	Metastases in the subcarinal or the ipsilateral mediastinal lymph nodes, including the ipsilateral internal mammary nodes
N3	Metastases in the contralateral mediastinal, contralateral internal mammary, ipsilateral or contralateral supraclavicular lymph nodes
Mx	Presence of distant metastases cannot be assessed
M0	No distant metastases
M1	Distant metastases present

effects. The standard World Health Organization analgesic ladder is often ineffective in patients with mesothelioma, and the early use of opioids often is required [91]. Neuropathic pain is best treated with anticonvulsants. Radiotherapy is a good treatment for localized pain (eg, from bone erosion) and needle tract metastases. It can be used to palliate symptoms arising from extrinsic compression or direct tumor invasion of the esophagus, superior vena cava, and spinal cord.

Indwelling epidural catheters have been used in patients with chest wall pain because of rib erosion by mesothelioma. The catheters are tunneled to a medication port under the skin on the contralateral rib cage. This is a method by which long-lasting analgesia may be given, with tolerable side effects [92].

Spinal cordectomy has been found to be an effective therapy for some patients with intractable chest wall pain. Percutaneous cervical cordotomy is performed, interrupting the spinothalamic tract at the C1-2 level [93,94]. This procedure causes contralateral loss of pain sensation. There is a low complication rate, with mild dysesthesia and mild weakness reported in a few patients. No gait or sphincter disturbance and no deterioration in respiratory control have been reported [95]. In one series, pain was reduced significantly in 83% to the extent that more than one third of the patients were able to discontinue opiate analgesia [93]. This is a highly skilled procedure and must be performed in the limited centers with expertise in the technique.

Pleurodesis

Greater than 95% of patients with mesothelioma develop a pleural effusion, often associated with symptomatic dyspnea [96]. Pleurodesis is an effective way of preventing the fluid reaccumulation, and this should be performed early in the disease course. Pleurodesis can be performed chemically by instillation of the agent via a chest tube or thoracoscopically (medical thoracoscopy or video-assisted thoracoscopic surgery). Common pleurodesing agents include talc, bleomycin, tetracycline, and doxycycline. Talc is the most commonly used agent, although its pros and cons are debated [97]. Pleurodesis with talc offers a greater efficacy than placebo or other sclerosant, and if this can be performed as part of thoracoscopy, the diagnostic and therapeutic procedure can be combined [98]. In a large randomized trial, talc pleurodesis by slurry was as effective as thoracoscopic poudrage for malignant pleural effusions [99].

Pleurodesis is unlikely to be successful when trapped lung develops [100]. This condition occurs when tumor encasement of the visceral pleura prevents lung re-expansion, prohibiting opposition of the pleural surfaces and pleural adhesion after inflammation. As malignant mesothelioma grows along the visceral pleura, trapped lung becomes more common as the disease advances. In these situations, an indwelling tunneled pleural catheter may be useful for ambulatory drainage of the pleural space when the patient is symptomatic [101]. Metastatic spread along the catheter tract is a rare but potential complication.

Radiotherapy

Palliative radiotherapy

Radiotherapy has an established role in symptom palliation [102–104]. Mesothelioma cells are relatively sensitive to radiotherapy, but the radiotherapy dose that can be given to attempt cure is limited, owing to the large target volume of the affected pleural surface, with toxic effects likely on the adjacent lung, heart, mediastinum, spinal cord, and liver with large radiation doses. The effect of radiotherapy alone on prolonging survival in mesothelioma is minimal, with response rates of 3% reported, with significant mortality and morbidity. More recently published work indicates that the technique of inverse planned stereotactic intensity modulated radiotherapy may have a role in the palliative treatment of mesothelioma [105]. This technique involves computer three-dimensional visualization of the dose distribution area; the treatment field of any beam direction is divided into subfields with different intensity levels. The combination of the subfields allows a homogeneous dose distribution in the target volume, and the normal surrounding tissue is protected more accurately. Field sizes of 20 × 27 cm were treated in 11 patients, with a total radiation dose of 40 to 50 Gy; this size included the tumor macroscopic volume and lymph nodes. Although skin reactions were seen, no lung toxicity was reported. This approach needs further evaluation, but may be beneficial particularly in patients with a small tumor load.

Prophylaxis against needle tract metastases

Because mesothelioma is characterized by direct local invasion, it often invades the tracts after pleural puncture, such as after pleural aspiration, biopsy, thoracostomy, and thoracoscopy (Fig. 5). Prophylactic radiotherapy has been found to be effective at preventing malignant seeding at these sites in two studies. In a randomized controlled trial of 40 patients, 40% in the control group developed needle tract spread, whereas none in the radiotherapy group did [106]. Radiotherapy was administered as 21 Gy in three fractions over 48 hours, 10 to 12 days after the procedures. A delay in radiotherapy of more than 2 months was found to be associated with increased

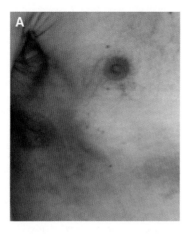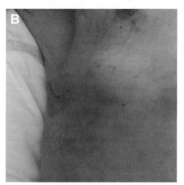

Fig. 5. (*A* and *B*) Photographs of a patient with mesothelioma with area of skin pigmentation in the axilla, from prophylactic radiotherapy, and a tract site metastasis on the anterior chest wall, anterior to the radiotherapy field.

chest wall recurrence in a nonrandomized study [107]. A study sought to establish whether single-fraction lower dose radiotherapy of 10 Gy was as effective at preventing procedure tract metastases in patients with mesothelioma [108]. Patients were randomized to no radiotherapy or low-dose, single-fraction radiotherapy given within 15 days of the chest procedure. There was no significant difference in the incidence of tract metastases between the two groups (metastasis rate 10% in the no radiotherapy group and 7% in the radiotherapy group; $P = .53$). Prophylactic radiotherapy using the 3-day protocol is recommended for all patients with mesothelioma after any pleural procedure.

Chemotherapy

Mesothelioma generally has been thought to be unresponsive to chemotherapy with most of the common anticancer drugs. Although response rates previously were observed in numerous phase II clinical trials, only pemetrexed and raltitrexed (see below) have been shown to improve survival. Chemotherapy results are disappointing because mesothelioma is relatively resistant to common chemotherapeutic agents, and delivery of adequate concentrations of drugs to the pleural tumor and the underlying tissue is often difficult. The objective response rate, with single-agent or combination chemotherapy, has rarely exceeded 40%. Treatment successes in the context of clinical trials can be measured in terms of survival, quality of life, or radiologic response, or often a combination of all three. Radiologic response now is based on the modified RECIST (response evaluation in solid tumors) criteria, which were adapted for mesothelioma and have been validated [77]. These criteria are applicable only to tumors that are radiologically measurable. There are limitations to radiologic staging of response because many patients may have disease in which measurement is not possible. Response is harder to measure in patients who have had pleurodesis because the pleural fibrosis can be difficult to differentiate from disease progression. In addition, radiologic responses do not necessarily translate into survival benefits.

Intrapleural chemotherapy

Intrapleural chemotherapy is the technique of administering chemotherapy to the pleural space via a chest tube, to provide maximum local effect and minimal systemic toxicity. Cisplatin administered into the pleural space was found to give higher peak levels and greater total exposure than intravenous cisplatin [109]. A study looking at clinical response to this form of treatment found, however, minimal objective tumor response [110]. This low response was postulated to be due to advanced disease with probable shallow penetration of the tumor and pleura. Attempts also have been made using hyperthermic intrapleural chemotherapy, such as intrapleural instillation of cisplatin and doxorubicin at 40°C to 41°C to enhance tumor killing. Although the technique is feasible, there is little clinical evidence to show any benefit [111].

Systemic chemotherapy

The single agents cisplatin, doxorubicin, and gemcitabine all have been tried in mesothelioma, with limited effects. Combination chemotherapy such as cisplatin and gemcitabine showed significant symptomatic improvement in patients with mesothelioma, although survival benefits were unclear [112,113]. The antifolate drugs previously were reported to have activity, with high-dose methotrexate giving a 37% response rate in mesothelioma [114]. A systematic review of the evidence for chemotherapy for mesothelioma found 83 studies in which cisplatin was found to be the most active single drug and cisplatin plus doxorubicin had the highest response rate (28.5%; 95% confidence interval 21.3–35.7%) [115]. This combination often has been used as the control arm for studies of chemotherapy. Gemcitabine in combination with cisplatin was shown to improve patient symptoms in one study [112], but subsequent trials showed significant toxicities, and the symptomatic benefits were more modest than initially expected [113].

Pemetrexed, a novel multitargeted antifolate, represents one of the most exciting advances in treatment of mesothelioma. Pemetrexed inhibits several enzymes in the de novo pathways of pyrimidine and purine biosynthesis, and its main site of action is thymidylate synthetase, a folate-dependent enzyme that catalyzes the transformation of deoxyuridine monophosphate to deoxythymidine monophosphate. Inhibition of thymidylate synthetase results in decreased thymidine pools, which are essential for DNA synthesis [116]. Its other sites of action are the inhibition of dihydrofolate reductase and glycinamide ribonucleotide formyltransferase. These multiple targets of action distinguish it from other antifolate compounds. It has undergone clinical development, and preliminary studies showed antitumor activity in several solid tumors, including mesothelioma; non–small cell lung cancer; and pancreas, colorectal, gastric, bladder, head and neck, cervix, and breast cancer [116,117]. The detailed pharmacology of pemetrexed has been reviewed elsewhere [118].

A multicenter randomized phase III trial of pemetrexed with cisplatin versus cisplatin alone in mesothelioma has been completed [119]. This study is the largest trial of any therapy in mesothelioma ($n = 448$) and the only one to have shown a survival benefit in the treatment arm. Suitable patients were patients with histologically confirmed mesothelioma (68% epithelioid type), with measurable disease, with predicted life expectancy of more than 12 weeks, and who were not candidates for curative surgery. Significant survival benefits were seen in the pemetrexed and cisplatin arm above those in the cisplatin-alone arm. Median survival was 12.1 months versus 9.3 months ($P = .02$). Median time to disease progression also was significantly improved, at 5.7 months versus 3.9 months ($P = .001$). Partial response rate to treatment was 41% versus 17%. No patients experienced a complete response. Quality of life, measured by the Lung Cancer Symptom Scale modified for mesothelioma [120], was increased significantly in the pemetrexed and cisplatin arm compared with cisplatin alone ($P < .017$) [121]. Pemetrexed is administered with folic acid and vitamin B_{12} supplementation to reduce toxicity [122] and with corticosteroids to reduce skin rashes [123]. Patients with impaired renal function (creatinine clearance <45 mL/min) should not receive pemetrexed because its safety is not established [124]. Also, patients with ascites or pleural effusions should have these drained before pemetrexed therapy, in the same way as with methotrexate therapy. This is in case clearance is delayed by the third-space fluid collection, which may lead to toxicity [125].

Pemetrexed represents an important advance in the management of patients with mesothelioma, but its precise role in mesothelioma management is still being explored. In the initial randomized trial, pemetrexed was administered to patients with advanced mesothelioma. The survival benefit was modest (3 months), but the benefit in symptom relief was attractive. At present, the role of pemetrexed in early-stage mesothelioma patients, with no or little symptoms, is not yet defined. Trials are under way to examine the role of pemetrexed as an adjunct therapy to surgery. In Europe, the Extended Access Program aims to evaluate pemetrexed alone or combined with cisplatin or carboplatin in more than 1500 enrolled patients. There are also international randomized studies comparing pemetrexed plus best supportive care versus best supportive care alone [126].

The combination of raltitrexed, another novel multi-targeted antifolate agent, with cisplatin also showed similar survival benefits when used as first-line chemotherapy for mesothelioma in another randomized controlled trial [127]. A phase II trial using these drugs as second-line chemotherapy in patients with mesothelioma who had failed to respond to first-line chemotherapy (regimens included pemetrexed and cisplatin) was performed to see if there was any additional benefit in using them; however, this trial showed no objective response and was stopped [128].

Multimodality treatment including surgery

Surgery to resect mesothelioma completely is difficult because of the infiltration of mesothelioma to structures underlying and adjacent to the pleura. Surgical options can be considered as being of three main types: the first to palliate breathlessness, by removal of pleural fluid and subsequent pleurodesis (discussed earlier); the second to debulk the mesothelioma mass; and the third, radical surgery, extrapleural pneumonectomy (EPP), to try to remove all the affected tissues. Both of the latter two operations have been used as single-modality treatments; there was no impact on survival owing to a high tumor recurrence rate [129,130]. These operations are now used in the context of multimodality therapy, as a cytoreductive strategy to reduce tumor bulk in the hope that it will render the tumor more amenable to other therapies, such as chemotherapy or radiotherapy or both.

The evidence supporting the use of radical surgery in mesothelioma is limited because appropriately designed prospective clinical trials are rare. Published work is mostly retrospective in nature, uncontrolled, and flawed with selection bias, making results difficult to interpret. Treatment groups have been poorly defined, and there have been large variations in treatment schedules, with few systematic attempts made to evaluate treatment strategies [131]. Significant controversy exists about whether multimodality therapy improves outcomes, and if so which are the optimal treatments and their sequence [90]. Adjuvant chemotherapy is thought to be more effective when the tumor bulk has been reduced, although this has not been proven. Radiotherapy can be used in higher doses because the underlying lung that limits dosing owing to toxicity has been removed, although hepatitis and carditis are still complications.

Pleurectomy and decortication

Thoracic debulking with pleurectomy is performed to remove the involved parietal and visceral pleura and possibly the diaphragm [132]. The lung is not removed. Complete tumor resection is difficult, if at all possible, by pleurectomy because the tumor often invades into deeper tissue, and the resection margin is usually small. Pleurectomy is not feasible if the pleural space is obliterated by tumor. Pleurectomy has not been associated with survival benefits, but carries a mortality rate of 1.5% to 5% and morbidity rate of 25% [133]. Its role in the treatment of mesothelioma is not established.

Extrapleural pneumonectomy

EPP is the radical debulking of locally advanced mesothelioma, in which all the pleura, lung, pericardium, and ipsilateral diaphragm are removed en bloc. Reconstruction of the diaphragm and pericardium with patches is necessary to prevent organ herniation [134,135]. This procedure is said to offer potential complete tumor resection, and postoperative radiotherapy can be given at high dose without toxicity concerns to the underlying lung.

It is estimated that less than 10% of mesothelioma patients are able to fulfill the selection criteria for EPP [136]. Even in this select group of patients, the surgical mortality rate is at least 5% (even by the most experienced surgical group), and significant complications occur in 50% [137]. Despite such risks, EPP does not provide a cure, and tumor inevitably recurs [138]. As a result, EPP with various post-operative adjunct therapies has been attempted.

Extrapleural pneumonectomy with chemotherapy

EPP combined with postoperative intrapleural cisplatin and later intravenous cisplatin and mitomycin failed to control local recurrence and was associated with significant side effects. Median survival was 13 months [139]. Surgery with immunochemotherapy with interferon-α, cisplatin, and tamoxifen and photodynamic therapy also provided no survival benefit [140].

Extrapleural pneumonectomy or pleurectomy with adjuvant high-dose radiotherapy

After EPP, adjuvant radiotherapy can be administered to eliminate any residual tumor. The field to which radiotherapy is given is smaller, making higher doses easier to administer. Patients received high-dose hemithoracic radiotherapy, 54 Gy, after EPP or pleurectomy and decortication [141]. This dose was well tolerated in general, and the median survival was 33.8 months for stage I and II tumors, but 10 months for stage III and IV tumors. Local and distant tumor relapse occurred. For early-stage disease, this regimen is associated with prolonged survival.

Extrapleural pneumonectomy with adjuvant chemotherapy and radiotherapy (trimodality therapy)

Patients receiving trimodality treatment are highly selected, with good performance status, normal hepatic and renal function, no significant comorbidity, and good cardiopulmonary reserve [142]. The tumor is confined within one hemithorax on CT and MRI, and the tumor equates to Butchart stage I disease. Laparoscopy may be done to study the undersurface of the diaphragm to ensure it is disease-free [138]. Echocardiogram is used to assess pericardial tumor invasion. Routine cervical mediastinoscopy is undertaken in some centers to assess lymph node involvement because this is poorly predicted on CT and MRI [143]. Extrapleural nodes with metastatic disease are related to poorer survival.

Trimodality therapy has shown some success in studies. The results of these highly publicized studies are biased and must be interpreted with caution [144]. There is a patient selection bias because few patients with mesothelioma have the limited disease and minimal comorbidity to be eligible for this therapy. Other variations in the regimens of chemoirradiation (eg, using neoadjuvant chemotherapy before EPP, followed by postoperative radiotherapy) are being tested [145]. Even with such aggressive trimodality regimens, the median overall survival in a series of 183 patients was reported as only 19 months (after excluding deaths from surgery), with 2-year and 5-year survival rates of 38% and 15% [137]. Epithelioid histology and negative node status are independent prognostic factors predicting improved survival [146]. Considering that these were highly selected patients with good performance status, early-stage disease, and no significant comorbidity, such survival figures are disappointing. Without a comparison group, the possibility that such treatment, with its complications, has adversely affected patient survival cannot be excluded. One study followed the patients who completed trimodality treatment. The median survival for 49 patients was 22 months (range 0–64 months) [42]. The median time from treatment to relapse after trimodality therapy was 20 months. Recurrence tended to occur in the ipsilateral hemithorax (67% of all recurrences). Other sites for recurrence included the contralateral hemithorax, the abdomen, and distant sites such as the central nervous system.

Because trimodality therapy does not provide cure and does not seem to prolong survival, it is essentially a palliative procedure. The aggressive nature and high complication rates cannot justify its use as a palliative procedure, however. Quality of life has never been assessed in patients who underwent EPP or trimodality therapy. It remains a valid concern that quality of life of these patients potentially may be reduced given the high adverse event rates with the treatment.

A randomized controlled trial is under way in the United Kingdom, comparing two groups of patients with mesothelioma: one having chemotherapy, EPP, and postoperative hemithoracic radiotherapy and the other having chemotherapy alone (Mesothelioma and Radical Surgery trial) [147]. It is hoped that the results will provide much needed information on the role of EPP in mesothelioma.

Pleurectomy followed by brachytherapy and radiotherapy

Pleurectomy followed by brachytherapy and radiotherapy was associated with a median survival of 21 months in a small, uncontrolled study of 41 patients [148]. Brachytherapy has not been evaluated further in the context of a randomized controlled trial in mesothelioma. It may be used in combination with other treatment modalities, such as photodynamic therapy, although its use has shown no survival advantage compared with groups receiving the other treatment alone [131,149].

Novel therapies

Gene therapy

Gene therapy is in the early stages of development. The theory is that the delivery of toxic or "suicide" genes into tumor cells would facilitate their destruction, by rendering the cell sensitive to a non-toxic substrate, which then generates cytotoxic metabolites and causes cell death. A phase I study administered a retroviral vector into the pleural space to deliver herpes simplex virus thymidine kinase into the cells [136,150,151]. This rendered the cell sensitive to ganciclovir, which was administered and converted to an extremely cytotoxic triphosphory-lated form by normal mammalian thymidine kinase, which led to cell death. The administration of the retroviral vector was safe, but gene transfer was patchy. The "bystander effect" is the transfer of toxic metabolites from transduced cells to nontransduced cells, which amplifies cytotoxic activity [152].

One interesting approach is the use of Ad.Inter-feron-beta. Use of this gene therapy in conjunction with other strategies (eg, surgery, neoadjuvant chemotherapy) is being tested. More detailed discussion on recent advances in gene therapy for mesothelioma can be found elsewhere [3,150].

Immunotherapy

Intrapleural administration of the cytokines inter-leukin (IL)-2 and interferon-γ has been investigated in mesothelioma [153]. IL-2 activates lymphokine activated killer cells and reverses the suppression of natural killer cells induced by asbestos fibers. Systemic administration of IL-2 showed limited efficacy and significant side effects [154]. Intra-pleural administration was used to provide high local concentration and low systemic toxicity. Half of the patients responded to IL-2 and had a complete or partial response, with a median survival of 28 ± 12 months [155]. Interferon-γ is a lymphokine produced by T lymphocytes in response to specific antigenic or mitogenic stimuli. It has antiproliferative effects and can activate macrophage antitumor cytotoxicity [156]. Interferon-γ alone induced a response in only 20% of patients [157]. Interferon-α with chemotherapy drugs and interferon-β also have been tried, but have not produced any significant responses [158,159].

Photodynamic therapy

Photodynamic therapy is a surface-orientated, photochemical-induced cytotoxic therapy, in which the tumor preferentially takes up agents that lead to cell toxicity when activated by light. The administration of porphyrin dye intravenously has been used, which is absorbed from the bloodstream. Non-malignant cells excrete the dye rapidly, whereas malignant cells do not. These retain the dye for 48 hours after administration. Single-wavelength light from a laser activates the dye, which produces oxygen free radicals and ultimately cell death. A phase III trial randomized patients to have photodynamic therapy as an adjunct to surgery or just surgery, but there was no survival benefit in the photodynamic therapy group [140,149,160].

Others

The role of angiogenic cytokines (eg, vascular endothelial growth factor) is well shown in tumor growth [161]. Antiangiogenic strategies are being tested in phase I/II clinical trials for management of mesothelioma [162]. The role of ranpirnase also is being examined [126]. Molecular-targeted therapies, such as bortezomid, mTOR inhibitors, and Met (receptor of hepatocyte growth factor) inhibitors, have generated interest and are being explored [163]. Many previous attempts have shown initial promise in small, uncontrolled trials, but the results did not survive more rigorous testing with larger size randomized studies. Multicenter collaboration is important to recruit patients to adequately powered clinical trials, to produce useful information for the advancement of patient care.

Summary

Malignant mesothelioma is increasing in incidence globally and has no known cure. Its unique clinical feature of local infiltration along tissue planes makes it a difficult neoplasm to manage. There have been few randomized controlled trials regarding treatment options, although these have increased in recent years, and results are eagerly awaited. Patient selection bias, variable inclusion methods, and different measurements of response and survival have hampered the interpretation of the existing trials, and controversy persists. Small nonrandomized trials of novel therapies have led to false hope and confusion. Pemetrexed has given hope in the area of chemotherapy, but the best timing of its use is unknown. Surgery is being used in some centers, but without quality data to support it. Good quality palliative care delivered by experienced professions in a coordinated team approach is strongly recommended. It is crucial that research institutions collaborate closely in future research to answer key clinical questions with appropriately powered randomized controlled trials, using practical study end points, such as quality-of-life measures and survival.

References

[1] Lanphear BP, Buncher CR. Latent period for malignant mesothelioma of occupational origin. J Occup Med 1992;34:718–21.

[2] Peto J, Hodgson JT, Matthews FE, Jones JR. Continuing increase in mesothelioma mortality in Britain. Lancet 1995;345:535–9.

[3] Sterman DH, Albelda SM. Advances in the diagnosis, evaluation, and management of malignant pleural mesothelioma. Respirology 2005;10:266–83.

[4] Musk AW, de Klerk NH. Epidemiology of malignant mesothelioma in Australia. Lung Cancer 2004; 45(Suppl 1):S21–3.

[5] Leigh J, Driscoll T. Malignant mesothelioma in Australia, 1945–2002. Int J Occup Environ Health 2003;9:206–17.

[6] Kjellstrom T, Smartt P. Increased mesothelioma incidence in New Zealand: the asbestos-cancer epidemic has started. N Z Med J 2000;113:485–90.

[7] Gaafar RM, Eldin NH. Epidemic of mesothelioma in Egypt. Lung Cancer 2005;49(Suppl 1):S17–20.

[8] Ulvestad B, Kjaerheim K, Moller B, Andersen A. Incidence trends of mesothelioma in Norway, 1965–1999. Int J Cancer 2003;107:94–8.

[9] Takahashi K, Karjalainen A. A cross-country comparative overview of the asbestos situation in ten Asian countries. Int J Occup Environ Health 2003;9: 244–8.

[10] Kazan-Allen L. Asbestos and mesothelioma: worldwide trends. Lung Cancer 2005;49(Suppl 1):S3–8.

[11] Wagner JC, Sleggs CA, Marchand P. Diffuse pleural mesothelioma and asbestos exposure in the North Western Cape Province. Br J Ind Med 1960; 17:260–71.

[12] Antman KH. Natural history and epidemiology of malignant mesothelioma. Chest 1993;103(4 Suppl): 373S–6S.

[13] Holt PF. Translocation of inhaled dust to the pleura. Environ Res 1983;31:212–20.

[14] de Klerk NH, Musk AW, Williams V, et al. Comparison of measures of exposure to asbestos in former crocidolite workers from Wittenoom Gorge, W. Australia. Am J Ind Med 1996;30:579–87.

[15] Pass HI, Pogrebniak HW. Malignant pleural mesothelioma. Curr Probl Surg 1993;30:921–1012.

[16] Lemen RA. Chrysotile asbestos as a cause of mesothelioma: application of the Hill causation model. Int J Occup Environ Health 2004;10:233–9.

[17] Bonn D. Asbestos—the legacy lives on. Lancet 1999; 353:1336.

[18] Chapman SJ, Cookson WO, Musk AW, Lee YC. Benign asbestos pleural diseases. Curr Opin Pulm Med 2003;9:266–71.

[19] Lee YC, Lane KB. Cytokines in pleural diseases. In: Light RW, Lee YC, editors. Textbook of pleural diseases. London: Arnold; 2003. p. 63–89.

[20] Jaurand MC, Kaplan H, Thiollet J, et al. Phagocytosis of chrysotile fibers by pleural mesothelial cells in culture. Am J Pathol 1979;94:529–38.

[21] Jaurand MC. Mechanisms of fiber-induced genotoxicity. Environ Health Perspect 1997;105(Suppl 5): 1073–84.

[22] Jaurand MC, Fleury-Feith J. Pathogenesis of malignant pleural mesothelioma. Respirology 2005;10:2–8.

[23] Lee YC, De Klerk NH, Henderson DW, Musk AW. Malignant mesothelioma. In: Hendrick DJ, Burge PS, Beckett WS, Chung A, editors. Occupational disorders of the lung: recognition, management and prevention. London: Saunders; 2002. p. 359–79.

[24] Testa JR, Jhanwar SC. Genetics of malignant mesothelioma. In: Light RW, Lee YC, editors. Textbook of pleural diseases. London: Arnold; 2003. p. 120–30.

[25] Roushdy-Hammady I, Siegel J, Emri S, et al. Genetic-susceptibility factor and malignant mesothelioma in the Cappadocian region of Turkey. Lancet 2001;357: 444–5.

[26] Ramos-Nino ME, Scapoli L, Martinelli M, et al. Microarray analysis and RNA silencing link fra-1 to cd44 and c-met expression in mesothelioma. Cancer Res 2003;63:3539–45.

[27] Gordon GJ, Jensen RV, Hsiao LL, et al. Translation of microarray data into clinically relevant cancer diagnostic tests using gene expression ratios in lung cancer and mesothelioma. Cancer Res 2002; 62:4963–7.

[28] Gordon GJ, Jensen RV, Hsiao LL, et al. Using gene expression ratios to predict outcome among pa-

tients with mesothelioma. J Natl Cancer Inst 2003;
95:598–605.

[29] Singhal S, Wiewrodt R, Malden LD, et al. Gene expression profiling of malignant mesothelioma. Clin Cancer Res 2003;9:3080–97.

[30] Gordon GJ, Rockwell GN, Jensen RV, et al. Identification of novel candidate oncogenes and tumor suppressors in malignant pleural mesothelioma using large-scale transcriptional profiling. Am J Pathol 2005;166:1827–40.

[31] Hegmans JP, Bard MP, Hemmes A, et al. Proteomic analysis of exosomes secreted by human mesothelioma cells. Am J Pathol 2004;164:1807–15.

[32] Lopez-Rios F, Illei PB, Rusch V, Ladanyi M. Evidence against a role for SV40 infection in human mesotheliomas and high risk of false-positive PCR results owing to presence of SV40 sequences in common laboratory plasmids. Lancet 2004;364:1157–66.

[33] Manfredi JJ, Dong J, Liu WJ, et al. Evidence against a role for SV40 in human mesothelioma. Cancer Res 2005;65:2602–9.

[34] Fleury-Feith J, Pilatte Y, Jaurand MC. Cells in the pleural cavity. In: Light RW, Lee YC, editors. Textbook of pleural diseases. London: Arnold; 2003. p. 17–34.

[35] Whitaker D, Henderson DW, Shilkin KB. The concept of mesothelioma in situ: implications for diagnosis and histogenesis. Semin Diagn Pathol 1992;9:151–61.

[36] Henderson DW, Shilkin KB, Whitaker D. Reactive mesothelial hyperplasia vs mesothelioma, including mesothelioma in situ: a brief review. Am J Clin Pathol 1998;110:397–404.

[37] Cury PM, Butcher DN, Corrin B, Nicholson AG. The use of histological and immunohistochemical markers to distinguish pleural malignant mesothelioma and in situ mesothelioma from reactive mesothelial hyperplasia and reactive pleural fibrosis. J Pathol 1999; 189:251–7.

[38] Corson JM. Pathology of diffuse malignant pleural mesothelioma. Semin Thorac Cardiovasc Surg 1997; 9:347–55.

[39] Sugarbaker DJ, Garcia JP, Richards WG, et al. Extrapleural pneumonectomy in the multimodality therapy of malignant pleural mesothelioma: results in 120 consecutive patients. Ann Surg 1996;224:288–94.

[40] Hulks G, Thomas JS, Waclawski E. Malignant pleural mesothelioma in western Glasgow 1980–6. Thorax 1989;44:496–500.

[41] King JA, Tucker JA, Wong SW. Mesothelioma: a study of 22 gases. South Med J 1997;90:199–205.

[42] Baldini EH, Recht A, Strauss GM, et al. Patterns of failure after trimodality therapy for malignant pleural mesothelioma. Ann Thorac Surg 1997;63:334–8.

[43] Wang NS. Pleural mesothelioma: an approach to diagnostic problems. Respirology 1996;1:259–71.

[44] Antman K, Shemin R, Ryan L, et al. Malignant mesothelioma: prognostic variables in a registry of 180 patients, the Dana-Farber Cancer Institute and Brigham and Women's Hospital experience over two decades, 1965–1985. J Clin Oncol 1988;6:147–53.

[45] Corson JM. Pathology of mesothelioma. Thorac Surg Clin 2004;14:447–60.

[46] Chahinian AP, Pajak TF, Holland JF, et al. Diffuse malignant mesothelioma: prospective evaluation of 69 patients. Ann Intern Med 1982;96(6 Pt 1):746–55.

[47] Leigh J, Davidson P, Hendrie L, Berry D. Malignant mesothelioma in Australia, 1945–2000. Am J Ind Med 2002;41:188–201.

[48] Lee YCG, Dean A, Thompson RI, Robinson BWS. Clinical and palliative care aspects of malignant mesothelioma. In: Robinson BWS, Chahinian P, editors. Mesothelioma. London: Martin Dunitz; 2002. p. 111–26.

[49] Sugarbaker PH, Welch LS, Mohamed F, Glehen O. A review of peritoneal mesothelioma at the Washington Cancer Institute. Surg Oncol Clin N Am 2003;12: 605–21.

[50] Vigneswaran WT, Stefanacci PR. Pericardial mesothelioma. Curr Treat Options Oncol 2000;1:299–302.

[51] Eren NT, Akar AR. Primary pericardial mesothelioma. Curr Treat Options Oncol 2002;3:369–73.

[52] Plas E, Riedl CR, Pfluger H. Malignant mesothelioma of the tunica vaginalis testis: review of the literature and assessment of prognostic parameters. Cancer 1998;83:2437–46.

[53] Wong CF, Fung SL, Yew WW, Fu KH. A case of malignant pleural mesothelioma with unexpectedly long survival without active treatment. Respiration 2002;69:166–8.

[54] Edwards JG, Abrams KR, Leverment JN, et al. Prognostic factors for malignant mesothelioma in 142 patients: validation of CALGB and EORTC prognostic scoring systems. Thorax 2000;55:731–5.

[55] Herndon JE, Green MR, Chahinian AP, et al. Factors predictive of survival among 337 patients with mesothelioma treated between 1984 and 1994 by the Cancer and Leukemia Group B. Chest 1998;113: 723–31.

[56] Mikulski SM, Costanzi JJ, Vogelzang NJ, et al. Phase II trial of a single weekly intravenous dose of ranpirnase in patients with unresectable malignant mesothelioma. J Clin Oncol 2002;20:274–81.

[57] Curran D, Sahmoud T, Therasse P, et al. Prognostic factors in patients with pleural mesothelioma: the European Organization for Research and Treatment of Cancer experience. J Clin Oncol 1998;16:145–52.

[58] Pisani RJ, Colby TV, Williams DE. Malignant mesothelioma of the pleura. Mayo Clin Proc 1988;63: 1234–44.

[59] Musk AW, Woodward SD. Conventional treatment and its effect on survival of malignant pleural mesothelioma in Western Australia. Aust N Z J Med 1982; 12:229–32.

[60] Ceresoli GL, Locati LD, Ferreri AJ, et al. Therapeutic outcome according to histologic subtype in 121 patients with malignant pleural mesothelioma. Lung Cancer 2001;34:279–87.

[61] Law MR, Gregor A, Hodson ME, et al. Malignant mesothelioma of the pleura: a study of 52 treated and 64 untreated patients. Thorax 1984;39:255–9.

[62] Boutin C, Rey F. Thoracoscopy in pleural malignant mesothelioma: a prospective study of 188 consecutive patients. Part 1: diagnosis. Cancer 1993;72:389–93.

[63] Renshaw AA, Dean BR, Antman KH, et al. The role of cytologic evaluation of pleural fluid in the diagnosis of malignant mesothelioma. Chest 1997;111:106–9.

[64] Attanoos RL, Gibbs AR. Pathology of malignant mesothelioma. Histopathology 1997;30:403–18.

[65] Edge JR, Choudhury SL. Malignant mesothelioma of the pleura in Barrow-in-Furness. Thorax 1978;33:26–30.

[66] Maskell NA, Gleeson FV, Davies RJ. Standard pleural biopsy versus CT-guided cutting-needle biopsy for diagnosis of malignant disease in pleural effusions: a randomised controlled trial. Lancet 2003;361:1326–30.

[67] King JE, Hasleton PS. Immunohistochemistry and the diagnosis of malignant mesothelioma. Histopathology 2001;38:471–6.

[68] Wick MR. Pleural cytology, tumor markers and immunohistochemistry. In: Light RW, Lee YC, editors. Textbook of pleural diseases. London: Arnold; 2003. p. 256–81.

[69] Robinson BW, Creaney J, Lake R, et al. Mesothelin-family proteins and diagnosis of mesothelioma. Lancet 2003;362:1612–6.

[70] Hassan R, Bera T, Pastan I. Mesothelin: a new target for immunotherapy. Clin Cancer Res 2004;10(12 Pt 1):3937–42.

[71] Pass HI, Lott D, Lonardo F, et al. Asbestos exposure, pleural mesothelioma, and serum osteopontin levels. N Engl J Med 2005;353:1564–73.

[72] Antman KH. Current concepts: malignant mesothelioma. N Engl J Med 1980;303:200–2.

[73] Ng CS, Munden RF, Libshitz HI. Malignant pleural mesothelioma: the spectrum of manifestations on CT in 70 cases. Clin Radiol 1999;54:415–21.

[74] Yilmaz UM, Utkaner G, Yalniz E, et al. Computed tomographic findings of environmental asbestos-related malignant pleural mesothelioma. Respirology 1998;3:33–8.

[75] Bittner RC, Felix R. Magnetic resonance (MR) imaging of the chest: state-of-the-art. Eur Respir J 1998;11:1392–404.

[76] McLoud TC. CT and MR in pleural disease. Clin Chest Med 1998;19:261–76.

[77] Byrne MJ, Nowak AK. Modified RECIST criteria for assessment of response in malignant pleural mesothelioma. Ann Oncol 2004;15:257–60.

[78] Nowak AK. CT, RECIST, and malignant pleural mesothelioma. Lung Cancer 2005;49(Suppl 1):S37–40.

[79] Knuuttila A, Halme M, Kivisaari L, et al. The clinical importance of magnetic resonance imaging versus computed tomography in malignant pleural mesothelioma. Lung Cancer 1998;22:215–25.

[80] Heelan RT, Rusch VW, Begg CB, et al. Staging of malignant pleural mesothelioma: comparison of CT and MR imaging. AJR Am J Roentgenol 1999;172:1039–47.

[81] Patz Jr EF, Shaffer K, Piwnica-Worms DR, et al. Malignant pleural mesothelioma: value of CT and MR imaging in predicting resectability. AJR Am J Roentgenol 1992;159:961–6.

[82] Wang ZJ, Reddy GP, Gotway MB, et al. Malignant pleural mesothelioma: evaluation with CT, MR imaging, and PET. Radiographics 2004;24:105–19.

[83] Benard F, Sterman D, Smith RJ, et al. Metabolic imaging of malignant pleural mesothelioma with fluorodeoxyglucose positron emission tomography. Chest 1998;114:713–22.

[84] Benard F, Sterman D, Smith RJ, et al. Prognostic value of FDG PET imaging in malignant pleural mesothelioma. J Nucl Med 1999;40:1241–5.

[85] Flores RM. Induction chemotherapy, extrapleural pneumonectomy, and radiotherapy in the treatment of malignant pleural mesothelioma: the Memorial Sloan-Kettering experience. Lung Cancer 2005;49(Suppl 1):S71–4.

[86] Steinert HC, Santos Dellea MM, Burger C, et al. Therapy response evaluation in malignant pleural mesothelioma with integrated PET-CT imaging. Lung Cancer 2005;49(Suppl 1):S33–5.

[87] Butchart EG, Ashcroft T, Barnsley WC, et al. Pleuropneumonectomy in the management of diffuse malignant mesothelioma of the pleura: experience with 29 patients. Thorax 1976;31:15–24.

[88] Boutin C, Rey F, Gouvernet J, et al. Thoracoscopy in pleural malignant mesothelioma: a prospective study of 188 consecutive patients. Part 2: prognosis and staging. Cancer 1993;72:394–404.

[89] Rusch VW. A proposed new international TNM staging system for malignant pleural mesothelioma: from the International Mesothelioma Interest Group. Chest 1995;108:1122–8.

[90] van Meerbeeck JP, Boyer M. Consensus report: pretreatment minimal staging and treatment of potentially resectable malignant pleural mesothelioma. Lung Cancer 2005;49(Suppl 1):S123–7.

[91] Robinson BW, Musk AW, Lake RA. Malignant mesothelioma. Lancet 2005;366:397–408.

[92] Jaklitsch MT, Grondin SC, Sugarbaker DJ. Treatment of malignant mesothelioma. World J Surg 2001;25:210–7.

[93] Jackson MB, Pounder D, Price C, et al. Percutaneous cervical cordotomy for the control of pain in patients with pleural mesothelioma. Thorax 1999;54:238–41.

[94] Kanpolat Y, Savas A, Ucar T, et al. CT-guided percutaneous selective cordotomy for treatment of intractable pain in patients with malignant pleural mesothelioma. Acta Neurochir (Wien) 2002;144:595–9.

[95] Price C, Pounder D, Jackson M, et al. Respiratory function after unilateral percutaneous cervical cordotomy. J Pain Symptom Manage 2003;25:459–63.

[96] Pass HI, Pogrebniak HW. Malignant pleural mesothelioma. Curr Probl Surg 1993;30:921–1012.

[97] West SD, Davies RJ, Lee YC. Pleurodesis for malignant pleural effusions: current controversies and variations in practices. Curr Opin Pulm Med 2004;10:
305–10.

[98] Shaw P, Agarwal R. Pleurodesis for malignant pleural effusions. Cochrane Database Syst Rev 2004;
1:CD002916.

[99] Dresler CM, Olak J, Herndon JE, et al. Phase III
intergroup study of talc poudrage vs talc slurry sclerosis for malignant pleural effusion. Chest 2005;
127:909–15.

[100] Lee YC, Light RW. Management of malignant pleural
effusions. Respirology 2004;9:148–56.

[101] Putnam Jr JB, Light RW, Rodriguez RM, et al. A
randomized comparison of indwelling pleural catheter
and doxycycline pleurodesis in the management of
malignant pleural effusions. Cancer 1999;86:1992–9.

[102] Ball DL, Cruickshank DG. The treatment of malignant mesothelioma of the pleura: review of a 5-year
experience, with special reference to radiotherapy.
Am J Clin Oncol 1990;13:4–9.

[103] Gordon Jr W, Antman KH, Greenberger JS, et al.
Radiation therapy in the management of patients with
mesothelioma. Int J Radiat Oncol Biol Phys 1982;
8:19–25.

[104] Alberts AS, Falkson G, Goedhals L, et al. Malignant
pleural mesothelioma: a disease unaffected by current
therapeutic maneuvers. J Clin Oncol 1988;6:527–35.

[105] Munter MW, Christian T, Anna N, et al. Inverse
planned stereotactic intensity modulated radiotherapy
(IMRT) in the palliative treatment of malignant
mesothelioma of the pleura: the Heidelberg experience. Lung Cancer 2005;49(Suppl 1):S83–6.

[106] Boutin C, Rey F, Viallat JR. Prevention of malignant
seeding after invasive diagnostic procedures in
patients with pleural mesothelioma: a randomized
trial of local radiotherapy. Chest 1995;108:754–8.

[107] Boutin C, Irisson M, Rathelot P, Petite JM. [Parietal
extension of diffuse malignant pleural mesothelioma
after biopsy: prevention by local radiotherapy]. Presse
Med 1983;12:1823.

[108] Bydder S, Phillips M, Joseph DJ, et al. A randomised
trial of single-dose radiotherapy to prevent procedure
tract metastasis by malignant mesothelioma. Br J
Cancer 2004;91:9–10.

[109] Rusch VW, Niedzwiecki D, Tao Y, et al. Intrapleural
cisplatin and mitomycin for malignant mesothelioma
following pleurectomy: pharmacokinetic studies.
J Clin Oncol 1992;10:1001–6.

[110] Markman M, Cleary S, Pfeifle C, et al. Cisplatin
administered by the intracavitary route as treatment
for malignant mesothelioma. Cancer 1986;58:18–21.

[111] van Ruth S, Baas P, Haas RL, et al. Cytoreductive
surgery combined with intraoperative hyperthermic
intrathoracic chemotherapy for stage I malignant pleural mesothelioma. Ann Surg Oncol 2003;10:176–82.

[112] Byrne MJ, Davidson JA, Musk AW, et al. Cisplatin
and gemcitabine treatment for malignant mesothelioma: a phase II study. J Clin Oncol 1999;17:25–30.

[113] Nowak AK, Byrne MJ, Williamson R, et al. A
multicentre phase II study of cisplatin and gemcitabine for malignant mesothelioma. Br J Cancer 2002;
87:491–6.

[114] Solheim OP, Saeter G, Finnanger AM, et al. High-
dose methotrexate in the treatment of malignant
mesothelioma of the pleura: a phase II study. Br J
Cancer 1992;65:956–60.

[115] Berghmans T, Paesmans M, Lalami Y, et al. Activity
of chemotherapy and immunotherapy on malignant
mesothelioma: a systematic review of the literature
with meta-analysis. Lung Cancer 2002;38:111–21.

[116] Hanauske AR, Chen V, Paoletti P, et al. Pemetrexed
disodium: a novel antifolate clinically active against
multiple solid tumors. Oncologist 2001;6:363–73.

[117] Hanna N, Shepherd FA, Fossella FV, et al. Randomized phase III trial of pemetrexed versus docetaxel in
patients with non-small-cell lung cancer previously
treated with chemotherapy. J Clin Oncol 2004;22:
1589–97.

[118] Curtin NJ, Hughes AN. Pemetrexed disodium, a
novel antifolate with multiple targets. Lancet Oncol
2001;2:298–306.

[119] Vogelzang NJ, Rusthoven JJ, Symanowski J, et al.
Phase III study of pemetrexed in combination with
cisplatin versus cisplatin alone in patients with malignant pleural mesothelioma. J Clin Oncol 2003;21:
2636–44.

[120] Hollen PJ, Gralla RJ, Liepa AM, et al. Adapting the
Lung Cancer Symptom Scale (LCSS) to mesothelioma: using the LCSS-Meso conceptual model for
validation. Cancer 2004;101:587–95.

[121] Bottomley A, Gaafa R, Manegold C, et al. Short-term
treatment-related symptoms and quality of life: results
from an international randomized phase III study of
cisplatin with or without raltitrexed in patients with
malignant pleural mesothelioma: an EORTC Lung-
Cancer Group and National Cancer Institute, Canada,
Intergroup Study. J Clin Oncol 2006;24:1435–42.

[122] Niyikiza C, Baker SD, Seitz DE, et al. Homocysteine
and methylmalonic acid: markers to predict and avoid
toxicity from pemetrexed therapy. Mol Cancer Ther
2002;1:545–52.

[123] Hazarika M, White Jr RM, Booth BP, et al. Pemetrexed in malignant pleural mesothelioma. Clin Cancer Res 2005;11:982–92.

[124] Adjei AA. Pemetrexed (Alimta): a novel multi-
targeted antifolate agent. Exp Rev Anticancer Ther
2003;3:145–56.

[125] Adjei AA. Pharmacology and mechanism of action
of pemetrexed. Clin Lung Cancer 2004;5(Suppl 2):
S51–5.

[126] Favaretto A. Overview on ongoing or planned clinical
trials in Europe. Lung Cancer 2005;49(Suppl 1):
S117–21.

[127] van Meerbeeck JP, Gaafar R, Manegold C, et al. Randomized phase III study of cisplatin with or without

raltitrexed in patients with malignant pleural meso-thelioma: an intergroup study of the European Organisation for Research and Treatment of Cancer Lung Cancer Group and the National Cancer Institute of Canada. J Clin Oncol 2005;23:6881–9.

[128] Porta C, Zimatore M, Bonomi L, et al. Raltitrexed-oxaliplatin combination chemotherapy is inactive as second-line treatment for malignant pleural mesothe-lioma patients. Lung Cancer 2005;48:429–34.

[129] DaValle MJ, Faber LP, Kittle CF, et al. Extrapleural pneumonectomy for diffuse, malignant mesothe-lioma. Ann Thorac Surg 1986;42:612–8.

[130] Rusch VW, Piantadosi S, Holmes EC. The role of extrapleural pneumonectomy in malignant pleural mesothelioma. A Lung Cancer Study Group trial. J Thorac Cardiovasc Surg 1991;102:1–9.

[131] van Ruth S, Baas P, Zoetmulder FA. Surgical treat-ment of malignant pleural mesothelioma: a review. Chest 2003;123:551–61.

[132] Aisner J. Current approach to malignant meso-thelioma of the pleura. Chest 1995;107(6 Suppl): 332S–44S.

[133] Rusch VW. Pleurectomy/decortication in the setting of multimodality treatment for diffuse malignant pleural mesothelioma. Semin Thorac Cardiovasc Surg 1997;9:367–72.

[134] Sugarbaker DJ, Mentzer SJ, Strauss G. Extrapleural pneumonectomy in the treatment of malignant pleural mesothelioma. Ann Thorac Surg 1992;54:941–6.

[135] Sugarbaker DJ, Mentzer SJ, DeCamp M, et al. Extrapleural pneumonectomy in the setting of a multimodality approach to malignant mesothelioma. Chest 1993;103(4 Suppl):377S–81S.

[136] Kaiser LR. New therapies in the treatment of malig-nant pleural mesothelioma. Semin Thorac Cardiovasc Surg 1997;9:383–90.

[137] Sugarbaker DJ, Flores RM, Jaklitsch MT, et al. Resection margins, extrapleural nodal status, and cell type determine postoperative long-term survival in trimodality therapy of malignant pleural mesothe-lioma: results in 183 patients. J Thorac Cardiovasc Surg 1999;117:54–63.

[138] Jaklitsch MT, Grondin SC, Sugarbaker DJ. Treatment of malignant mesothelioma. World J Surg 2001;25: 210–7.

[139] Rice TW, Adelstein DJ, Kirby TJ, et al. Aggressive multimodality therapy for malignant pleural meso-thelioma. Ann Thorac Surg 1994;58:24–9.

[140] Pass HI, Temeck BK, Kranda K, et al. Phase III randomized trial of surgery with or without intra-operative photodynamic therapy and postoperative immunochemotherapy for malignant pleural meso-thelioma. Ann Surg Oncol 1997;4:628–33.

[141] Rusch VW, Rosenzweig K, Venkatraman E, et al. A phase II trial of surgical resection and adjuvant high-dose hemithoracic radiation for malignant pleural mesothelioma. J Thorac Cardiovasc Surg 2001;122: 788–95.

[142] Sugarbaker DJ, Jaklitsch MT, Bueno R, et al.

Prevention, early detection, and management of com-plications after 328 consecutive extrapleural pneu-monectomies. J Thorac Cardiovasc Surg 2004;128: 138–46.

[143] Pilling JE, Stewart DJ, Martin-Ucar AE, et al. The case for routine cervical mediastinoscopy prior to radical surgery for malignant pleural mesothelioma. Eur J Cardiothorac Surg 2004;25:497–501.

[144] Sugarbaker DJ, Jaklitsch MT, Liptay MJ. Mesothe-lioma and radical multimodality therapy: who bene-fits? Chest 1995;107(6 Suppl):345S–50S.

[145] Stahel RA, Weder W, Ballabeni P, et al. Neoadjuvant chemotherapy followed by extrapleural pneumonec-tomy in malignant pleural mesothelioma: a multi-centre phase II trial of the SAKK. Proc Am Soc Clin Oncol 2004;23:626a.

[146] Sugarbaker DJ, Strauss GM, Lynch TJ, et al. Node status has prognostic significance in the multimodal-ity therapy of diffuse, malignant mesothelioma. J Clin Oncol 1993;11:1172–8.

[147] Treasure T, Waller D, Swift S, Peto J. Radical surgery for mesothelioma. BMJ 2004;328:237–8.

[148] Hilaris BS, Nori D, Kwong E, et al. Pleurectomy and intraoperative brachytherapy and postoperative radiation in the treatment of malignant pleural mesothelioma. Int J Radiat Oncol Biol Phys 1984; 10:325–31.

[149] Friedberg JS, Mick R, Stevenson J, et al. A phase I study of Foscan-mediated photodynamic therapy and surgery in patients with mesothelioma. Ann Thorac Surg 2003;75:952–9.

[150] Albelda SM, Sterman DH. Gene therapy in pleural diseases. In: Light RW, Lee YC, editors. Textbook of pleural diseases. London: Arnold; 2003. p. 526–35.

[151] Sterman DH, Kaiser LR, Albelda SM. Gene therapy for malignant pleural mesothelioma. Hematol Oncol Clin North Am 1998;12:553–68.

[152] Elshami AA, Saavedra A, Zhang H, et al. Gap junc-tions play a role in the 'bystander effect' of the herpes simplex virus thymidine kinase/ganciclovir system in vitro. Gene Ther 1996;3:85–92.

[153] Goey SH, Eggermont AM, Punt CJ, et al. Intrapleural administration of interleukin 2 in pleural meso-thelioma: a phase I–II study. Br J Cancer 1995;72: 1283–8.

[154] Astoul P. Pleural mesothelioma. Curr Opin Pulm Med 1999;5:259–68.

[155] Astoul P, Picat-Joossen D, Viallat JR, et al. Intrapleu-ral administration of interleukin-2 for the treatment of patients with malignant pleural mesothelioma: a Phase II study. Cancer 1998;83:2099–104.

[156] Sterman DH, Kaiser LR, Albelda SM. Advances in the treatment of malignant pleural mesothelioma. Chest 1999;116:504–20.

[157] Boutin C, Nussbaum E, Monnet I, et al. Intrapleural treatment with recombinant gamma-interferon in early stage malignant pleural mesothelioma. Cancer 1994;74:2460–7.

[158] Upham JW, Musk AW, van Hazel G, et al. Interferon

alpha and doxorubicin in malignant mesothelioma: a
phase II study. Aust N Z J Med 1993;23:683 – 7.

[159] Pass HW, Temeck BK, Kranda K, et al. A phase II
trial investigating primary immunochemotherapy for
malignant pleural mesothelioma and the feasibility of
adjuvant immunochemotherapy after maximal cyto-
reduction. Ann Surg Oncol 1995;2:214 – 20.

[160] Pass HI, Temeck BK, Kranda K, et al. Preoperative
tumor volume is associated with outcome in malignant pleural mesothelioma. J Thorac Cardiovasc Surg
1998;115:310 – 7.

[161] Grove CS, Lee YC. Vascular endothelial growth
factor: the key mediator in pleural effusion formation.
Curr Opin Pulm Med 2002;8:294 – 301.

[162] Catalano A, Gianni W, Procopio A. Experimental
therapy of malignant mesothelioma: new perspectives
from anti-angiogenic treatments. Crit Rev Oncol
Hematol 2004;50:101 – 9.

[163] Vogelzang NJ, Porta C, Mutti L. New agents in the
management of advanced mesothelioma. Semin
Oncol 2005;32:336 – 50.

CLINICS
IN CHEST
MEDICINE

Clin Chest Med 27 (2006) 355 – 368

ELSEVIER
SAUNDERS

Pleural Disease in Lymphangioleiomyomatosis

Khalid F. Almoosa, MD[a],*, Francis X. McCormack, MD[a],
Steven A. Sahn, MD[b]

[a]Department of Internal Medicine, Division of Pulmonary, Critical Care, and Sleep Medicine,
University of Cincinnati College of Medicine, 231 Albert Sabin Way, 6004 MSB, PO Box 670564, Cincinnati,
OH 45267-0564, USA
[b]Division of Pulmonary and Critical Care Medicine, Department of Allergy and Clinical Immunology,
Medical University of South Carolina, Charleston, SC, USA

Lymphangioleiomyomatosis (LAM) is a rare lung disease of unknown etiology that is characterized by the proliferation and infiltration of the pulmonary interstitium with atypical smooth muscle cells [1–3]. The first case description was published in 1919 in a child with tuberous sclerosis complex (TSC) who presented with bilateral spontaneous pneumothorax [4]. TSC is an inherited neurocutaneous disorder with variable penetrance characterized by the development of multiorgan hamartomas, cognitive impairment, and seizures [5–9]. In 1966, Cornog and Enterline [10] attempted to bring order to the LAM literature by clarifying the nomenclature and describing characteristic histologic features in a group of patients. Whether LAM is associated with TSC or not, it occurs almost exclusively in women of reproductive age and leads to the development of numerous pulmonary parenchymal cysts (Figs. 1 and 2). The pathologic findings of TSC-LAM are similar to those found in sporadic LAM and include profuse smooth muscle infiltration of all lung structures—airways, blood vessels, lymphatics, and interstitium [7,9]. In either TSC-LAM or sporadic LAM, progressive respiratory insufficiency and pleural complications, specifically pneumothorax and chylothorax, are the clinical hallmarks. Because most of the initial episodes of pneumothorax or chylothorax occur before the diagnosis of LAM is established, their occurrence is often the

sentinel event that leads the clinician to consider the diagnosis of LAM. Because pleural complications are important for the recognition of LAM and constitute unique challenges for clinical management, this article presents an overview of pleural complications in LAM. There is a paucity of data on this topic, and most of this article is based on published case series and survey reports.

Pneumothorax

Pneumothorax is defined as the abnormal presence of air in the pleural cavity. Pneumothorax can occur traumatically by the introduction of ambient air after penetration of the chest wall and pleura or spontaneously. Spontaneous pneumothorax can occur in patients without clinically apparent underlying lung disease (primary spontaneous pneumothorax) or in patients with pulmonary disorders (secondary spontaneous pneumothorax). Secondary spontaneous pneumothorax can occur with virtually any pulmonary disease, but is more common in specific obstructive, interstitial, and infectious lung diseases, such as chronic obstructive pulmonary disease, cystic fibrosis, Langerhans' cell histiocytosis, and *Pneumocystis jiroveci* pneumonia [11–16].

Incidence, recurrence, and clinical presentation

The incidence of pneumothorax in LAM is one of the highest among diseases associated with secondary

---

* Corresponding author.
E-mail address: khalid.almoosa@uc.edu (K.F. Almoosa).

0272-5231/06/$ – see front matter © 2006 Elsevier Inc. All rights reserved.
doi:10.1016/j.ccm.2006.01.005

chestmed.theclinics.com

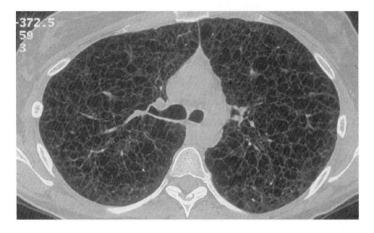

Fig. 1. Chest CT scan of a patient with LAM shows characteristic bilateral cysts of various sizes.

spontaneous pneumothorax (range 39–76%) (Table 1). Pneumothorax frequently is the presenting event that leads to the diagnosis of LAM in affected patients [17–19]. Chu et al [17] reported that pneumothorax was the presenting event leading to the diagnosis of LAM in 15 (63%) of 24 patients with a pneumothorax. Corrin et al [18] reported that 6 (21%) of 28 patients had pneumothorax as a presenting manifestation of LAM. Oh et al [19] reported that 10 (48%) of 21 patients they evaluated had a pneumothorax at presentation; 7 of these 10 patients had recurrent pneumothoraces before the diagnosis of LAM was established. Rarely, bilateral spontaneous pneumothoraces have been reported to be the presenting feature of LAM [20,21]. In a large retrospective study of pneumothorax using the database of the LAM Foundation, Almoosa et al [21] reported that the prevalence of pneumothorax among 395 LAM patients during the course of their disease

was 66% (260 patients). Of the 193 patients who responded to a secondary questionnaire specifically inquiring into the details of their pneumothoraces, most (80%) had developed at least one pneumothorax before their diagnosis of LAM was established (Fig. 3). These patients averaged 2.6 pneumothoraces before diagnosis.

One of the most remarkable characteristics of pneumothorax in LAM is the rate of recurrence (Table 1). Most case series report that most LAM patients developed a recurrent pneumothorax [22–24]. Urban et al [24] reported a recurrence rate of 68% among 69 patients, whereas Taylor et al [23] reported a recurrence in 81% of 32 patients. Not all studies discriminated between ipsilateral and contralateral recurrence, however. In the LAM Foundation study [21], recurrence occurred in 140 (73%) of 193 patients who developed at least one pneumothorax. These recurrences were ipsilateral (71%) and contralateral

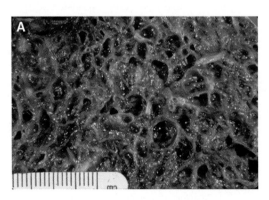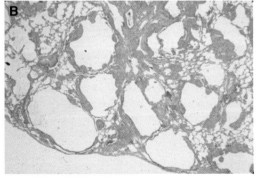

Fig. 2. Gross (A) (From McCormack FX, Sullivan EJ. Lymphangioleiomyomatosis. In: Mason RJ, Murray JF, Courtney V, et al, editors. Murray and Nadel's textbook of respiratory medicine. Fourth Edition. Philadelphia: Harcourt Health Sciences Group; 2005. p. 1706; with permission.) and microscopic (B) appearance of LAM lungs. Multiple cysts throughout both lungs are characteristic of LAM.

Table 1
Prevalence, recurrence rate, and pleurodesis for Pneumothorax during course of lymphangioleiomyomatosis

Author [reference]	No. patients	Incidence of PTX (%)	Recurrence of PTX (%)	No. patients who had pleurodesis (%)
Corrin et al [18]	28	12 (43)	n/a	NA
Taylor et al [23]	32	17 (53)	26 (81)	NA
Kitaichi et al [37]	46	18 (39)	NA	NA
Chu et al [17]	35	24 (69)	NA	19 (54)
Oh et al [19]	21	13 (76)	NA	7 (33)
Urban et al [24]	69	32 (46)	47 (68)	40 (58)
Johnson and Tattersfield [22]	50	30 (60)	23 (46)	NA
Ryu et al [67]	230	128 (56)	NA	NA
Almoosa et al [21]	193	NA	140 (73)	154

Abbreviations: NA, not available; PTX, pneumothorax.

(74%), occurring an average of 21.7 and 30 months after the initial pneumothorax, respectively. Compared with the incidence of recurrence of pneumothorax in other diseases, LAM has the highest rate (Table 2), although the absolute number of pneumothoraces in this patient group is small because of the rarity of the disease. Consistent with the conclusions of the Delphi consensus conference on pneumothorax management, early aggressive intervention is suggested to avoid the morbidity and risk of subsequent pneumothoraces in patients with compromised lung function, although firm evidence to support this approach is lacking [25].

An important alternative diagnosis that must be considered for recurrent pneumothorax in nonsmoking women of childbearing age is catamenial pneumothorax, a spontaneous pneumothorax that occurs during or within 24 to 48 hours of menstruation and is usually, but not always, associated with thoracic endometriosis [26–28]. A high-resolution CT scan that reveals normal lung parenchyma suggests catamenial pneumothorax, whereas the presence of cysts suggests LAM.

The most common presenting symptoms of pneumothorax are dyspnea and chest pain. In the LAM Foundation study [21], most pneumothorax occurred at rest or with minimal activity (81%). Less commonly, pneumothorax occurred during exertion, such as lifting or during exercise. Four patients developed a pneumothorax during pulmonary function testing, where most described feeling a "pop" in the chest. Cough and hemoptysis also may occur in association with pneumothorax in a few cases.

Bilateral simultaneous pneumothorax is an acute and potentially fatal situation that occurs rarely in patients with underlying lung disease. A few case series have described bilateral simultaneous pneumothorax, and most have occurred in patients with

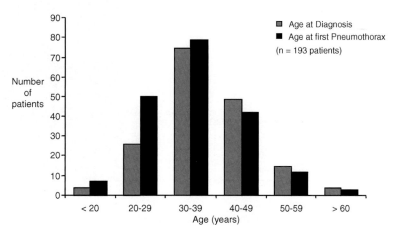

Fig. 3. Age at onset of initial pneumothorax compared with diagnosis of LAM. Most women developed their first pneumothorax before a diagnosis of LAM was established. (*From* Almoosa KF, Ryu JH, Mendez J, et al. Management of pneumothorax in lymphangioleiomyomatosis: effects on recurrence and lung transplantation complications. Chest 2006;129:1277; with permission.)

Table 2
Prevalence and recurrence rates of secondary spontaneous pneumothorax

	Prevalence	Recurrence
PSP	4.3–12/100,000	16–52%
CF (>18 years old)	16–20%	50–78%
LCH	10–28%	25–50%
COPD	26/100,000	39–47%
LAM	64–66%	62–76%

Abbreviations: CF, cystic fibrosis; COPD, chronic obstructive pulmonary disease; LCH, Langerhan's cell histiocytosis; PSP, *Pneumocystis jiroveci* pneumonia.

chronic obstructive pulmonary disease, pulmonary or pleural metastases, Hodgkin's disease, tuberculosis, Langerhans' cell histiocytosis, undefined interstitial lung disease, cystic fibrosis, and LAM [29–31]. Despite the rarity of LAM, it is routinely mentioned in case reports discussing bilateral simultaneous pneumothorax [20,29]. The LAM Foundation study identified 8 (4%) of 193 patients who developed bilateral simultaneous pneumothorax during the course of their disease, with several patients experiencing recurrent bilateral simultaneous pneumothorax [21].

Pathophysiology

The cardinal pathologic feature of LAM is the proliferation of immature smooth muscle cells along the peribronchial, perivascular, and perilymphatic structures [18,32,33]. Compression and obstruction of these conduits result in the development of airflow obstruction and pneumothorax, hemoptysis and alveolar hemorrhage, and chyloptysis and chylothorax, respectively. There is little or no associated inflammation or fibrosis in LAM. Although it is known that smooth muscle cells can infiltrate the pleura, a systematic pathologic study of pleural involvement in LAM has not been reported [34].

Some investigators have suggested that bronchial obstruction by overgrowth of LAM cells is responsible for the obstructive pattern and air trapping (Fig. 4) [2,18,32,33]. It has been postulated that this process ultimately leads to the formation of diffuse, bilateral, thin-walled pulmonary cysts, ranging in size from a few millimeters to a few centimeters in diameter, which are the pathologic and radiographic hallmark of LAM [18,33]. Biopsy specimens also have revealed the presence of a mixed proximal acinar and irregular emphysematous pattern, however, which may be present in areas associated with less affected bronchioles. This finding has led to other theories for the pathogenesis of airflow obstruction, such as the

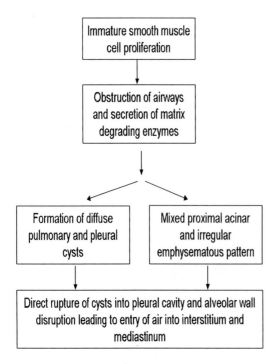

Fig. 4. Pathogenesis of pneumothorax in LAM.

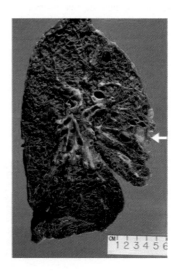

Fig. 5. Lung of LAM patient showing multiple cysts, some of which abut the pleura (*arrow*). (*From* Almoosa KF, Ryu JH, Mendez J, et al. Management of pneumothorax in lymphangioleiomyomatosis: effects on recurrence and lung transplantation complications. Chest 2006;129:1277; with permission.)

destruction of supportive fibers by matrix degrading enzymes resulting in an emphysematous pattern and cyst formation [35,36]. Notwithstanding their origin, these cysts often involve the pleural surface (Fig. 5), and a pneumothorax can occur from their direct rupture into the pleural space or through alveolar wall disruption that allows air to enter the lung interstitium and mediastinum and eventually cause rupture of the mediastinal pleura (Fig. 6).

Radiologic features

The patient's history first suggests the diagnosis of pneumothorax in LAM, and the diagnosis most commonly is confirmed by a standard chest radiograph [17,19,37] showing the classic visceral pleural line that runs parallel to the inner thoracic wall [14]. In some cases, the cystic changes in LAM are apparent on a chest radiograph only when partial collapse secondary to pneumothorax enhances the contrast between lung tissue and airspace. CT more clearly defines the pneumothorax and may show the classic findings of LAM pathology in the unaffected lung [17,24,37]. These findings include reticulonodular shadows, cysts or bullae, and hyperinflation. Incidental small pneumothoraces occasionally are discovered on CT scans performed for other purposes (see Fig. 6B). Pleurodesis complicates the diagnosis and management of pneumothorax in LAM patients. Patients may present with persistent chest pain, shortness of breath, or subcutaneous emphysema in the absence of a radiographically apparent pneumothorax on chest radiograph. CT may show a small loculated pneumothorax in these instances.

Treatment

All LAM patients should be counseled on the symptoms associated with pneumothorax and given explicit instructions to seek medical care when a

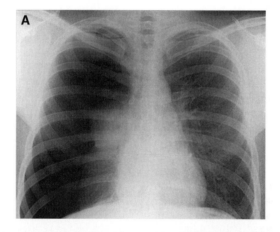

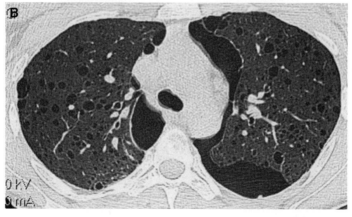

Fig. 6. Chest radiograph (*A*) and CT scan (*B*) show pneumothorax in two patients with LAM. The pneumothorax on chest CT scan was discovered incidentally.

pneumothorax is suspected. The American College of Chest Physicians Delphi Consensus Statement published in 2001 offers recommendations on the optimal approach to the management of spontaneous pneumothorax [23,25]. It states that for small or large secondary spontaneous pneumothoraces, whether stable or unstable, chest tube thoracostomy and hospitalization are recommended. For recurrence prevention, most members of the panel suggested a pleurodesis intervention because of the potential lethality of recurrent pneumothoraces in patients with compromised lung function. The preferred intervention for the lung diseases studied in that report was surgical because it was associated with a lower recurrence rate compared with the instillation of a sclerosant [38]. The authors evaluated failure rates for chemical and surgical pleurodesis in LAM [21].

Nonsurgical treatment options for pneumothorax can be divided into lung expansion therapy (ie, conservative, including observation, simple aspiration, and tube thoracostomy) and interventional therapy (ie, chemical pleurodesis). Surgical options include mechanical pleurodesis, talc poudrage at thoracoscopy and thoracotomy, and partial or complete pleurectomy. For secondary spontaneous pneumothorax in general, surgical interventions have been associated with lower recurrence rates than nonsurgical techniques [39,40]. Limited data address this issue in LAM. Only two studies reported success rates of different interventions for pneumothorax. The LAM Foundation study [21] reported lower failure rates with chemical pleurodesis (27%) and surgery (32%) compared with conservative interventions (66%). Johnson and Tattersfield [22] reported that approximately half (23 of 47, 49%) of the patients treated had a recurrence, with most occurring in patients treated conservatively (20 of 30, 66%) compared with the surgical intervention group (3 of 17, 18%). Although the reason for the poor treatment response for LAM compared with other lung diseases is unclear, it is possible that the dramatic profusion of blebs on the lung surface could limit the apposition of the visceral and parietal pleurae after mechanical abrasion or chemical sclerosant instillation and lead to incomplete fusion.

One of the major conclusions of the LAM Foundation study was that current experience with pneumothorax in LAM supports an early interventional procedure—chemical pleurodesis or surgery—after the first pneumothorax. This recommendation was made because of the high incidence of pneumothorax recurrence and associated morbidity, including a lifelong average of 1 month in the hospital for pneumothorax management in LAM patients who develop an initial pneumothorax (Fig. 7). Most initial pneumothoraces in LAM patients occur before the diagnosis of LAM, however [21,22,24,37]. Patients often experience several pneumothoraces before a diagnosis is established and an intervention is performed. The paucity of data and published literature on this issue is a major impediment to the development of recommendations with a high degree of clinical confidence.

Patient perspectives on interventions for pneumothorax in LAM also have been addressed. In a study by Young et al [41], 314 patients registered with the LAM Foundation were given a questionnaire inquiring into their perspectives regarding different treatment options. Although 41% believed that a previous pneumothorax contributed to the decline in their lung function, and one third made lifestyle modifications to prevent pneumothorax, only 12% worried about

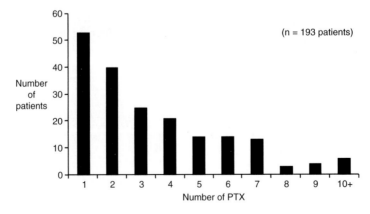

Fig. 7. Recurrence of pneumothorax (PTX) in LAM. Most LAM patients developed multiple pneumothoraces during their lifetime. (*From* Sullivan EJ. Lymphangioleiomyomatosis: a review. Chest 1998;114:1689–703; with permission.)

developing a pneumothorax. Although most patients agreed that pleurodesis helps prevent pneumothorax recurrence, only 25% thought it was appropriate for the first pneumothorax, and only 60% believed it was appropriate for a recurrence. This finding may be related to concerns of extensive and inadequately treated pain associated with chest tube thoracostomy that were reported by the subjects. This study suggests that views between physicians and patients differ regarding the optimal therapy for pneumothorax in LAM, and that patients favor a more conservative approach initially. It remains to be determined whether optimal pain management may change these views.

Effect of treatment on lung transplantation

Interventional approaches for pneumothorax in LAM may affect candidacy and outcomes of lung transplantation. As obstructive lung disease progresses in this population of young, otherwise healthy women, lung transplantation frequently is considered. It is well accepted that prior chemical or surgical pleurodesis increases the risk of perioperative bleeding in any lung transplant recipient [42,43]. LAM patients are prone to pleural complications and often present for consideration for lung transplantation after unilateral or bilateral pleurodesis. It is especially important to understand the consequences of pleural interventions in LAM patients to minimize the impact of pleural manangement decisions on eligibility for lung transplantation.

Few studies have evaluated specifically the outcomes of lung transplantation in LAM patients who have had a pleural symphysis procedure (Table 3). Boehler et al [44] conducted a retrospective survey of 34 LAM patients who underwent lung transplantation at 16 centers in the United States and Europe. Of patients, 27 received single-lung transplants, 6 received bilateral transplants, and 1 received a heart-lung transplant. Of 34 patients, 13 (38%) had previous pleurectomy or pleurodesis. Also, 18 (53%) of 34 patients had extensive pleural adhesions, which

were judged to be of moderate severity in 8 and severe in 10 cases. In addition, 13 (72%) of 18 cases of pleural adhesions were believed to be secondary to the underlying disease because they occurred in patients who had not had previous pleural interventions, whereas the remaining 5 (28%) were due to prior pleurectomy. Moderate-to-severe hemorrhage occurred in four patients, leading to intraoperative death in one patient and repeat thoracotomy in two patients. Overall, post-transplantation survival in this cohort of LAM patients was similar to other chronic lung disease populations. The authors concluded that although perioperative complications do occur in LAM patients who had pleural procedures, lung transplantation remains an important option that improves long-term outcomes.

A study by Pechet et al [45] retrospectively evaluated seven single and seven bilateral lung transplant recipients for LAM. All 14 patients had multiple previous pleurodeses for pleural complications of LAM, and 6 patients had at least one thoracotomy for pleurectomy or bullectomy. Extensive pleural adhesions were present in 10 (71%) of 14 patients, and 7 (50%) experienced blood loss greater than 1000 mL intraoperatively. There were no perioperative deaths. The authors concluded that although perioperative morbidity is common in LAM patients undergoing lung transplantation, early and late survival is comparable to that of lung transplant patients for other diseases.

In the LAM Foundation study [21], 85 registered LAM Foundation patients who received a lung transplant were sent a questionnaire focused on the impact of pleural symphysis on complications arising in the perioperative period. Data from 80 recipients of 81 transplants (1 patient had a re-transplant) were evaluated. In 45 (56%) of 80 patients, chemical or surgical pleurodesis had been performed before the transplant for a pneumothorax or a chylothorax. In 12 (27%) of 45 patients, the side of previous pleural procedure influenced the side of the lung transplant. Fourteen (18%) of 80 patients reported pleural-related bleeding complications perioperatively, 13 (93%) of

Table 3
Lung transplantation, pleurodesis, and perioperative bleeding in lymphangioleiomyomatosis

Author [reference]	No. patients transplanted	No. patients with previous pleurodesis (%)	No. patients with adhesions seen during surgery	No. patients with perioperative bleeding
Pechet et al [45]	14 (7 single, 7 bilateral)	14 (100)	10	7
Boehler et al [44]	34 (27 single, 6 bilateral, 1 heart-lung)	13 (38)	18	4
Almoosa et al [21]	81 (38 single, 43 bilateral)	45 (56)	NA	14

Abbreviation: NA, not available.

whom had previous pleural procedures. Half (7 of 14) of these complications required a return to surgery, and most occurred in patients with previous bilateral pleural procedures. The average length of stay in the group with prior pleural procedures tended to be greater than the group without prior procedures (33.5 ± 5.4 days versus 26.4 ± 6.2 days), although the different was not statistically significant. There were no perioperative deaths. These results indicate that although perioperative complications, bleeding in particular, are common in patients with prior pleural interventions, they are generally manageable.

An ongoing study is evaluating the bias of transplant centers regarding candidacy for transplant in LAM patients who have had previous pleurodesis (Chris Lyons, personal communication, 2005). Of 52 centers evaluated, 22 responded, of which 40% considered previous bilateral pleurodesis with talc or pleurectomy a contraindication to transplant. Paradoxically, most centers (55%) agreed that talc was the preferred agent for pleurodesis for pneumothorax recurrence. In the LAM Foundation study, 43% of patients had bilateral pleurodesis before transplant [21]. This study suggests considerable controversy exists regarding the optimal management for pleural disease in LAM.

Specific situations of pneumothorax in lymphangioleiomyomatosis

The risk of developing a pneumothorax in LAM patients may be increased further during certain activities or specific situations. Air travel poses a potential risk for patients with underlying lung disease. The decrease in partial pressure of oxygen that accompanies the fall in cabin pressure during commercial flights results in several physiologic responses, including hyperventilation, pulmonary vasoconstriction, and an altered ventilation-perfusion ratio, which may place increased demand on the respiratory system [46,47]. Patients with chronic obstructive pulmonary disease may experience hypoxemia during air travel [47,48], and pneumothorax during flight has been reported in patients with underlying lung disease [49–52]. There are no data, however, on the incidence or risk of pneumothorax in LAM patients during flight. Data collected through the LAM Foundation on the incidence of pneumothorax during commercial flight reported a total of 8 (2%) cases of pneumothorax among 395 registered patients (Eugene Sullivan, MD, personal communication, 2005). Without knowing the number of flights, the distances traveled, or the altitudes reached during all trips taken by these patients, no firm conclusions regarding the

risk of flight on the development of pneumothorax in LAM can be reached.

Pregnancy may contribute to an increased risk of pleural complications in LAM. Several investigators have speculated that the elevated hormonal levels associated with pregnancy may accelerate the progression of LAM. The changes in lung volumes and pressures that occur with pregnancy may increase the risk of pleural complications. No published reports specifically describe the prevalence of pneumothorax in pregnant LAM patients. A few subjects reported in two separate LAM cases series developed a pneumothorax during pregnancy, however. Johnson and Tattersfield [22] reported that 7 (14%) of 50 LAM patients studied were pregnant, 3 (43%) of whom developed a pneumothorax during pregnancy. In the 21 patients evaluated by Oh et al [19], all 3 patients who were pregnant developed a pneumothorax during pregnancy. In view of this paucity of data, the LAM Foundation conducted a survey among registered patients inquiring into the incidence and management of pneumothorax during pregnancy (Janet Maurer, MD, MBA, personal communication, 2005). Of the 239 registered women who had at least one pregnancy, 53 (22%) reported complications associated with their pregnancy and received a second questionnaire. Among the 41 respondents, there were a total of 80 pregnancies. Twenty-one patients had a total of 122 pneumothoraces that complicated 49 pregnancies. Of these patients, 16 (76%) experienced their initial pneumothorax during pregnancy, and in 7 it led to the diagnosis of LAM. Ten (48%) of 21 patients eventually required surgical management of pneumothorax, and 13 (62%) pregnancies were delivered by cesarean section because of pneumothorax. Twenty (95%) patients reported that the occurrence of pneumothorax discouraged them from future pregnancies, and 30 (73%) of 41 believed that pregnancy accelerated their pulmonary deterioration. These data suggest that pneumothorax is common in pregnant LAM patients and may influence the mode of delivery and decisions about future pregnancies. In addition, most patients thought that pregnancy accelerated the deterioration of their pulmonary function.

Chylothorax

Chylothorax is defined as the accumulation of chyle in the pleural space [53]. It results from disruption or obstruction of the thoracic duct or its tributaries in the thorax by tumor, trauma, or surgery, leading to leakage of chyle into the thoracic cavity

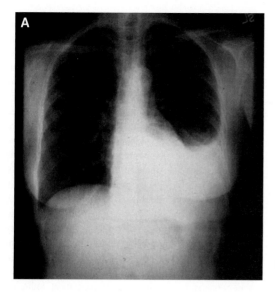
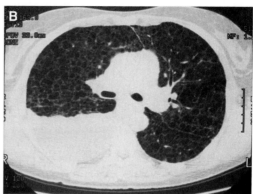

Fig. 8. Chest radiograph (*A*) and CT scan (*B*) (*From* McCormack FX, Sullivan EJ. Lymphangioleiomyomatosis. In: Mason RJ, Murray JF, Courtney V, et al, editors. Murray and Nadel's textbook of respiratory medicine. Fourth Edition. Philadelphia: Harcourt Health Sciences Group; 2005. p. 1708; with permission.) shows chylothoraces in two LAM patients.

[53,54]. Chylothorax also may complicate medical disorders, such as superior vena cava syndrome, lymphatic disorders such as lymphangiomatosis, and yellow nail syndrome [53,55–57]. Chylothorax is a well-recognized complication of LAM (Fig. 8) [17–19,22–24,37,58–67].

Prevalence and clinical presentation

Table 4 summarizes the prevalence of chylothorax in LAM patients based on published reports. Chylothorax is a less common pleural complication of LAM than pneumothorax, with a prevalence of about 20% to 30% among all reported cases. Most

Table 4
Prevalence of chylothorax during course of lymphangioleiomyomatosis

Author [reference]	No. patients	Prevalence of chylothorax (%)
Corrin et al [18]	28	11 (39)
Taylor et al [23]	32	9 (28)
Kitaichi et al [37]	46	3 (7)
Chu et al [17]	35	8 (23)
Oh et al [19]	21	0
Urban et al [24]	69	20 (29)
Johnson and Tattersfield [22]	50	11 (22)
Ryu et al [69]	79	8 (10)
Ryu et al [67]	230	48 (21)
Total	**590**	**118 (20)**

chylothoraces are unilateral with no side preference, and most are large enough to require intervention [58,64,65,68–70]. Reports often describe the occurrence of a pneumothorax or a chylothorax complicating LAM, but these two complications rarely seem to occur simultaneously. Abdominal involvement in patients with chylothorax also may be present, manifesting as chylous ascites and lymphadenopathy [66,71–73]. The clinical presentation of chylothorax almost invariably includes progressive dyspnea, but this may be a manifestation of the underlying lung disease and the pleural effusion. Chest pain, cough, and chyloptysis also may occur. In a retrospective review of 79 LAM patients, Ryu et al [69] identified 8 (10%) who developed a chylothorax. The average age at presentation of chylothorax in these LAM patients was 41.1 years compared with the average age for diagnosis of LAM of 34 years. The occurrence of chylothorax in these patients did not correlate with the extent of lung involvement.

Pathophysiology and diagnosis

Chylothorax in LAM most likely results from obstruction of lymphatic vessels by infiltration of smooth muscle cells. Lymphangiography has shown that obstruction occurs at several different levels, causing chyle leakage to occur on the surface of the lung, pleura, and mediastinum [18,70,74]. A histologic section of the thoracic duct in a LAM patient typically reveals a grossly enlarged duct containing proliferating smooth muscle cells [75]. Evidence suggests that lymphangiogenesis plays a role in disease progression. Kumasaka et al [76] used immunohistochemistry to identify VEGFR-3, a vascular endothelial growth factor (VEGF) receptor and specific marker for lymphatic endothelial cells, and VEGF-C, a lymphatic-specific VEGF, in specimens obtained from autopsy and surgical cases. They concluded that lymphatics were extremely abundant in pulmonary and extrapulmonary LAM, and lymphangiogenesis was abundant in vascular walls and interstitium surrounding the area where LAM cells were proliferating. In addition, a significant correlation was noted between the degree of lymphangiogenesis in LAM or VEGF-C expression on LAM cells and the LAM histologic score, which represents the histologic severity of pulmonary LAM, a prognostic indicator. Chylothorax also may develop through transdiaphragmatic flow of chylous ascites. Thoracic and abdominal lymphadenopathy may be present [17] and reveal proliferating smooth muscle cells [75]. Globular collections of HMB 45–positive cells can be found in the pleural fluid [77,78]. In a subsequent study, Kumasaka et al [79] further showed that these clusters of LAM cells are enveloped by VEGF-positive lymphatic endothelial cells, and that the shedding of these structures into the lymphatic circulation may play a central role in the dissemination of LAM lesions.

The diagnosis of chylothorax should be entertained when a LAM patient presents with a pleural effusion on a chest radiograph. Although most pleural effusions in LAM are chylothoraces [2,17,70,80], diagnostic thoracentesis should be performed to confirm the diagnosis. A triglyceride level greater than 110 mg/dL makes the diagnosis highly likely, and the presence of chylomicrons on lipoprotein electrophoresis is confirmatory if the triglyceride concentration is less than 110 mg/dL. Radionuclide or contrast lymphangiography may be used to locate the site of thoracic duct obstruction [81,82].

Treatment

Management of chylothorax in LAM is no different than for other diseases [53,54,83]. Although the treatment of the underlying cause may help in treating chylothorax in other diseases, it is problematic in LAM because there is no effective therapy for LAM. Management is based on clinical experience and anecdotal reports. Nonoperative management, consisting of aspiration or thoracostomy tube drainage, often is done initially to re-expand the lung and improve symptoms. Because there is a high risk of nutritional

depletion with persistent drainage, careful monitoring of the patient's weight, serum prealbumin and albumin, total protein, absolute lymphocyte count, and electrolyte levels is essential [54,84]. The nutritional approach to chylothorax involves substitution of long-chain dietary fat with medium-chain triglycerides, which do not become incorporated into chylomicrons. Dietary supplements can be oral or intravenous. Hyperalimentation with medium-chain triglyceride supplementation can shorten the duration of the chylous effusion [22,70,85], although variable degrees of success have been reported in adults [86]. Similarly, total parenteral nutrition has been used to replete nutrients and decrease chyle formation in persistently draining effusions and is generally more effective than dietary modification [87]. Improvements in the formulation and delivery of total parenteral nutrition have improved the safety and reliability of this mode of supplementation, although it remains costly [88].

Nonoperative drainage may be useful initially to improve symptoms, but many patients eventually require a chemical or surgical pleurodesis procedure [22,69]. This intervention seems to be more successful at preventing recurrences of chylothorax than drainage alone [10,70,89–91]. In the series by Ryu et al [69], four of five patients with recurrent chylothorax were treated successfully with pleurodesis. Thoracic duct ligation [10,70,92,93] and the placement of a LeVeen shunt [24] have been attempted, with variable success.

Hormonal therapy has been used to treat LAM lung disease with mixed results [94–97]. Some studies have reported that medroxyprogesterone therapy has been useful in treating chylothorax that complicates LAM [23,37,69]. Taylor et al [23] found that most patients whose LAM improved with medroxyprogesterone therapy had chylothorax or chylous ascites present. The authors postulated that the presence of chylothorax seemed to be a marker for clinical response and might reflect a reversible element in the LAM-affected lung. Octreotide, a long-acting somatostatin analogue, also has been reported to be effective in treating persistent chylothorax in several case reports [98–102]. Octreotide reduces the thoracic duct flow and triglyceride levels and may be particularly effective when combined with a reduction in oral intake.

Summary

LAM is a rare, gender-restricted interstitial lung disease that causes significant morbidity and mortality. Pneumothorax or chylothorax occurs during the course of illness in most patients. The incidence of secondary spontaneous pneumothorax in LAM is among the highest of all chronic lung diseases and may result in considerable morbidity. The effect of pneumothorax and chylothorax on disease progression and prognosis is unknown, however. Most patients require a definitive chemical or surgical pleurodesis procedure for pneumothorax and chylothorax to prevent recurrences. The optimal procedure and timing of therapy is unknown, however, and the failure rate for pleurodesis is high. The management of pneumothorax and chylothorax in LAM has important consequences for subsequent lung transplantation. The frequency of pneumothorax in LAM and the cohesiveness of the LAM patient community facilitate the study of pleural disease. Properly designed clinical studies are needed to answer important questions in the diagnosis and treatment of pleural complications in LAM.

References

[1] Kalassian KG, Doyle R, Kao P, et al. Lymphangioleiomyomatosis: new insights. Am J Respir Crit Care Med 1997;155:1183–6.

[2] Sullivan EJ. Lymphangioleiomyomatosis: a review. Chest 1998;114:1689–703.

[3] Tattersfield AE, Harrison TW. Step 3 of the asthma guidelines. Thorax 1999;54:753–4.

[4] Lutembacher R. Dysembryomes metatypique des reins: carcinose submiliare aigue du poumon avec emphyseme generalise et double pneumothorax. Ann Med 1918;5:435–50.

[5] Castro M, Shepherd CW, Gomez MR, et al. Pulmonary tuberous sclerosis. Chest 1995;107:189–95.

[6] Dwyer JM, Hickie JB, Garvan J. Pulmonary tuberous sclerosis: report of three patients and a review of the literature. QJM 1971;40:115–25.

[7] Hauck RW, Konig G, Permanetter W, et al. Tuberous sclerosis with pulmonary involvement. Respiration (Herrlisheim) 1990;57:289–92.

[8] Uzzo RG, Libby DM, Vaughan Jr ED, Levey SH. Coexisting lymphangioleiomyomatosis and bilateral angiomyolipomas in a patient with tuberous sclerosis. J Urol 1994;151:1612–5.

[9] Valensi QJ. Pulmonary lymphangiomyoma, a probable forme frust of tuberous sclerosis: a case report and survey of the literature. Am Rev Respir Dis 1973; 108:1411–5.

[10] Cornog Jr JL, Enterline HT. Lymphangiomyoma, a benign lesion of chyliferous lymphatics synonymous with lymphangiopericytoma. Cancer 1966;19:1909–30.

[11] Flume PA. Pneumothorax in cystic fibrosis. Chest 2003;123:217–21.

[12] Mitchell-Heggs PF. Spontaneous pneumothorax in cystic fibrosis. Thorax 1970;25:256–7.

[13] Penketh AR, Knight RK, Hodson ME, Batten JC. Management of pneumothorax in adults with cystic fibrosis. Thorax 1982;37:850–3.

[14] Sahn SA, Heffner JE. Spontaneous pneumothorax. N Engl J Med 2000;342:868–74.

[15] Sassoon CS. The etiology and treatment of spontaneous pneumothorax. Curr Opin Pulm Med 1995;1: 331–8.

[16] Yoshida S, Yamagishi T, Fukutake K, et al. [Thoracotomy as treatment for pneumothorax associated with Pneumocystic carinii pneumonia in a patient with hemophilia A and the acquired immunodeficiency syndrome]. Nihon Kyobu Shikkan Gakkai Zasshi 1995;33:1464–8.

[17] Chu SC, Horiba K, Usuki J, et al. Comprehensive evaluation of 35 patients with lymphangioleiomyomatosis. Chest 1999;115:1041–52.

[18] Corrin B, Liebow AA, Friedman PJ. Pulmonary lymphangiomyomatosis: a review. Am J Pathol 1975; 79:348–82.

[19] Oh YM, Mo EK, Jang SH, et al. Pulmonary lymphangioleiomyomatosis in Korea. Thorax 1999;54: 618–21.

[20] Berkman N, Bloom A, Cohen P, et al. Bilateral spontaneous pneumothorax as the presenting feature in lymphangioleiomyomatosis. Respir Med 1995;89: 381–3.

[21] Almoosa KF, Ryu J, Mendez J, et al. Management of pneumothorax in lymphangioleiomyomatosis: effects on recurrence and lung transplantation complications. Chest 2006, in press.

[22] Johnson SR, Tattersfield AE. Clinical experience of lymphangioleiomyomatosis in the UK. Thorax 2000; 55:1052–7.

[23] Taylor JR, Ryu J, Colby TV, Raffin TA. Lymphangioleiomyomatosis: clinical course in 32 patients. N Engl J Med 1990;323:1254–60.

[24] Urban T, Lazor R, Lacronique J, et al. Pulmonary lymphangioleiomyomatosis: a study of 69 patients. Groupe d'Etudes et de Recherche sur les Maladies "Orphelines" Pulmonaires (GERM"O"P). Medicine (Baltimore) 1999;78:321–37.

[25] Baumann MH, Strange C, Heffner JE, et al. Management of spontaneous pneumothorax: an American College of Chest Physicians Delphi consensus statement. Chest 2001;119:590–602.

[26] Johnson MM. Catamenial pneumothorax and other thoracic manifestations of endometriosis. Clin Chest Med 2004;25:311–9.

[27] Korom S, Canyurt H, Missbach A, et al. Catamenial pneumothorax revisited: clinical approach and systematic review of the literature. J Thorac Cardiovasc Surg 2004;128:502–8.

[28] Peikert T, Gillespie DJ, Cassivi SD. Catamenial pneumothorax. Mayo Clin Proc 2005;80:677–80.

[29] Graf-Deuel E, Knoblauch A. Simultaneous bilateral spontaneous pneumothorax. Chest 1994;105:1142–6.

[30] Sayar A, Turna A, Metin M, et al. Simultaneous bilateral spontaneous pneumothorax report of 12 cases and review of the literature. Acta Chir Belg 2004;104: 572–6.

[31] Sunam G, Gok M, Ceran S, Solak H. Bilateral pneumothorax: a retrospective analysis of 40 patients. Surg Today 2004;34:817–21.

[32] Sobonya RE, Quan SF, Fleishman JS. Pulmonary lymphangioleiomyomatosis: quantitative analysis of lesions producing airflow limitation. Hum Pathol 1985;16:1122–8.

[33] Carrington CB, Cugell DW, Gaensler EA, et al. Lymphangioleiomyomatosis: physiologic-pathologic-radiologic correlations. Am Rev Respir Dis 1977; 116:977–95.

[34] Louis H, Los H, Lagendijk JH, et al. [Spontaneous pneumothorax in young women: possible lymphangioleiomyomatosis]. Ned Tijdschr Geneeskd 1997; 141:1924–8.

[35] Fukuda Y, Kawamoto M, Yamamoto A, et al. Role of elastic fiber degradation in emphysema-like lesions of pulmonary lymphangiomyomatosis. Hum Pathol 1990;21:1252–61.

[36] Hayashi T, Fleming MV, Stetler-Stevenson WG, et al. Immunohistochemical study of matrix metalloproteinases (MMPs) and their tissue inhibitors (TIMPs) in pulmonary lymphangioleiomyomatosis (LAM). Hum Pathol 1997;28:1071–8.

[37] Kitaichi M, Nishimura K, Itoh H, et al. Pulmonary lymphangioleiomyomatosis: a report of 46 patients including a clinicopathologic study of prognostic factors. Am J Respir Crit Care Med 1995;151(2 Pt 1): 527–33.

[38] Baumann MH, Strange C. Treatment of spontaneous pneumothorax: a more aggressive approach? Chest 1997;112:789–804.

[39] Hatz RA, Kaps MF, Meimarakis G, et al. Long-term results after video-assisted thoracoscopic surgery for first-time and recurrent spontaneous pneumothorax. Ann Thorac Surg 2000;70:253–7.

[40] Massard G, Thomas P, Wihlm JM. Minimally invasive management for first and recurrent pneumothorax. Ann Thorac Surg 1998;66:592–9.

[41] Young LR, Almoosa KF, Pollock-BarZiv S, et al. Patient perspectives on management of pneumothorax in lymphangioleiomyomatosis. Chest 2006, in press.

[42] Curtis HJ, Bourke SJ, Dark JH, et al. Lung transplantation outcome in cystic fibrosis patients with previous pneumothorax. J Heart Lung Transplant 2005;24:865–9.

[43] Judson MA, Sahn SA. The pleural space and organ transplantation. Am J Respir Crit Care Med 1996; 153:1153–65.

[44] Boehler A, Speich R, Russi EW, et al. Lung transplantation for lymphangioleiomyomatosis. N Engl J Med 1996;335:1275–80.

[45] Pechet TT, Meyers BF, Guthrie TJ, et al. Lung transplantation for lymphangioleiomyomatosis. J Heart Lung Transplant 2004;23:301–8.

[46] Mortazavi A, Eisenberg MJ, Langleben D, et al. Altitude-related hypoxia: risk assessment and management for passengers on commercial aircraft. Aviat Space Environ Med 2003;74:922–7.

[47] Gendreau MA, DeJohn C. Responding to medical events during commercial airline flights. N Engl J Med 2002;346:1067–73.

[48] Christensen CC, Ryg M, Refvem OK, et al. Development of severe hypoxaemia in chronic obstructive pulmonary disease patients at 2,438 m (8,000 ft) altitude. Eur Respir J 2000;15:635–9.

[49] Cheatham ML, Safcsak K. Air travel following traumatic pneumothorax: when is it safe? Am Surg 1999; 65:1160–4.

[50] Flux M, Dille JR. Inflight spontaneous pneumothorax: a case report. Aerosp Med 1969;40:660–2.

[51] Haid MM, Paladini P, Maccherini M, et al. Air transport and the fate of pneumothorax in pleural adhesions. Thorax 1992;47:833–4.

[52] Ho BL. A case report of spontaneous pneumothorax during flight. Aviat Space Environ Med 1975;46: 840–1.

[53] Doerr CH, Miller DL, Ryu JH. Chylothorax. Semin Respir Crit Care Med 2001;22:617–26.

[54] Valentine VG, Raffin TA. The management of chylothorax. Chest 1992;102:586–91.

[55] Doerr CH, Allen MS, Nichols III FC, et al. Etiology of chylothorax in 203 patients. Mayo Clin Proc 2005; 80:867–70.

[56] Tanaka E, Matsumoto K, Shindo T, et al. Implantation of a pleurovenous shunt for massive chylothorax in a patient with yellow nail syndrome. Thorax 2005;60: 254–5.

[57] Valmary J, Delbrouck P, Herning R, et al. [Yellow nail syndrome with chylous effusions]. Rev Med Interne 1988;9:425–8.

[58] Adachi H, Hashimoto T, Komiyama M, et al. [Lymphangioleiomyomatosis (LAM) causing chylothorax]. Nihon Kokyuki Gakkai Zasshi 2004;42:80–3.

[59] Bjorn-Hansen L, Larsen KE. [Lymphangioleiomyomatosis as the cause of chylothorax]. Ugeskr Laeger 1988;150:28–9.

[60] Buhl L, Larsen KE, Bjorn-Hansen L. Lymphangioleiomyomatosis: is fine needle aspiration cytodiagnosis possible? Acta Cytol 1988;32:559–62.

[61] Chuang ML, Tsai YH, Pang LC. Early chylopneumothorax in a patient with pulmonary lymphangioleiomyomatosis. J Formos Med Assoc 1993;92: 278–82.

[62] Gong JH, Gao L, Zhang LY. [Pulmonary lymphangiomyomatosis: report of a case]. Zhonghua Nei Ke Za Zhi 1993;32:313–5.

[63] Itami M, Teshima S, Asakuma Y, et al. Pulmonary lymphangiomyomatosis diagnosed by effusion cytology: a case report. Acta Cytol 1997;41:522–8.

[64] Kaptanoglu M, Hatipoglu A, Kutluay L, et al. Bilateral chylothorax caused by pleuropulmonary lymphangiomyomatosis: a challenging problem in thoracic surgery. Scand Cardiovasc J 2001;35:151–4.

[65] Morimoto N, Hirasaki S, Kamei T, et al. Pulmonary lymphangiomyomatosis (LAM) developing chylothorax. Intern Med 2000;39:738–41.

[66] Yamauchi M, Nakahara H, Uyama K, et al. Cytologic finding of chyloascites in lymphangioleiomyomatosis: a case report. Acta Cytol 2000;44:1081–4.

[67] Ryu JH, Moss J, Beck GJ, et al. The NHLBI Lymphangioleiomyomatosis Registry: characteristics of 230 patients at enrollment. Am J Respir Crit Care Med 2006;173(1):105–11.

[68] Miller WT, Cornog Jr JL, Sullivan MA. Lymphangiomyomatosis: a clinical-roentgenologic-pathologic syndrome. Am J Roentgenol Radium Ther Nucl Med 1971;111:565–72.

[69] Ryu JH, Doerr CH, Fisher SD, et al. Chylothorax in lymphangioleiomyomatosis. Chest 2003;123:623–7.

[70] Silverstein EF, Ellis K, Wolff M, et al. Pulmonary lymphangiomyomatosis. Am J Roentgenol Radium Ther Nucl Med 1974;120:832–50.

[71] Avila NA, Kelly JA, Chu SC, et al. Lymphangioleiomyomatosis: abdominopelvic CT and US findings. Radiology 2000;216:147–53.

[72] Pallisa E, Sanz P, Roman A, et al. Lymphangioleiomyomatosis: pulmonary and abdominal findings with pathologic correlation. Radiographics 2002; 22(Spec No):S185–98.

[73] Schneider AR, Jacobi V, Achenbach HJ, Caspary WF. [Lymphangioleiomyomatosis (LAM): a rare cause of ascites and pleural effusion]. Dtsch Med Wochenschr 2004;129:1375–8.

[74] Merchant RN, Pearson MG, Rankin RN, et al. Computerized tomography in the diagnosis of lymphangioleiomyomatosis. Am Rev Respir Dis 1985;131: 295–7.

[75] Graham ML, Spelsberg TC, Dines DE, et al. Pulmonary lymphangiomyomatosis: with particular reference to steroid-receptor assay studies and pathologic correlation. Mayo Clin Proc 1984;59:3–11.

[76] Kumasaka T, Seyama K, Mitani K, et al. Lymphangiogenesis in lymphangioleiomyomatosis: its implication in the progression of lymphangioleiomyomatosis. Am J Surg Pathol 2004;28:1007–16.

[77] Longacre TA, Hendrickson MR, Kapp DS, et al. Lymphangioleiomyomatosis of the uterus simulating high-stage endometrial stromal sarcoma. Gynecol Oncol 1996;63:404–10.

[78] Matsui K, Tatsuguchi A, Valencia J, et al. Extrapulmonary lymphangioleiomyomatosis (LAM): clinicopathologic features in 22 cases. Hum Pathol 2000; 31:1242–8.

[79] Kumasaka T, Seyama K, Mitani K, et al. Lymphangiogenesis-mediated shedding of LAM cell clusters as a mechanism for dissemination in lymphangioleiomyomatosis. Am J Surg Pathol 2005;29:1356–66.

[80] Johnson S. Rare diseases. 1. Lymphangioleiomyomatosis: clinical features, management and basic mechanisms. Thorax 1999;54:254–64.

[81] Teba L, Dedhia HV, Bowen R, et al. Chylothorax review. Crit Care Med 1985;13:49–52.

[82] Thambo JB, Jimenez M, Jougon J, et al. [Diagnostic and therapeutic value of lymphography in persistent postoperative chylothorax]. Arch Mal Coeur Vaiss 2004;97:546–8.

[83] Paes ML, Powell H. Chylothorax: an update. Br J Hosp Med 1994;51:482–90.

[84] Johnstone DW, Feins RH. Chylothorax. Chest Surg Clin N Am 1994;4:617–28.

[85] Hashim SA, Roholt HB, Babayan VK, et al. Treatment of chyluria and chylothorax with medium-chain triglyceride. N Engl J Med 1964;270:756–61.

[86] Jensen GL, Mascioli EA, Meyer LP, et al. Dietary modification of chyle composition in chylothorax. Gastroenterology 1989;97:761–5.

[87] Ramos W, Faintuch J. Nutritional management of thoracic duct fistulas: a comparative study of parenteral versus enteral nutrition. JPEN J Parenter Enteral Nutr 1986;10:519–21.

[88] Sassoon CS, Light RW. Chylothorax and pseudochylothorax. Clin Chest Med 1985;6:163–71.

[89] Hughes E, Hodder RV. Pulmonary lymphangiomyomatosis complicating pregnancy. A case report. J Reprod Med 1987;32:553–7.

[90] Lieberman J, Agliozzo CM. Intrapleural nitrogen mustard for treating chylous effusion of pulmonary lymphangioleiomyomatosis. Cancer 1974;33: 1505–11.

[91] Luna CM, Gene R, Jolly EC, et al. Pulmonary lymphangiomyomatosis associated with tuberous sclerosis: treatment with tamoxifen and tetracycline-pleurodesis. Chest 1985;88:473–5.

[92] Pamukcoglu T. Lymphangiomyoma of the thoracic duct with honeycomb lungs. Am Rev Respir Dis 1968;97:295–301.

[93] Bush JK, McLean RL, Sieker HO. Diffuse lung disease due to lymphangiomyoma. Am J Med 1969;46: 645–54.

[94] Johnson SR, Tattersfield AE. Decline in lung function in lymphangioleiomyomatosis: relation to menopause and progesterone treatment. Am J Respir Crit Care Med 1999;160:628–33.

[95] Rossi GA, Balbi B, Oddera S, et al. Response to treatment with an analog of the luteinizing-hormone-releasing hormone in a patient with pulmonary lymphangiomyomatosis. Am Rev Respir Dis 1991;143: 174–6.

[96] Seyama K, Kira S, Takahashi H, et al. Longitudinal follow-up study of 11 patients with pulmonary lymphangioleiomyomatosis: diverse clinical courses of LAM allow some patients to be treated without anti-hormone therapy. Respirology 2001;6: 331–40.

[97] Taveira-DaSilva AM, Stylianou MP, Hedin CJ, et al. Decline in lung function in patients with lymphangioleiomyomatosis treated with or without progesterone. Chest 2004;126:1867–74.

[98] Al Zubairy SA, Al Jazairi AS. Octreotide as a therapeutic option for management of chylothorax. Ann Pharmacother 2003;37:679–82.

[99] Demos NJ, Kozel J, Scerbo JE. Somatostatin in the treatment of chylothorax. Chest 2001;119:964–6.

[100] Evans J, Clark MF, Mincher L, et al. Chylous effusions complicating lymphoma: a serious event with octreotide as a treatment option. Hematol Oncol 2003;21:77–81.

[101] Gabbieri D, Bavutti L, Zaca F, et al. Conservative treatment of postoperative chylothorax with octreotide. Ital Heart J 2004;5:479–82.

[102] Leelahanon S, Petlek W, Sontimuang W, et al. Can octreotide be the first line treatment for chylothorax? J Med Assoc Thai 2003;86(Suppl 3):S741–5.

ELSEVIER
SAUNDERS

Clin Chest Med 27 (2006) 369 – 381

CLINICS
IN CHEST
MEDICINE

Management of Spontaneous Pneumothorax

Michael H. Baumann, MD

Division of Pulmonary, Critical Care, and Sleep Medicine, University of Mississippi Medical Center, 2500 North State Street, Jackson, MS 39216, USA

Pneumothoraces are classified as spontaneous or nonspontaneous [1–4]. Spontaneous pneumothoraces (SP) occur without an obvious preceding cause, including trauma. Nonspontaneous pneumothoraces are due to trauma and may be iatrogenic. SP occurring in a patient with no underlying lung disease is termed "primary spontaneous pneumothorax" (PSP). "Secondary spontaneous pneumothoraces" (SSP) develop in the presence of an underlying lung condition, including chronic obstructive pulmonary disease (COPD), cystic fibrosis, or *Pneumocystis jerovici* (formerly *Pneumocystis carinii*) pneumonia.

Incidence, recurrence rates, and mortality

More than 20,000 new cases of SP occur each year in the United States [5] at a cost of more than $130 million [6]. The incidence of PSP versus SSP in the United States is roughly equal [5]. The combined rate of PSP and SSP patients appearing for evaluation in the United Kingdom is approximately 24 patients per 100,000 population per year [7]. The US age-adjusted incidence of PSP is 7.4 and 1.2 per 100,000 per year for men and women, respectively. For SSP, the incidence is 6.3 and 2 per 100,000 per year for men and women, respectively [5].

Recurrence rates are a central consideration when selecting management choices. Reported recurrence rates for PSP and SSP vary widely in the literature partly as a result of differences in follow-up duration

and treatment choices [3,6,8–10]. The largest randomized controlled trial assessing SP recurrence prevention by chest tube–directed tetracycline noted recurrence rates of 31.8% in PSP and 43% in SSP patients not undergoing recurrence prevention. Most recurrences in PSP and SSP patients, without recurrence intervention, occur in the first 6 months. Notably, there were 86 patients in the SSP group, but only 22 in the PSP group without tetracycline recurrence prevention efforts [11]. A compilation of 11 studies (including the aforementioned large study) may present a more accurate assessment of PSP recurrence and highlights the reported recurrence variability. These compilation data noted a recurrence rate range of 16% to 52% with a mean recurrence rate of 30% in PSP patients without definitive prevention [12]. Independent risk predictors for recurrent SP include the presence of pulmonary fibrosis, age 60 years or older, and increased height-to-weight ratio [10].

Death rarely occurs in the setting of PSP [6,13]. In SP patients aged 15 to 34 years, a group most likely representing largely PSP patients, the mortality rate is reported to be 0.09% for men and 0.06% for women [7]. By contrast, SSP occurrence is far more life-threatening as a result of compromise of pulmonary reserve from the underlying precipitating lung disease. COPD is a common cause of SSP [4], with age-matched COPD patients having a 3.5-fold increase in relative mortality with SP occurrence [9]. COPD-related SSP reported morality rates vary from 1% to 17% [11,14–16]. One study noted that 5% of COPD-related SP patients died before definitive treatment [16]. Mortality in SP patients age 55 years or older, likely representing mostly SSP patients, is 1.8% in men and 3.3% in women [7].

E-mail address: mbaumann@medicine.umsmed.edu

0272-5231/06/$ – see front matter © 2006 Elsevier Inc. All rights reserved.
doi:10.1016/j.ccm.2005.12.006

History, clinical presentation, physical examination, and diagnosis

Most commonly, PSP patients present with ipsilateral pleuritic chest pain and dyspnea [4,17,18]. Asymptomatic patients with PSP may be found during routine medical examination and during evaluation for other diseases [19,20]. Most episodes occur while the patient is at rest [4,18,21]. An ectomorphic body type and smoking are associated with the development of PSP [17]. A study of primarily male PSP patients noted that patients are on average taller (2 inches taller) and thinner (10 lb underweight) compared with reference averages of height and weight [22]. Tachycardia is the most common physical finding [4]. The larger the pneumothorax, the more likely findings may include decreased movement of the chest wall, hyperresonance to percussion, diminished fremitus, and decreased breath sounds on the affected side [4].

Although SSP may be precipitated by a myriad of underlying lung diseases, dyspnea, often severe and out of proportion to the size of the pneumothorax, is nearly universal [4,14–17]. COPD is the most common cause of SSP [4,17]. In COPD patients with SSP, hypoxemia and hypotension may be severe [14–16]. Physical examination detection of pneumothorax relying on findings of ipsilateral decreased breath sounds and tactile fremitus and hyperresonance may be unreliable because these findings already may exist owing to the patient's underlying COPD [16].

Given the nonspecific signs and symptoms associated with a pneumothorax, diagnosis requires suspicion and a low threshold for obtaining a confirmatory chest radiograph [23]. Identification of the visceral pleural line displaced from the chest wall on an upright chest radiograph is the key to diagnosis [4]. Use of an expiratory chest radiograph adds little diagnostic sensitivity over a routine inspiratory film [24,25]. More recent guidelines do not recommend expiratory chest films for the routine diagnosis of pneumothorax [26]. The most important differential diagnosis, particularly in patients with SSP secondary to COPD (emphysema), is the distinction of a pneumothorax from a large thin-walled, air-containing cyst or giant bulla [16]. CT may be required to differentiate a pneumothorax from a giant bulla [26,27].

Some clinicians advocate using the chest radiograph to calculate the percentage size of the pneumothorax to determine a management strategy [3,8]. Although estimation of size by such formulas may be accurate in PSP [28], abnormal collapse of the lung in the presence of emphysema-induced SSP [15] may preclude accurate calculations. Minimal underlying lung disease in PSP patients allowing uniform collapse may permit formulas to predict the percentage of lung collapse. More accurate CT estimates of pneumothorax collapse compared with the chest radiograph highlight, however, the poor prediction of chest radiograph–calculated pneumothorax size and concerns for asymmetric collapse of the lung in SP patients [29]. These vagaries highlight the need to focus not on calculating the size of the SP, but instead on the patient's clinical status to determine management interventions [6,26,29,30].

Pathophysiology

Primary spontaneous pneumothorax

On closer scrutiny, the definition of PSP as SP that occurs in a patient with no underlying lung disease may be misleading and confusing. Perhaps a better definition would be that PSP are SP occurring in patients without an immediately obvious underlying lung disease [31]. A strong etiologic association has been made between emphysema-like changes (ELC) (blebs and bullae) and the occurrence of PSP; the strongest evidence for that association may be found by CT [31]. Bense and colleagues [32] found on CT that 81% of non–α_1-antitrypsin-deficient PSP patients have ELC, whereas normal controls had no such changes. CT showed that ELC often are bilateral and located predominantly in the upper lung zones [32–36]. ELC may predict the likelihood of PSP occurrence [32]. Warner and colleagues [36] prospectively found a CT-derived ELC score in the ipsilateral lung to be significantly greater in PSP patients with recurrence. Sihoe and colleagues [37,38] noted a significant association of CT-detected lung bullae in the contralateral lung after unilateral PSP and a higher rate of subsequent pneumothorax occurrence in the contralateral hemithorax. At least two CT studies cast doubt on the potential association of ELC and the development of PSP [35,39]. The study by Mitlehner and colleagues [35] was uncontrolled, and the CT evaluation was suboptimal. The second study by Smit and colleagues [39] employed a potentially flawed study premise that a higher incidence of ELC should be noted in patients with recurrence compared with patients with a first-time PSP [31,40]. The surgical literature provides additional support for the potential etiologic association between ELC and PSP occurrence. In reports separating PSP from SSP patients, ELC are found in at least 75% [41] to 84% [42] of PSP patients undergoing video-assisted thoracoscopic surgery (VATS).

The ectomorphic physique often noted in PSP patients is present from childhood and driven primarily by the patient's greater than average height, which is particularly prominent in the early teen years. The patient's rapid increase in vertical size of the thorax may affect intrathoracic pressure at the lung apex and drive subpleural cyst formation (ELC formation) [43]. Familial patterns of inheritance, although uncommon, continue to be reported in patients with PSP [44]. Included in reports is an autosomal dominant pattern with the case made that such affected patients may have an unrecognized connective tissue disorder [45]. This begs the question: Could such disorders drive ELC formation? An X-linked recessive pattern of disease also is reported; however, episodes of PSP per patient seem more common in an autosomal dominant form with incomplete penetrance [46]. Other genetic associations have been reported more recently, including FBN1 gene mutations as causative [47], certain causative HLA haplotypes [48], and an autosomal recessive inheritance pattern [49]. Given these continuing reports, questions regarding familial occurrences should be a routine part of the history in patients with PSP.

Smoking has been implicated strongly in the pathogenesis of PSP and is associated with a ninefold or greater risk of developing a first PSP [50]. Respiratory bronchiolitis in smokers may be the pathologic driving process in PSP [51]. Respiratory bronchiolitis is found in more than 88% of smokers operated on for PSP when blebs, bullae, or areas of air leaks were surgically resected. Despite the known association, more than 80% of PSP patients informed of the risk of smoking continue smoking [52].

Despite the strong evidence that ELC cause PSP, other authors make the case that ELC are not the sole cause or are not causative at all [12,39,53–55]. Core to this argument is that an air leak is not observed at the site of a ruptured ELC in every patient undergoing surgical intervention. The incidence is noted to vary widely from 3.6% to 73%. Additionally, air leakage can be present in lung areas where no ELC are seen. This observation has led to the concept of "pleural porosity" as a factor in air leakage in PSP [53,54]. Fluorescein-enhanced autofluorescence thoracoscopy has been reported as a tool to identify areas of potentially abnormal pleural surfaces not associated with ELC. Further study is needed to determine if autofluorescing areas truly represent areas of abnormality [56].

Such debate is not merely academic. Optimal recurrence prevention intervention must address potential etiologic issues effectively. As discussed subsequently, various recurrence prevention options

are available, with surgical options often focused on removal of ELC (blebs and bullae). The evidence to date for ELC as the cause of PSP is circumstantial, and ELC may not be the sole etiologic factor. ELC are the most immediately obvious cause of PSP, however, and cannot and should not be ignored, unless compelling evidence develops to the contrary [31].

Secondary spontaneous pneumothorax

SSP may be associated with a host of underlying lung diseases, with COPD often cited as the most common [4,17]. Acquired immunodeficiency syndrome–related pneumothoraces, particularly from underlying *P jerovici* pneumonia, in urban areas have a high frequency [23,57]. Patients with SSP from locations with a high tuberculosis prevalence should have underlying tuberculosis considered as a cause [44]. In Spain, 23% of SSP patients reviewed had active pulmonary tuberculosis as the cause [58].

A review of SP lists multiple other causes of SSP in a tabular fashion by frequency of occurrence [4]. Airway diseases, including COPD, cystic fibrosis, and status asthmaticus, lead the list followed by infectious lung diseases, including *P jerovici* pneumonia and necrotizing pneumonias. Less common causes include interstitial lung diseases, such as sarcoidosis, Langerhans cell granulomatosis, and lymphangioleiomyomatosis. Connective tissue disorders, cancer, and thoracic endometriosis (catamenial pneumothorax) also should be considered as potential causes of SSP. With such an extensive list of potential causes of SSP, the clinician should view the occurrence of a non–trauma-related pneumothorax as a challenge to find the underlying etiologic disorder.

Guidelines and consensus statements

Clinicians have a heterogeneous approach to the management of SP [59]. The American College of Chest Physicians (ACCP) [30] and British Thoracic Society (BTS) [26] published separate guidelines for the management of SP that provide a uniform approach to the care of these patients. The approaches outlined by the ACCP and BTS guidelines are complementary with only rare areas of divergence. Both sets of guidelines have limitations. At publication of the ACCP guidelines, there were only eight randomized controlled trials dealing with any aspect of SP care. The writing group used the Delphi process to limit bias in reaching consensus regarding management [30]. The BTS evidence-grading system lacks rigor, and the guidelines represent "a blend of published evidence and clinical experience" [26] without a clear outline of how expert opinion was obtained in an unbiased fashion [60]. Regardless, these two statements provide a map to uniformity of care for SP patients.

Physician compliance with the earlier 1993 version of the BTS guidelines [61] has been quite limited. Less than 21% of patients with SP were treated as directed by these guidelines in Liverpool [62]. Frequent noncompliance with guideline recommendations regarding the use of aspiration and chest tube clamping were noted in Northern Ireland [63]. Two later publications, predating the newest BTS guidelines, continued to note noncompliance [64,65]. Perhaps this noncompliance with the earlier BTS guidelines reflects recognized poor clinician adoption of evidence-based practice [66]. Alternately, this noncompliance may represent issues surrounding dissemination of and education about these specific guidelines. No compliance data regarding the ACCP or newer BTS guidelines are available, but similar noncompliance issues would be expected. Improving local guideline implementation strategies continues to be a challenge to evidence-based guideline adoption and success.

Management

The goals of pneumothorax therapy are to eliminate the intrapleural air collection and to attempt recurrence prevention [4,6]. Oxygen supplementation, observation, simple aspiration, and chest tube placement without sclerosis do not address recurrence risks [6]. Chest tube placement with pleurodesis and various surgical interventions, including thoracotomy or VATS, offer recurrence prevention. Management hinges on pneumothorax size; severity of symptoms; whether an air leak is present; and the type of pneumothorax, primary or secondary.

The following discussion focuses on guideline-directed approaches to therapy as outlined by the ACCP and BTS guidelines [26,30]. Salient differences in the two guidelines and new developments are highlighted. The ACCP guidelines specifically note that their recommendations pertain to adult patients with PSP and patients with SSP associated with COPD [30]. The BTS guidelines are not as explicit. The ACCP notes that their recommendations regarding SSP have relevance to SSP affecting patients with underlying lung disorders other than COPD. The same is true of the recommendations and suggestions that follow. Regardless of these recommendations and suggestions, treatment must be individualized to the patient's unique issues, and open discussion of the various treatment options is encouraged. Figs. 1 and 2 summarize salient management points for PSP and SSP patients.

Size of the pneumothorax, clinical stability, and computed tomography

As discussed earlier, the size of the pneumothorax has been used in the past to direct the selection of therapeutic options. Emphasis instead should be placed on the patient's clinical status, not solely on the radiographic size of the pneumothorax, when making a therapeutic choice [6]. The ACCP and BTS guidelines use a combination of pneumothorax size and the patient's clinical status to direct management [26,30]. There are slight guideline differences in what is considered a small versus a large pneumothorax. The ACCP considers a small pneumothorax to be less than 3 cm in collapse; the BTS notes small to be less than 2 cm in collapse. Large pneumothoraces are considered to 3 cm or greater in collapse by the ACCP or 2 cm or greater in collapseby the BTS. Neither the ACCP nor the BTS guideline uses a percentage of lung collapse to direct therapy [26,30]. The ACCP defines clinical stability as respiratory rate less than 24 breaths/min, heart rate greater than 60 or less than 120 beats/min, normal blood pressure for the patient, room air oxygen saturation greater than 90%, and the ability to speak in whole sentences between breaths [30]. The BTS highlights the absence of "breathlessness" as a marker of stability [26].

As reviewed previously, CT may reveal a potential underlying pathophysiologic cause of SP. The ACCP does not recommend routine CT, however, for first-time PSP or SSP patients. CT may be useful in SSP patients with a recurrence, for management of a persistent air leak, and for planning surgical intervention [30].

Oxygen

A pneumothorax changes arterial PaO_2 and alveolar-arterial oxygen difference owing to alterations in anatomic shunt, ventilation-perfusion relationships, and dead space [67,68]. Ventilation-perfusion relationships may become worse with an increase in shunt after pleural air evacuation, with improvement in these derangements delayed for 90 minutes [68]. These derangements emphasize the role for oxygen supplementation in SP patients.

Oxygen supplementation also enhances the rate of pleural air absorption. The rate of pleural air absorption without oxygen supplementation is about

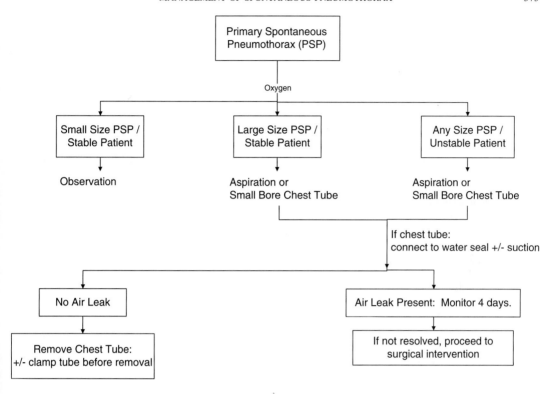

Fig. 1. Management of primary spontaneous pneumothorax.

1.25% per day of the involved hemithorax [69]. A 25% pneumothorax takes about 20 days to reabsorb. Oxygen supplementation enhances this basal rate by three to four fold, with the greatest increase found in patients with larger pneumothoraces [70,71]. Oxygen supplementation in these studies varied from nasal cannula oxygen delivery at 3 L/min to high-flow masks. Oxygen supplementation creates a gas pressure gradient between the pleural space and the tissue capillaries surrounding the pleural space. This gradient enhances the absorption of pleural nitrogen preferentially followed by other gases in the space [70,71]. The BTS guidelines specifically note that SP patients admitted for care should receive high-flow (10 L/min) oxygen with appropriate caution in patients with COPD, who may be prone to hypercapnia [26].

Observation

Primary spontaneous pneumothorax
   Observation of a patient with PSP or SSP is an option, but does not provide recurrence prevention.

Given the low mortality rate in patients with PSP (see earlier), observation in carefully selected patients is reasonable because pleural air absorption occurs with time. The ACCP and the BTS guidelines note observation as a preferred treatment for clinically stable PSP patients with small pneumothoraces. The ACCP guidelines suggest observing the patient in a controlled setting for 3 to 6 hours and discharging home if the repeat chest radiograph excludes progression [30]. This observation period helps ensure that the patient has a "closed pneumothorax," [26] one without active air leak, a point made by the BTS guidelines. PSP patients should be considered for admission for observation if they live a long distance from medical care or if follow-up care may be unreliable. Follow-up should occur within 2 days [30].

Secondary spontaneous pneumothorax
   The ACCP and the BTS guidelines reserve observation for clinically stable SSP patients with small pneumothoraces and preferentially in the hospital setting [6,26].

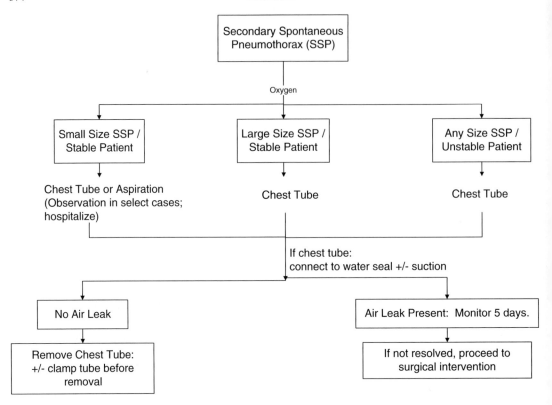

Surgical Recurrence Prevention at the First SSP Occurrence

Fig. 2. Management of secondary spontaneous pneumothorax.

Simple aspiration

Pleural air drainage may be pursued using various approaches. One such approach is simple aspiration entailing the placement of a small catheter (often an intravenous catheter) with subsequent air aspiration and removal of the device. Refinements of this technique and multiple commercially available small-bore catheters that may be removed immediately or left in place have confused the terminology. When such a catheter is left in place, simple aspiration has been transfigured into placement of a chest tube [6]. A review of five articles that focused on the use of aspiration noted an average success rate of 53% to 58% in SP patients. On average, success for PSP is greater (75%) than for SSP (37%) [6].

Primary spontaneous pneumothorax

Simple aspiration is reserved only for PSP patients who have failed observation (initially clinically stable and with a small PSP) according to the ACCP approach. By contrast, the BTS approach embraces simple aspiration as the "first line treatment for all primary pneumothoraces requiring intervention" [26]. The BTS guidelines seem to base this decision primarily on three randomized controlled trials [72–74]. Two of these studies [72,73] were available at development of the earlier ACCP document and have significant methodologic flaws [60,75].

The third study is a prospective, multicenter pilot study and the most methodologically sound [74]. This study compared aspiration (16G intravenous catheter) or chest tube drainage (16F or 20F) in PSP patients and noted no difference in immediate success, 1-week success, or urgent readmissions. This study had "only a less than 25% probability of not missing meaningful differences between endpoints" between the two groups [74] and provides preliminary data inferring possible equivalence of aspiration and chest tube placement in PSP patients. The study also noted that a failed initial aspiration is often unsuccessful on a second attempt [53], although the BTS guidelines note that repeat aspiration is reasonable if the air volume removed on the first aspiration is less than 2.5 L [26]. This pilot study is a valuable addition to the literature, but has several methodologic flaws, including different definitions of success between the two groups, different aspiration management approaches by location, an apparent difference in prevalence of smokers in each group, and the chest tube group not being offered discharge to home with a Heimlich valve or similar device. A meta-analysis including the three aforementioned prospective aspiration studies [72–74] noted that the efficacy data are inconclusive, but found shorter hospitalization in the simple aspiration group [76]. Notably, the authors of the meta-analysis [76] seemed unaware that the study by Noppen and colleagues [72–74] required hospitalization for the chest tube group. Further study is required to uncover any superiority of aspiration compared with chest tube placement. Such a study seems moot, however, given the availability of commercial all-in-one chest tube kits for placement of small-bore chest tubes (8F–16F) that can be used for initial aspiration and easily left in place if a continued air leak exists [60].

The BTS guidelines recognize this blurred line between simple aspiration and placement of a small-bore chest tube and discuss the concept of catheter aspiration of a pneumothorax (CASP) [26]. "In centers where the experience and equipment is available, consideration should be given to using small-bore catheter aspiration kits (CASP) to aspirate pneumothoraces as the catheter may be left in place until full re-expansion of the lung is confirmed" [26]. The debate over aspiration versus chest tube placement, at least small-bore tubes, is moot. Increasing United Kingdom adoption of the CASP concept was reflected in an abstract highlighting the success of CASP in hospitals at Leeds and York [77].

Secondary spontaneous pneumothorax
The ACCP found little role for aspiration in the management of SSP patients [30]. Simple aspiration is less likely to succeed in SSP than PSP [6] and is recommended by the BTS only in small pneumothoraces in minimally breathless patients younger than age 50 years [26]. Patients with large SSP and who are older than 50 years seem to be at greater risk of failure with aspiration [26]. If SSP patients are managed by aspiration, such patients should be admitted for observation [26,30].

Chest tube placement

Primary spontaneous pneumothorax
The ACCP advocates chest tube placement in clinically stable or unstable PSP patients with large pneumothoraces. Most stable patients and all unstable

patients should be hospitalized [30]. Alternatively, the BTS advocates chest tube placement only if initial aspiration is unsuccessful in controlling the patient's symptoms [26].

Secondary spontaneous pneumothorax
Clinically stable patients with a small SSP, if hospitalized, may be observed or have a chest tube placed depending on the extent of their symptoms and course of their pneumothorax. Clinically stable SSP patients with a large pneumothorax or any unstable SSP patient should have a chest tube placed according to the ACCP [30]. Similarly, the BTS recommends chest tube placement in SSP patients except in patients who are not breathless and have a very small (<1 cm or apical) pneumothorax [26].

Chest tube size and suction

The ACCP and the BTS generally eschew larger chest tubes in the management of PSP and SSP patients. The ACCP emphasizes, however, considering the potential for large air leaks or the use of mechanical ventilation, which may drive a large air leak. For a stable PSP patient with a large pneumothorax, the ACCP advocates 14F to 22F size or smaller chest tubes; alternately, if the patient is unstable and has a large pneumothorax, a larger (24F–28F) tube may be used if the patient is suspected to have a large bronchopleural fistula (air leak) or is at risk for positive-pressure ventilation. For a SSP patient who is at risk for a large air leak or may require mechanical ventilation (with consequent increased risk for a large air leak), a 24F to 28F tube is suggested. Stable SSP patients without risks for large air leaks may be managed by 14F to 22F size or smaller chest tubes [30]. The BTS notes that there is no evidence that larger tubes (20F–24F) are any better than small tubes (10F–14F) in the management of pneumothoraces and does not recommend the use of a large (20F–24F) tube. Replacement of a smaller bore chest tube with a larger one may be necessary, however, if there is a persistent air leak [26].

Given the emphasis on the use of smaller bore catheters by the ACCP and the BTS, the variability in airflow rates accommodated by the commercially available small-bore catheter kits must be recognized. Airflow through a chest tube is determined primarily by the radius of the tube and less so by the length ($v = \Pi^2 r^5 P/fl$, where v = flow, r = radius, l = length, P = pressure, and f = friction factor). Small-bore catheters commonly available in the United States assessed at -20 cm H_2O water pressure are found to have widely varying flow rates. Lowest mean flow rates are found with thoracentesis catheters (with side ports) used as pneumothorax catheters, such as the Arrow thoracentesis kit (8F, 12 cm length, 3.4 L/min; Arrow International, Reading, Pennsylvania) and Argyle Safety Thoracentesis (8F, 10-cm length, 2.6 L/min; Sherwood Medical, Tullamore, Ireland). Arrow drainage catheters (14F, 23-cm length, pigtail or straight) have significantly greater mean flow rates (both 16.8 L/min) compared with the 14F (29-cm length, 12.8 L/min) and 16F (41-cm length, 14.8 L/min) Cook devices (Cook, Bloomington, Indiana) [78].

After a chest tube is in place, little evidence is available regarding the role of suction. So and Yu [79] found no advantage to early suction drainage in a group of 53 episodes of SP, with similar results for PSP and SSP patients. Minami and colleagues [80] found a 77% success rate (full lung re-expansion and no air leak) not using chest tube suction in 71 SP episodes. Additionally, suction has been found to have no effect on the likelihood of lung collapse after chest tube removal [81]. The variability in suction use recommendations by the ACCP and BTS likely derives from the limited available evidence. For a PSP patient, the ACCP suggests using a water-seal device without suction initially with subsequent suction if the lung fails to re-expand. For SSP patients, the approach is less directive; the chest tube is attached to a water-seal device with or without suction. If the lung treated without suction fails to re-expand, however, suction should be applied [30]. The BTS is more proscriptive, stating that suction should not be applied in SP patients immediately after chest tube placement, but can be added after 48 hours for persistent air leak or failure of lung re-expansion. High-volume, low-pressure (-10 to -20 cm H_2O) suction is recommended [26]. The ACCP notes that a Heimlich valve–like device may be used in SP patients in lieu of a water-seal device, but notes a preference for water-seal devices in most patients with a SSP [30].

The data on the risk of suction precipitating re-expansion pulmonary edema are anecdotal. Re-expansion pulmonary edema may occur in the absence of suction [82,83] and may occur in the contralateral lung [83]. Multiple logistic regression reveals young age and extent of lung collapse as independent risks for re-expansion pulmonary edema in SP patients [84].

Just as commercially available small-bore catheters have variable flow rates, commercially available pleural drainage units differ in flow rates accommodated. Of tested pleural drainage units available in the United States, the Argyle Aqua-Seal (Sherwood

Medical) has the highest mean flow rate at -20 cm H_2O water pressure (41.1 L/min) with the Argyle Sentinel Seal (Sherwood Medical) having the lowest rate (10.8 L/min) [78].

Chest tube removal

Chest tube removal may be considered after a pneumothorax-related air leak has resolved. Tubes should be removed in a staged sequence to ensure that any air leak has resolved before removal. A radiograph showing lung re-expansion and no clinical evidence of an air leak is requisite [23]. The ACCP and the BTS suggest a similar staged tube removal [26,30]. The ACCP specifically notes that any suction applied should be discontinued first. The ACCP and the BTS guidelines differ, however, in their use of clamping before chest tube removal. This difference seems to reflect an ongoing debate between US and non-US practitioners [85,86]. US pulmonologists commonly incorporate clamping during chest tube removal, whereas US thoracic surgeons [59] and British physicians do not [86]. The ACCP consensus group was divided regarding the use of clamping, with 47% and 59% of the group advocating clamping before chest tube removal in PSP and SSP [30]. Practitioners opposed to clamping note concerns for the development of unnoticed lung collapse [86]. Supporters of clamping note that air leaks may not be obvious in the air leak indicator chamber, and clamping with proper instructions may detect a small air leak precluding chest tube replacement owing to an overlooked air leak [85]. The BTS guidelines state that a chest tube that is not bubbling usually should not be clamped. If a chest tube is clamped, it should be under the supervision of a respiratory physician or thoracic surgeon, and the patient should be managed on a ward with experienced nursing staff [26]. This debate is expected to continue until a prospective study answers the question. The question is not moot because timely discovery, by whatever means, of a persistent air leak shortens the patient's length of stay and prevents chest tube replacement if such leaks are missed.

The question of whether to remove a chest tube at end expiration or end inspiration has been answered. Bell and colleagues [87] randomized 102 chest tube removals in 69 trauma patients and found no difference in post–chest tube removal pneumothoraces rates. The presence of hemothorax, thoracotomy or thoracoscopy, previous lung disease, or chest tube duration did not affect the pneumothorax recurrence rate. These findings, although in the trauma patient population, likely can be extrapolated to the SP patient population.

How long to monitor a persistent air leak

An ongoing air leak is apparent in 18% of PSP patients and 40% of SSP patients 48 hours after chest tube placement [88]. How long to monitor an air leak before pursuing a definitive intervention becomes a major management question. In the United States, more than 75% of physicians monitor an air leak for 5 to 10 days before recommending a definitive corrective course of action [59]. This variability in timing is understandable given that the published suggested monitoring time periods range from 2 to 14 days [88–91]. The ACCP statement suggests observation of a persistent air leak for 4 days for PSP and 5 days for SSP before a definitive intervention. Alternately, the BTS suggests referral to a respiratory physician if a pneumothorax fails to re-expand or an air leak persists after 2 days and "early" (3–5 days) solicitation of a thoracic surgical opinion [26]. Prolonged SP air leak monitoring may increase cost of care and decrease thoracoscopy success proportional to the preoperative delay [92].

Recurrence prevention and air leak intervention

The ACCP and the BTS advocate surgical interventions for recurrence prevention and persistent air leak intervention [26,30]. Acknowledging that the relative merits of thoracoscopy and thoracotomy have not been clearly defined, the ACCP suggests a thoracoscopic approach for recurrence prevention and to correct a persistent air leak for PSP and SSP patients. Parietal pleural abrasion limited to the upper half of the hemithorax and intraoperative bullectomy are recommended for PSP recurrence prevention. Bullectomy accompanied by parietal pleurectomy or parietal pleural abrasion limited to the upper half of the hemithorax is the preferred approach to prevent recurrence in SSP patients [30]. The BTS notes that open thoracotomy and pleurectomy remains the procedure with the lowest recurrence rate for difficult or recurrent pneumothoraces. Minimally invasive procedures, thoracoscopy (VATS), pleural abrasion, and surgical talc pleurodesis all are effective alternative strategies. There seems to be a slight advantage to pleurectomy over pleural abrasion with a recurrence rate of 0.4% for pleurectomy and 2.3% for pleural abrasion [26].

Although likely considered an aggressive surgical approach by many clinicians, a report by Watanabe and colleagues [93] may be worthy of future study and consideration. Based on the bilateral nature of the bullous lesions in PSP, four patients with unilateral PSP underwent single-stage bilateral VATS with no complications and a postoperative hospital stay of 2 to 4 days. Supporting this report is a series of 15 patients with contralateral SP or bilateral simultaneous SP occurrences safely and effectively treated with single-stage bilateral VATS [94]. Given that contralateral occurrence rates range from 5.2% [11] to 14.6% [95] in a combined PSP and SSP population, this may be a valid consideration. In 1957, Barnofsky and colleagues [96] reported bilateral thoracotomy for unilateral SP.

Chest tube–directed recurrence prevention using pleurodesis agents is a second-line approach after a surgical approach for PSP and SSP patients. Patients refusing or not capable of tolerating a surgical approach may be offered chest tube–directed pleurodesis according to the ACCP. Despite ongoing debate regarding talc safety [97,98], talc and doxycycline are the preferred pleurodesis agents [30]. Similarly, the BTS notes chemical pleurodesis should be attempted only if the patient is unwilling or unable to undergo surgery. Despite problems with tetracycline availability and acknowledging the talc safety debate, tetracycline is the recommended agent [26]. More recent work confirms that small talc particle size may be the driving mechanism in the rare instances of talc-associated respiratory failure [99], making use of appropriately size graded talc optimal.

Timing of recurrence prevention

Except for patients with persistent air leaks requiring early intervention, 85% of ACCP panelists recommend recurrence prevention procedures for PSP patients at the second pneumothorax occurrence. Of panelists, 81% recommend a recurrence prevention procedure after the first SSP occurrence [30]. The BTS highlights the traditional indications for surgical SP recurrence prevention, including a second ipsilateral pneumothorax, first contralateral pneumothorax, and bilateral pneumothorax [26].

Both sets of guidelines note that professionals at pneumothorax risk, such as pilots and divers, need prompt operative recurrence prevention [26,30]. Patients without an "active intervention" should be warned against flying until a follow-up chest radiograph confirms full pneumothorax resolution. Commercial airlines "arbitrarily" advise air travelers to wait 6 weeks between having a pneumothorax and an airline flight. Patients with SSP should be advised to avoid air travel for 1 year if no definitive surgical procedure has been performed. After SP, diving should be discouraged permanently, unless a definitive prevention strategy, such as surgical pleurectomy, has been performed [26].

Decision analysis studies in PSP patients make a persuasive case for a more cost-effective approach to PSP that includes thoracoscopic surgery as the treatment of choice for first episodes of PSP [100,101]. The quality-adjusted life expectancy for a thoracoscopic intervention at first PSP occurrence failing simple aspiration treatment exceeded five other strategies, including pleural drainage followed by thoracoscopic surgery for recurrence, pleural drainage followed by thoracoscopic surgery for second occurrence, pleurodesis followed by thoracoscopic surgery for recurrence, pleurodesis followed by thoracoscopic surgery for second recurrence, and pleural drainage followed by pleurodesis for the first recurrence and thoracoscopic surgery for the second recurrence [101]. Although thoracoscopic surgery at the first episode of PSP failing simple aspiration treatment increased costs compared with other strategies, it may be an acceptable approach based on cost-effectiveness [100]. Similarly, an additional decision analysis supports a thoracoscopic approach for the second episode of SP (no differentiation of PSP and SSP), noting substantial cost savings with only a minimal decrease in effectiveness compared with more conservative management [102].

Summary and future study

Management of patients with SP continues to present challenges to the clinician. More recent guidelines have helped provide a common pathway for care in these patients and highlight the many areas in need of additional study. Areas foremost in need of additional study include establishing the role of VATS versus traditional surgical approaches (including type of intraoperative interventions) for pneumothorax recurrence prevention and air leak management, exploring the appropriate timing of recurrence prevention and air leak management, and defining the optimal pleurodesis agent. Given the flexibility of small-bore catheters and the concept of CASP, less effort should be expended in the ongoing debate of simple aspiration versus chest tube placement. Defining chest tube management issues, including the role of suction and the appropriate timing and steps to chest tube removal, could have a significant impact on patient length of stay and cost.

References

[1] Baumann MH, Noppen M. Pneumothorax. Respirology 2004;9:157–64.

[2] Baumann MH. Non-spontaneous pneumothorax. In: Light RW, Lee YCG, editors. Textbook of pleural diseases. London: Arnold; 2003. p. 464–74.

[3] Light RW. Pleural diseases. 4th edition. Baltimore: Williams & Wilkins; 2001.

[4] Sahn SA, Heffner JE. Spontaneous pneumothorax. N Engl J Med 2000;342:868–74.

[5] Melton LJ, Hepper NGG, Offord KP. Incidence of spontaneous pneumothorax in Olmsted County, Minnesota: 1950–1974. Am Rev Respir Dis 1974; 120:1379–82.

[6] Baumann MH, Strange C. Treatment of spontaneous pneumothorax: a more aggressive approach? Chest 1997;112:789–804.

[7] Gupta D, Hansell A, Nichols T, et al. Epidemiology of pneumothorax in England. Thorax 2000;55:666–71.

[8] Light RW, Broaddus VC. Pneumothorax, chylothorax, hemothorax, and fibrothorax. In: Murray JF, Nadel JA, Mason RJ, Boushey HA, editors. Textbook of respiratory medicine. 3rd edition. Philadelphia: Saunders; 2000. p. 2043–66.

[9] Videm V, Pillgram-Larsen J, Ellingsen O, et al. Spontaneous pneumothorax in chronic obstructive pulmonary disease: complications, treatment and recurrences. Eur J Respir Dis 1987;71:365–71.

[10] Lippert H, Lund O, Blegvad S, Larsen H. Independent risk factors for cumulative recurrence rate after first spontaneous pneumothorax. Eur Respir J 1991; 4:324–31.

[11] Light RW, O'Harra VS, Moritz TE, et al. Intrapleural tetracycline for the prevention of recurrent spontaneous pneumothorax: results of a Department of Veterans Affairs cooperative study. JAMA 1990;264: 2224–30.

[12] Schramel F, Postmus P, Vanderschueren R. Current aspects of spontaneous pneumothorax. Eur Respir J 1997;10:1372–9.

[13] O'Rourke JP, Yee ES. Civilian spontaneous pneumothorax: treatment options and long-term results. Chest 1989;96:1302–6.

[14] Shields TW, Oilschlager GA. Spontaneous pneumothorax in patients 40 years of age and older. Ann Thorac Surg 1966;2:377–83.

[15] George RB, Herbert SJ, Shames JM, et al. Pneumothorax complicating emphysema. JAMA 1975;234: 389–93.

[16] Dines DE, Clagett OT, Payne WS. Spontaneous pneumothorax in emphysema. Mayo Clin Proc 1970; 45:481–7.

[17] Light RW. Management of spontaneous pneumothorax. Am Rev Respir Dis 1993;148:245–8.

[18] Seremetis M. The management of spontaneous pneumothorax. Chest 1970;57:65–8.

[19] Maeda A, Ishioka S, Yoshihara M, et al. Primary spontaneous pneumothorax detected during a medical checkup. Chest 1999;116:847–8.

[20] Kadokura M, Nonaka M, Yamamoto S, et al. Five cases of asymptomatic spontaneous pneumothorax. Ann Thorac Cardiovasc Surg 1999;5:187–90.

[21] Bense L, Wiman LG, Hedenstierna G. Onset of symptoms in spontaneous pneumothorax: correlation with physical activity. Eur J Respir Dis 1987;71: 181–6.

[22] Withers J, Fishback M, Kiehl P, Hannon J. Spontaneous pneumothorax: suggested etiology and comparison of treatment methods. Am J Surg 1964;108: 772–6.

[23] Baumann MH. Pneumothorax. Semin Respir Crit Care Med 2001;22:647–55.

[24] Bradley M, Williams C, Walshaw M. The value of routine expiratory chest films in the diagnosis of pneumothorax. Arch Emerg Med 1991;8:115–6.

[25] Schramel FMNH, Golding RP, Haakman CDE, et al. Expiratory chest radiographs do not improve visibility of small apical pneumothoraces by enhanced contrast. Eur Respir J 1996;9:406–9.

[26] Henry M, Arnold T, Harvey JE. BTS guidelines for the management of spontaneous pneumothorax. Thorax 2003;58(Suppl II):39–52.

[27] Bourgouin P, Cousineau G, Lemire P, Herbert G. Computed tomography used to exclude pneumothorax in bullous lung disease. J Can Assoc Radiol 1985;36:341–2.

[28] Noppen M, Alexander P, Driesen P, et al. Quantification of the size of pneumothorax: accuracy of the Light index. Respiration (Herrlisheim) 2001;68: 396–9.

[29] Engdahl O, Toft T, Boe J. Chest radiograph—a poor method for determining size of a pneumothorax. Chest 1993;103:26–9.

[30] Baumann MH, Strange C, Heffner JE, et al. Management of spontaneous pneumothorax: an American College of Chest Physicians Delphi consensus statement. Chest 2001;119:590–602.

[31] Baumann MH. Do blebs cause primary spontaneous pneumothorax? Pro: blebs do cause primary spontaneous pneumothorax. J Bronchol 2002;9:313–8.

[32] Bense L, Lewander R, Eklund G, Hedenstierna G, Wiman L. Nonsmoking, non-alpha 1-antitrypsin deficiency-induced emphysema in nonsmokers with healed spontaneous pneumothorax, identified by computed tomography of the lungs. Chest 1993;103: 433–8.

[33] Schramel F, Zanen P. Blebs and/or bullae are of no importance and have no predictive value for recurrences in patients with primary spontaneous pneumothorax. Chest 2001;119:1976–7.

[34] Lesur O, Delorme N, Fromaget J, et al. Computed tomography in the etiologic assessment of idiopathic spontaneous pneumothorax. Chest 1990;98:341–7.

[35] Mitlehner W, Friedrich M, Dissmann W. Value of computed tomography in the detection of bullae and blebs in patients with primary spontaneous pneumothorax. Respiration (Herrlisheim) 1992;59:221–7.

[36] Warner B, Bailey W, Shipley T. Value of computed tomography of the lung in the management of primary spontaneous pneumothorax. Am J Surg 1991; 162:39–42.

[37] Yim APC, Lee TW, Ng CSH, et al. CT scanning and bilateral surgery for unilateral primary pneumothorax? Chest 2001;119:1294.

[38] Sihoe ADL, Yim APC, Lee TW, et al. Can CT scanning be used to select patients with unilateral primary spontaneous pneumothorax for bilateral surgery? Chest 2000;118:380–3.

[39] Smit HJM, Wienk MATP, Schreurs AJM, et al. Do bullae indicate a predisposition to recurrent pneumothorax? Br J Radiol 2000;73:356–9.

[40] Yim APC, Lee TW, Ng CSH, et al. Blebs and/or bullae are of no importance and have no predictive value for recurrences in patients with primary spontaneous pneumothorax. Chest 2001;119:1977.

[41] Yim APC, Ho J, Chung SS, Ng DCY. Video-assisted thoracoscopic surgery for primary spontaneous pneumothorax. N Z J Surg 1994;64:667–70.

[42] Inderbitzi RGC, Leiser A, Furrer M, Althaus U. Three years' experience in video-assisted thoracic surgery (VATS) for spontaneous pneumothorax. J Thorac Cardiovasc Surg 1994;107:1410–5.

[43] Fujino S, Inoue S, Tezuka N, et al. Physical development of surgically treated patients with primary spontaneous pneumothorax. Chest 1999;116: 899–902.

[44] Baumann MH. Treatment of spontaneous pneumothorax. Curr Opin Pulm Med 2000;6:275–80.

[45] Morrison P, Lowry R, Nevin N. Familial primary spontaneous pneumothorax consistent with true autosomal dominant inheritance. Thorax 1998;53:151–2.

[46] Abolnik IZ, Lossos IS, Zlotogora J, Brauer R. On the inheritance of primary spontaneous pneumothorax. Am J Med Genet 1991;40:155–8.

[47] Cardy CM, Maskell NA, Handford PA, et al. Familial spontaneous pneumothorax and FBN1 mutations. Am J Respir Crit Care Med 2004;169:1260–2.

[48] Yamada A, Takeda Y, Hayashi S, Shimizu K. Familial spontaneous pneumothorax in three generations and its HLA. Jpn J Throac Cardiovasc Surg 2003;51: 456–8.

[49] Koivisto PA, Mustonen A. Primary spontaneous pneumothorax in two siblings suggests autosomal recessive inheritance. Chest 2001;119:1610–2.

[50] Bense L, Eklund G, Wiman L-G. Smoking and increased risk of contracting spontaneous pneumothorax. Chest 1987;92:1009–12.

[51] Cottin V, Streichenberger N, Gamondes J-P, et al. Respiratory bronchiolitis in smokers with spontaneous pneumothorax. Eur Respir J 1998;12:702–4.

[52] Smit H, Chatrou M, Postmus P. The impact of spontaneous pneumothorax, and its treatment, on the smoking behaviour of young adult smokers. Respir Med 1998;92:1132–6.

[53] Noppen M. Management of primary spontaneous pneumothorax. Curr Opin Pulm Med 2003;9:272–5.

[54] Noppen M. Do blebs cause primary spontaneous pneumothorax? Con: blebs do not cause primary spontaneous pneumothorax. J Bronchol 2002;9: 319–23.

[55] Noppen M. Management of primary spontaneous pneumothorax: does cause matter? Monaldi Arch Chest Dis 2001;56:344–8.

[56] Noppen M, Stratakos G, Verbanck S, et al. Fluorescein-enhanced autofluorescence thoracoscopy in primary spontaneous pneumothorax. Am J Respir Crit Care Med 2004;170:680–2.

[57] Wait MA, Estrera A. Changing clinical spectrum of spontaneous pneumothorax. Am J Surg 1992;164: 528–31.

[58] Blanco-Perez J, Bordon J, Pineiro-Amigo L, et al. Pneumothorax in active pulmonary tuberculosis: resurgence of an old complication? Respir Med 1998;92:1269–73.

[59] Baumann MH, Strange C. The clinician's perspective on pneumothorax management. Chest 1997;112: 822–8.

[60] Baumann MH. Top ten list in pleural disease. Chest 2003;124:2352–5.

[61] Miller AC, Harvey JE. Guidelines for the management of spontaneous pneumothorax. BMJ 1993;307:114–6.

[62] Soulsby T. British Thoracic Society guidelines for the management of spontaneous pneumothorax: do we comply with them and do they work? J Accid Emerg Med 1998;15:317–21.

[63] Courtney P, McKane W. Audit of the management of spontaneous pneumothorax. Ulster Med J 1998;67: 41–3.

[64] Yeoh JH, Ansari S, Campbell IA. Management of spontaneous pneumothorax—a Welsh survey. Postgrad Med J 2000;76:496–500.

[65] Mendis D, El-Shanawany T, Mathur A, Redington AE. Management of spontaneous pneumothorax: are the British Thoracic Society guidelines being followed? Postgrad Med J 2002;78:80–4.

[66] Grol R, Wensing M. What drives change? Barriers to and incentives for achieving evidence-based practice. Med J Aust 2004;180(6 Suppl):S57–60.

[67] Moran JF, Jones RH, Wolfe WG. Regional pulmonary function during experimental unilateral pneumothorax in the awake state. J Thorac Cardiovasc Surg 1977;74:396–402.

[68] Norris RM, Jones JG, Bishop JM. Respiratory gas exchange in patients with spontaneous pneumothorax. Thorax 1968;23:427–33.

[69] Kircher LT, Swartzel RL. Spontaneous pneumothorax and its treatment. JAMA 1954;155:24–9.

[70] Chadha TS, Cohn MA. Noninvasive treatment of pneumothorax with oxygen inhalation. Respiration (Herrlisheim) 1983;44:147–52.

[71] Northfield TC. Oxygen therapy for spontaneous pneumothorax. BMJ 1971;4:86–8.

[72] Andrivet P, Djedaini K, Teboul J-L, et al. Spontaneous pneumothorax: comparison of thoracic drainage vs immediate or delayed needle aspiration. Chest 1995;108:335–40.

[73] Harvey J. Comparison of simple aspiration with intercostal drainage in the management of spontaneous pneumothorax. Thorax 1993;48:430–1.

[74] Noppen M, Alexander P, Driesen P, et al. Manual aspiration versus chest tube drainage in first episodes of primary spontaneous pneumothorax. Am J Respir Crit Care Med 2002;165:1240–4.

[75] Baumann MH, Strange C. Pneumothorax: what's wrong with simple aspiration? Chest 2001;120: 1041–2.

[76] Devanand A, Koh MS, Ong TH, et al. Simple aspiration versus chest-tube insertion in the management of primary spontaneous pneumothorax: a systematic review. Respir Med 2004;98:579–90.

[77] Horsley AR, White JS. Complication rates of small bore seldinger chest drains on medical wards [abstract]. Am J Resp Crit Care Med 2005;2:A537.

[78] Baumann MH, Patel PB, Roney CW, Petrini MF. Comparison of function of commercially available pleural drainage units and catheters. Chest 2003;123: 1878–86.

[79] So S, Yu D. Catheter drainage of spontaneous pneumothorax: suction or no suction, early or late removal? Thorax 1982;37:46–8.

[80] Minami H, Saka H, Senda K, et al. Small caliber catheter drainage for spontaneous pneumothorax. Am J Med Sci 1992;304:345–7.

[81] Sharma TN, Agnihotri S, Jain N, et al. Intercostal tube thoracostomy in pneumothorax: factors influencing re-expansion of the lung. Indian J Chest Dis All Sci 1988;30:32–5.

[82] Shaw TJ, Caterine JM. Recurrent re-expansion pulmonary edema. Chest 1984;86:784–6.

[83] Mahfood S, Hix WR, Aaron BL, et al. Reexpansion pulmonary edema. Ann Thorac Surg 1988;45:340–5.

[84] Matsuura Y, Nomimura T, Murakami H, et al. Clinical analysis of reexpansion pulmonary edema. Chest 1991;100:1562–6.

[85] Baumann MH, Strange C. Treatment of spontaneous pneumothorax: the clinicians' perspective on pneumothorax management. Chest 1998;113:1424–5.

[86] Miller AC. Treatment of spontaneous pneumothorax: the clinician's perspective on pneumothorax management. Chest 1998;113:1423–4.

[87] Bell RL, Ovadia P, Abdullah F, et al. Chest tube removal: end-inspiration or end-expiration? J Trauma 2001;50:674–7.

[88] Schoenenberger RA, Haefeli WE, Weiss P, Ritz RF. Timing of invasive procedures in therapy for primary and secondary spontaneous pneumothoraces. Arch Surg 1991;126:764–6.

[89] Chee CBE, Abisheganaden J, Yeo JKS, et al. Persistent air-leak in spontaneous pneumothorax—clinical course and outcome. Respir Med 1998;92: 757–61.

[90] Mathur R, Cullen J, Kinnear WJM, Johnston IDA. Time course of resolution of persistent air leak in spontaneous pneumothorax. Respir Med 1995;89: 129–32.

[91] Jain SK, Al-Kattan KM, Hamdy M. Spontaneous pneumothorax: determinants of surgical intervention. J Cardiovasc Surg (Torino) 1998;39:107–11.

[92] Waller DA, McConnell SA, Rajesh PB. Delayed referral reduces the success of video-assisted thoracoscopic surgery for spontaneous pneumothorax. Respir Med 1998;92:246–9.

[93] Watanabe S, Sakasegawa K, Kariatsumari K, et al. Bilateral video-assisted thoracoscopic surgery in the supine position for primary spontaneous pneumothorax. Thorac Cardiovasc Surg 2004;52:42–4.

[94] Ayed AK. Bilateral video-assisted thoracoscopic surgery for bilateral spontaneous pneumothorax. Chest 2002;122:2234–7.

[95] Ikeda M, Uno A, Yamane Y, Hagiwara N. Median sternotomy with bilateral bullous resection for unilateral spontaneous pneumothorax, with special reference to operative indications. J Thorac Cardiovasc Surg 1988;96:615–20.

[96] Baronofsky ID, Warden HG, Kaufman JL, et al. Bilateral therapy for unilateral spontaneous pneumothorax. J Thorac Surg 1957;34:310–22.

[97] Light RW. Talc should not be used for pleurodesis. Am J Respir Crit Care Med 2000;162:2024–6.

[98] Sahn SA. Talc should be used for pleurodesis. Am J Respir Crit Care 2000;162:2023–4.

[99] Maskell NA, Lee YCG, Gleeson FV, et al. Randomized trials describing lung inflammation after pleurodesis with talc of varying particle size. Am J Respir Crit Care Med 2004;170:377–82.

[100] Morimoto T, Shimbo T, Noguchi Y, et al. Effects of time of thoracoscopic surgery for primary spontaneous pneumothorax on prognosis and costs. Am J Surg 2004;187:767–74.

[101] Morimoto T, Fukui T, Koyama H, et al. Optimal strategy for the first episode of primary spontaneous pneumothorax in young men: a decision analysis. J Gen Intern Med 2002;17:193–202.

[102] Falcoz P-E, Binquet C, Clement F, et al. Management of the second episode of spontaneous pneumothorax: a decision analysis. Ann Thorac Surg 2003;76:1843–8.

**ELSEVIER
SAUNDERS**

Clin Chest Med 27 (2006) 383–393

**CLINICS
IN CHEST
MEDICINE**

Index

Note: Page numbers of article titles are in **boldface** type.

A

Abscess(es)
  intra-abdominal, 312

Adenomatoid tumor
  of pleura, 167–168

Adjuvant high-dose radiotherapy
  with extrapleural pneumonectomy
    for mesothelioma, 347

Analgesia
  for mesothelioma, 342–343

Antibiotic(s)
  for parapneumonic effusion, 259–260

Asbestos
  diffuse pleural thickening due to, 197–198
  mesothelioma due to, 335–336
  pleural fibrosis due to, 184

Asbestos pleural effusion, 314

Aspiration
  in spontaneous pneumothorax management,
    374–375
  pleural
    in mesothelioma diagnosis, 339

Atelectasis
  rounded
    in diffuse pleural thickening, 198–199

B

Bacterial infections
  of pleura, 160

Barogenic rupture, 296

Basic fibroblast growth factor
  in pleural fibrosis pathogenesis, 182

Bayesian approach
  to pleural fluid analysis in discriminating between
    transudates and exudates, 247–250

Biliopleural fistula, 298–299

Bilirubin
  pleural fluid
    in discriminating between transudates and
    exudates, 243

Biopsy
  pleural
    in mesothelioma diagnosis, 339–340

Biopsy(ies)
  pleural
    in pleural disease, 208–209

Blood markers
  in mesothelioma diagnosis, 340

Brachytherapy
  radiotherapy and
    after pleurectomy
      for mesothelioma, 347

Bronchopleural fistula
  imaging of, 207

Bronchoscopy
  in persistent undiagnosed pleural effusion
    evaluation, 317

C

CABG surgery. See *Coronary artery bypass graft
(CABG) surgery.*

Calcifying fibrous pseudotumor
  of pleura, 166–167

Catamenial pneumothorax, 174

Catheter(s)
  central venous
    extravascular migration of, 290–291. See also
    *Central venous catheter, extravascular
    migration of.*

0272-5231/06/$ – see front matter © 2006 Elsevier Inc. All rights reserved.
doi:10.1016/S0272-5231(06)00062-1

chestmed.theclinics.com

Changing Your Address?

Make sure your subscription changes too! When you notify us of your new address, you can help make our job easier by including an exact copy of your Clinics label number with your old address (see illustration below.) This number identifies you to our computer system and will speed the processing of your address change. Please be sure this label number accompanies your old address and your corrected address—you can send an old Clinics label with your number on it or just copy it exactly and send it to the address listed below.

We appreciate your help in our attempt to give you continuous coverage. Thank you.

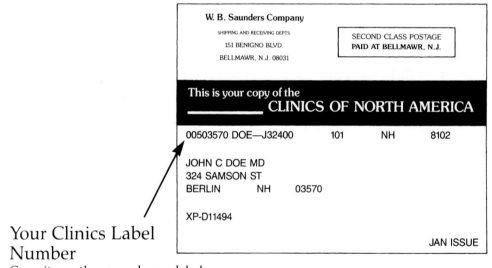

Your Clinics Label Number

Copy it exactly or send your label
along with your address to:
W.B. Saunders Company, Customer Service
Orlando, FL 32887-4800
Call Toll Free 1-800-654-2452

Please allow four to six weeks for delivery of new subscriptions and for processing address changes.